MANAGING THE
LONG-TERM CARE FACILITY

MANAGING THE LONG-TERM CARE FACILITY

PRACTICAL APPROACHES TO PROVIDING QUALITY CARE

Rebecca Perley, Editor

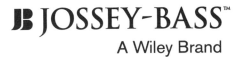

JOSSEY-BASS™

A Wiley Brand

Published by Jossey-Bass
A Wiley Brand
One Montgomery Street, Suite 1000, San Francisco, CA 94104-4594—www.josseybass.com

Jossey-Bass books and products are available through most bookstores. To contact Jossey-Bass directly call our Customer Care Department within the U.S. at 800-956-7739, outside the U.S. at 317-572-3986, or fax 317-572-4002.

Wiley publishes in a variety of print and electronic formats and by print-on-demand. Some material included with standard print versions of this book may not be included in e-books or in print-on-demand. If this book refers to media such as a CD or DVD that is not included in the version you purchased, you may download this material at http://booksupport.wiley.com. For more information about Wiley products, visit www.wiley.com.

Library of Congress Catalouging-in-Publication Data

Managing the long-term care facility : practical approaches to providing quality care / Rebecca Perley, editor.—First edition.

    p. ; cm.

    Includes bibliographical references and index.

    ISBN 978-1-118-65478-1 (pbk.)—ISBN 978-1-118-65474-3 (ePDF)—ISBN 978-1-118-65498-9 (epub)

    I. Perley, Rebecca, 1965–, editor.

    [DNLM: 1. Homes for the Aged—organization & administration—United States. 2. Continuity of Patient Care—United States. 3. Facility Design and Construction—United States. 4. Long-Term Care—organization & administration—United States. 5. Nursing Homes—organization & administration—United States. 6. Patient-Centered Care—United States. WT 27 AA1]

    RA999.A35

    362.16068—dc23

                          2015036509

Cover design: Wiley
Leaves image on the cover: © Evlakhov Valeriy/Shutterstock
Green background on the cover: © ZaZa Studio/Shutterstock

Printed in the United States of America
FIRST EDITION
PB Printing 10 9 8 7 6 5 4 3 2 1

CONTENTS

Chapter 13 Facility-Centered Clinical Operations · · · · · · · · 397

Paige Hector

Chapter 14 Facility Operations and Performance Improvement . . 427

Rebecca Perley, Jim Kinsey, Paige Hector, and Jill Harrison

TABLES, FIGURES, AND EXHIBITS

Tables

Figures

Exhibits

M*anaging the Long-Term Care Facility: Practical Approaches to Providing Quality Care* provides a comprehensive introduction to the growing field that encompasses the long-term care continuum. This area of health care is increasingly important due to the changing demographics of our society. The number of Americans age 65 and over is projected to grow from an estimated 43.1 million in 2012 to 83.7 million by the year 2050, per the U.S. Census Bureau. As people age and their health status changes, many will need long-term care services.

This book focuses on the importance of moving away from an institutional approach in long-term care to a more caring, empathetic, and nurturing one that fosters an empowering environment for persons needing services and those working in the field. Practical approaches to achieving quality of care and quality of life in the long-term care continuum are presented. It also offers information on every aspect of operating a long-term care facility that is proactive and robust, with suggestions that the facility administrator can implement immediately.

Readers will find this book a valuable resource that aids students and professionals in preparing for a career in long-term care. The text will supplement healthcare administration, health and human services, gerontology, nursing, and business and medical programs, in both domestic and international markets. Nursing home administrators, administrators-in-training, and preceptors will find this book an effective training tool in the nursing facility setting.

Another unique aspect to this book is the intentional use of different terms for the same person, object, or concept. The vernacular changes depending on the type of long-term care environment presented in the chapter. The interchangeable terms used in the book are listed below.

- Resident, patient, family member, and responsible party
- Incontinence product, brief
- Facility, community, skilled nursing facility, organization, nursing facility, nursing home facility

- Unit, neighborhood, household
- Patient-centered care, resident-centered care
- Community-based, client-centered, consumer-driven, consumer-based
- Staff, caregivers, team
- Physician, provider, medical provider
- Nursing home administrator, NHA, facility administrator

Chapter Overviews

Chapter 1: Public Policy: Historical Overview of Long-Term Care

Chapter 1 discusses public and private control mechanisms created to control escalating costs, ensure adequate access, and improve quality of care for long-term care services. Current policies emphasizing sociodemographic and culturally sensitive home- and community-based services are also reviewed.

Chapter 2: Long-Term Care Continuum

Chapter 2 describes that the levels of care range from aging in place in private homes to community resident environments, assisted living, and skilled nursing facilities. There is a renewed interest in enabling individuals to age in place in their homes as long as feasible, sometimes with the aid of community support programs.

Chapter 3: Resident Advocates, Diversity, and Resident-Centered Care

Chapter 3 explains that the goal of a nursing home is to provide the best possible care for the people who live there and to nourish the spirits of residents and staff. Working with resident advocates, recognizing the needs of a diverse population, and incorporating resident-centered care result in outcomes that are more effective and more compassionate.

Chapter 4: Physical Environment of Long-Term Care

Chapter 4 describes that the physical environment of long-term care settings should be designed around the different needs of individuals. The environment should be monitored by the facility administrator to ensure that regulatory standards are met or exceeded.

Chapter 5: Human Resources: Managing Employees in Long-Term Care

Chapter 5 discusses ways the human resource department manages both employee needs and organizational goals through proper administration of the recruiting, screening, hiring, orientation, and performance management processes. Human resource strategies for facility administrators are presented to effectively manage a rapidly changing workforce that serves a diverse and growing resident population.

Chapter 6: Reimbursement in the Long-Term Care Environment

Chapter 6 introduces financial and reimbursement concepts, issues, and methodologies that healthcare providers working in long-term care need to know. It includes information on the various payer sources, such as government, private insurance, and private pay arrangements, that typically fund the provision of long-term care services.

Chapter 7: Compliance and Risk Management

Chapter 7 maintains that the facility administrator must be current on changes in state and federal regulations and company employment policies and procedures and incorporate them into day-to-day facility operations. The long-term care provider can furnish better care and improve the success of the organization when a dynamic compliance and risk management program is in place.

Chapter 8: Legal and Ethical Issues

Chapter 8 explores the numerous legal and ethical responsibilities of the long-term care provider when serving one of the most vulnerable segments of society. Although the federal and state governments have attempted to legislate ethical conduct by prohibiting certain actions, this does not eliminate the obligation of the community to "do what is right."

Chapter 9: Marketing and Public Relations

Chapter 9 emphasizes the marketing of long-term care residential services in either assisted living or skilled nursing facilities. In most regions, there is intense competition among long-term care facilities for privately insured or self-pay clients, for whom reimbursement rates are higher. The key is to develop and nurture relationships with referral agents who can influence and direct prospective customers to the facility.

Chapter 10: Health Information Systems

Chapter 10 explains how health information technology has the potential to improve care in the areas of cost, quality, access, and efficiency. Specific anticipated benefits include ease of access to information, time saving, better coordination of care, improved quality management reporting, health information exchange between providers, and improved resident safety.

Chapter 11: Biological and Psychosocial Aspects of Aging: Implications for Long-Term Care

Chapter 11 discusses the biopsychosocial changes that occur with normal aging. Understanding basic principles of gerontology and geriatric care can prevent misdiagnosis of certain behaviors as pathological conditions; suggest simple, cost-effective interventions that can contribute to disease prevention; enhance quality of life; prevent unnecessary hospitalizations; and encourage the use of alternative, non-pharmacological treatments in some circumstances.

Chapter 12: Resident-Centered Clinical Operations

Chapter 12 maintains that clinical operations in the nursing facility are complex; as a leader, the administrator incorporates policies and procedures and regulations into daily operations and coaches all staff to employ critical thinking skills. The administrator helps ensure that care plans and documentation not only meet the needs of the residents but also demonstrate good clinical judgment.

Chapter 13: Facility-Centered Clinical Operations

Chapter 13 ascertains that managing clinical operations in the nursing facility is a challenging process. Utilizing systems and processes and dividing tasks into daily, weekly, and monthly categories help the administrator and the interdisciplinary team achieve success, facilitate communication, reduce survey and operational deficiencies, and improve resident outcomes.

Chapter 14: Facility Operations and Performance Improvement

Chapter 14 focuses on the nursing and business practices that are necessary to operate a well-managed and high-quality nursing home facility. The nursing home administrator's importance to the success of the organization and the quality of care and quality of life in the facility is emphasized. A review of state and or federal regulations and the survey process are discussed in detail.

Chapter 15: Financial Issues and Tools

Chapter 15 provides information on how financial data is collected, summarized, and reported. Included is a discussion on the budgeting process, revenue enhancement strategies, various provider types, and financial tools that can positively impact the organization.

Chapter 16: International Comparisons and Future Trends in Long-Term Care

Chapter 16 explores the concept that as the world population ages, the need for long-term care is increasing dramatically. A discussion of the importance of identifying an appropriate and timely private and public financing mechanism to protect our frailest population, as growth in the demand and spending increases, is included in the chapter.

Chapter Features

Learning Objectives

Each chapter begins with learning objectives to assist the student in understanding the goals of the chapter.

Introduction

Directly following the learning objectives is an introduction that helps orient the student to the remaining content in the chapter.

Chapter Summary

The summary covers the main points discussed and is located at the end of each chapter.

Key Terms

Key terms are available at the end of each chapter to review critical information. All key terms are bolded to assist the reader in locating them within the text.

Review Questions

Review questions are located at the end of the chapter to test knowledge of concepts presented in the text.

Case Studies

Case studies, available in each chapter, offer students the opportunity to apply their knowledge to real-world situations.

References

References are located at the close of the chapter to identify sources of specific material. These references also offer aid to the reader to find additional information on the subject.

Instructor Support Materials

An instructor's supplement, including PowerPoint lecture slides, glossary of important terms or phrases, and chapter-by-chapter test questions, is available at www.wiley.com/go/perley. Additional materials, such as videos, podcasts, and readings, can be found at www.josseybasspublichealth .com. Comments about this book are invited and can be sent to publichealth@wiley.com.

ACKNOWLEDGMENTS

I would like to thank Seth Schwartz, Editor, and the late Andy Pasternack, Senior Editor, from Jossey-Bass/Wiley for the guidance and support they provided me during this gratifying experience.

The following contributors are acknowledged for their expertise and commitment to this book. They are Andrew Alden, Jeffrey Anderzhon, Erlyana Erlyana, Janice Frates, Eduardo Gonzalez, Jill Harrison, Paige Hector, Abby Kazley, Jim Kinsey, Marian Last, Rebecca Lowell, Ken Merchant, Robert Miller, Susie Mix, Sarah Moser, Carissa Podesta, Jean Schuldberg, Sonja Talley, Barbara White, and Ann Wyatt.

My special appreciation goes to Paige Hector, a colleague and friend, for her invaluable support, astute input, and patience. I would also like to thank Mel Hector for his insightful recommendations.

Acknowledgment to Erlyana Erlyana for her expertise and savvy guidance.

A special thank you to Jim Kinsey, who provided valuable insight regarding the person-centered care model for this book.

I would also like to thank proposal reviewers Kathleen Abrahamson, Robert R. Kulesher, Roberto Muñiz, and Jen A. Porter for providing valuable feedback on the original book proposal. In addition, Steve Karnes, Roberto Muñiz, and Anne P. Stich provided thoughtful and constructive comments on the complete draft manuscript.

Thank you to Joshua Luke and Courtney Downey for their draft work on organizational structure.

Appreciation, acknowledgment, and thanks to my family and friends for their support and patience throughout this endeavor.

Rebecca Perley is owner and CEO of AIT Exam Prep, a company that prepares administrators-in-training to pass the California and federal nursing home administrator licensure exams. She is a member of the Executive Faculty in the Health Care Administration Department of California State University, Long Beach, and has been a guest lecturer for the State of California, Nursing Home Administrator Program.

Ms. Perley earned her bachelor of science in business administration at the University of Southern California and her master of science in healthcare administration at California State University, Long Beach. She is a licensed California nursing home administrator, with experience in skilled nursing facility management and the coauthor of *Nursing Home Administrator Guide to an Amazing Career*.

ABOUT THE CONTRIBUTORS

Abby Swanson Kazley, PhD, is an associate professor of healthcare management and leadership at the Medical University of South Carolina. In addition to teaching healthcare management and strategic management, she conducts research examining the prevalence and outcomes of health information technology. Specifically, she has examined national EHR and CPOE use and their relationship to quality, efficiency, cost, and patient satisfaction. Dr. Kazley earned her PhD in health services organization and research at Virginia Commonwealth University.

Andrew Lee Alden, MArch, Associate AIA, is a senior planner/designer for Eppstein Uhen Architects, Milwaukee, Wisconsin. He gained an understanding of older adults from a childhood surrounded by a large extended family. As a result he developed a strong motivation to specialize in design for aging, with an emphasis on environments that are innovative and resident-centered. He is active in local and national organizations dedicated to improving the lives of older adults through the built environment. A strong believer in the value of linking research and practice, he teaches, conducts post-occupancy evaluations, publishes articles, and presents at conferences.

Ann Wyatt is currently the project coordinator for the Alzheimer's Association, New York City Chapter, working with three nursing homes to establish innovative palliative care programs for people with advanced dementia. She has been a nursing home administrator and is an MSW. As associate director of the Office of Long-Term Care, New York City Health and Hospitals Corporation, she helped to oversee OBRA implementation for HHC's nearly 3,000 skilled nursing beds. She was a founding board member of the National Citizens Coalition for Nursing Home Reform, of the Village Nursing Home, Inc., of Music and Memory, Inc. (the iPod project), and of Ibasho.

Barbara White, DrPH, APRN, is an adult/gerontological nurse practitioner and associate professor of nursing at California State University, Long Beach, the director of the Gerontology program, which offers both a certificate and a master of science in gerontology, and the director of the Osher Lifelong Learning Institute on campus. She has coauthored two textbooks: *The Nurse Practitioner in Long-Term Care: Guidelines for*

Clinical Practice and *Critical Care Assessment Handbook*, which include geriatric care considerations.

Carissa Podesta, Esq., received her bachelor of arts in international relations from the University of California at Davis in 1997. She received her juris doctor from the George Washington University, in Washington DC, in 2000 and is an active member of the California State Bar. After law school, she practiced employment litigation in Los Angeles and Orange County, California. In 2006, she transitioned to an in-house attorney role for the skilled nursing, assisted living, home health, and hospice subsidiaries of The Ensign Group, Inc. During her eight years at Ensign, she served as the organization's vice president of human resources, chief compliance officer, and associate general counsel. While at Ensign, she worked exclusively on human resources and compliance-related legal matters involving long-term care.

A. Eduardo Gonzalez has 20-plus years in long-term care, having worked as a nursing home administrator, assisted living administrator, regional VP, CEO, owner/operator, and consultant. He holds licenses as a preceptor, residential care facility and nursing home administrator in the State of California. He offers webinars and seminars about current issues in long-term care operations and has authored three operational manuals on corporate compliance for skilled nursing facilities, corporate compliance for residential care facilities, and HIPAA. He has also been published as a guest columnist in both *Long-Term Care Living Magazine* and *McKnight's Magazine*.

Erlyana Erlyana is an associate professor in the Health Care Administration Department at California State University, Long Beach. She joined the school in fall 2009. Her research interests include access to care for underserved populations, social determinants of healthcare utilization, disparities in health, managed care, and comparative health systems. Dr. Erlyana received her MD from University of Atmajaya, Indonesia, and earned a PhD in public administration with a concentration in health service administration from University of Southern California.

Janice Frates, PhD, LCSW, is a professor emeritus of healthcare administration at California State University, Long Beach. Her research, projects, and publications cover a broad range of health policy and marketing topics, such as Medicaid, managed care, health insurance coverage for the uninsured, business marketing intelligence, and social marketing for organ donation. After retiring from university teaching, Dr. Frates reactivated her clinical social work license and opened a private practice with a focus on care management for elderly and disabled individuals.

Jean Schuldberg, EdD, MSW, professor at California State University, Chico (CSU, Chico) in the School of Social Work, is the director of the

Master of Social Work (MSW) program. She is also the codirector of the CSU, Chico Hartford Partnership Program for Aging Education (HPPAE), a program that trains MSW students as leaders in service to older adults and their families. Additionally, she is the coordinator of the Mental Health Stipend Program, which focuses on educating students in public behavioral health with an emphasis on the recovery/wellness model. Schuldberg has practiced social work for over 30 years in settings that provide medical and mental health services for older adults. In April 2013, she was appointed by Governor J. Brown to serve on the California Commission on Aging.

Jeffrey Anderzhon, FAIA, specializes in environments for the elderly and is senior architect for Eppstein Uhen Architects. He holds a BArch degree from Illinois Institute of Technology and was awarded its 2008 Alumni Professional Achievement Award. He is a member of the College of Fellows, American Institute of Architects, and coauthor of the books *Design for Aging Post-Occupancy Evaluations* and *Design for Aging: International Case Studies of Building and Program*, as well as numerous articles on environments for the elderly. He is a frequent speaker, nationally and internationally, on environments and their relationship to quality of life for the elderly.

Jill Harrison, PhD, works in health services for Planetree, an international nonprofit membership organization that provides education and training in person-centered care for organizations across the healthcare continuum. She completed her postdoctoral fellowship, funded by the Agency for Healthcare Research and Quality (AHRQ), at Brown University's Center for Gerontology and Health Care Research. She received her doctorate in sociology from Virginia Tech.

Jim Kinsey is the director of member experience at Planetree, a not-for-profit organization that provides education and information in a collaborative community of healthcare organizations, facilitating efforts to create patient-centered care in healing environments. In his role Jim leads a team of Planetree advisors, who are responsible for assessing organizations' patient- and resident-centered care practices, measuring their progress, and coaching/educating them to implement an authentic patient/resident-centered culture based on the Planetree components. Jim is also a nurse, with high-risk acute, subacute, and long-term care experience. He coauthored Planetree's *Long-Term Care Improvement Guide* and is a sought-after speaker and educator for topics associated with patient- and resident-centered care.

Ken Merchant is a consultant specializing in training and education issues in the healthcare field. He has helped to create nursing and allied health training programs throughout California by creating employer/government/training provider partnerships. A graduate of the

University of California Davis, and an Army veteran, he has served as the executive director of the Quality Care Health Foundation, and was appointed by Governor Schwarzenegger to serve on the Board of Vocational Nursing and Psychiatric Technicians. He is currently the chief operating officer of the College of Medical Arts, a chain of private postsecondary schools that specializes in training nursing home workers.

Marian Last is chair of the California Commission on Aging. She retired from the City of El Monte, where she directed a multipurpose senior center, offering wellness, integrated care management, nutrition, and advocacy programs. Cofounder of a family services and sexual assault center, Marian was a consultant to the USC Gerontology Center and a delegate to White House Conference on Aging. She continues her involvement with multiple boards and advisory committees and was appointed by Governor Schwarzenegger and reappointed by Governor Brown as a Commissioner on Aging. Marian holds degrees from Pitzer College and California State University, Long Beach. She is a licensed marriage and family therapist and is nationally board certified by the American Psychotherapy Association as a counselor.

Paige Hector, LMSW, is a clinical educator and consultant who gives workshops and seminars across the country on diverse topics, including clinical operations for the interprofessional team, meaningful use of data, advance care planning, refusal of care, documentation, and care plans. In 2014 she was named the National Association of Social Workers' representative to the Joint Commission's Professional and Technical Advisory Committee (PTAC) for Nursing and Rehabilitation Centers. In the spring of 2015 she participated in the White House Conference on Aging. She serves on the Board of Directors of the Arizona Geriatrics Society. She is a member of the Social Work Long-Term Care Research Network, a national group of social work leaders, and a CMS Social Work Research Call Group. Paige earned a master of social work degree from Arizona State University.

Rebecca Lowell is the principal of Lowell Law Center and is of Counsel to Beach | Whitman | Cowdrey, a member of the California Bar Association, CAHF, and AHLA. Ms. Lowell received her Juris Doctorate from Golden Gate University and a Certificate in Dispute Resolution from Pepperdine's Straus Institute for Dispute Resolution in 1995. Since becoming an attorney in 1995, Ms. Lowell has worked exclusively in the health care field, assisting with the development and implementation of corporate compliance programs and successfully defending health care providers through all facets of civil litigation and administrative hearings. Additionally, Ms. Lowell has developed expertise in regulatory compliance, appealing negative findings issued by state and federal agencies. She has been a frequent lecturer and program presenter on corporate compliance, health care litigation, long-term care and elder abuse topics.

Robert J. Miller, PhD, has been involved in healthcare systems development and administration for 30 years in the private and public sectors. He joined Arizona Emergency Medical Systems in 1981. While there he implemented the state's first standardized emergency department patient record system, which facilitated data collection for categorizing hospitals' emergency capabilities. He has served in a variety of C-level positions and is currently vice president for a national healthcare consulting firm. Dr. Miller received his PhD from Arizona State University in biological anthropology. He has taught at the undergraduate and graduate levels and served on numerous committees and advisory groups, including the Agency for International Development in Costa Rica.

Sarah C. Moser, EDAC, holds a Master of Architecture degree and a certificate in Architecture for Health and Wellness from the University of Kansas, where she was awarded the AIA Henry Adams Medal for Excellence in Architecture. She has a passion for evidence-based design and design research, particularly for healthcare environments and environments for aging. Sarah is fascinated by the effect of the built environment on physiological and cognitive processes, and specializes in leveraging design to promote user health and well-being.

Sonja M. Talley, MA, SHRM-SCP, SPHR, is a certified human resources (HR) professional, with 20 years management experience in health care, engineering/construction, government services, and education. She currently provides consulting services across all areas of HR as the principal consultant of her company CORE HR Solutions, LLC. She serves the Arizona Society for Human Resources Management (AZSHRM) State Council as State Director. Sonja's education includes a BA in business administration and a master's in human resources. Her current doctoral research adds a cultural lens to generational work value differences across and within generations in the U.S. workforce.

Susie Mix, MBA, is founder and owner of Mix Solutions, with over 18 years of experience in healthcare administration and a unique and extensive knowledge of the managed care industry. She has been an administrator, case manager, marketing director, contract negotiator, and consultant. She is still a licensed nursing home administrator and life agent. Her company serves skilled nursing facilities as well as hospitals and home health agencies for contracting, consulting, and training. She holds a BS in healthcare administration and an MBA from California State University, Long Beach, where she also developed and taught long-term care administration and serves as an intern preceptor to students interested in long-term care careers.

CHAPTER 1

PUBLIC POLICY

Historical Overview of Long-Term Care

Erlyana Erlyana
Jean Schuldberg
Marian Last

The U.S. and world population will continue to grow; the world population is currently growing at the rate of 1.14% per year. The number of older people in the population is also expected to increase both in number and in proportion. Between 2000 and 2010, the faster growth rates were seen at older ages (U.S. Census Bureau, 2011). Starting in 2011, approximately 10,000 Americans turn 65 every day. By 2050, when the last of the boomers reach age 85, about 20% of the U.S. population will be 65 or older, up from 13% today. As a result, the need for long-term care will also increase significantly. Of these 89 million people, about 27 million are expected to need some form of long-term care (SCAN Foundation, 2012). With this increasing need, it is important to ask whether there will be an adequate supply of services to meet our country's need and demand. The basic questions include the following: What is long-term care? Can we improve or maintain the quality of care provided? How should we prepare to finance those needs? Does the market respond adequately to the needs of its people? Should the government be involved in this matter to ensure that enough care of adequate quality is available? What policies are best to put in place and/or maintain the long-term care needs of our aging population?

LEARNING OBJECTIVES

- Describe the U.S. demographic profile transition.

- Identify key demographic trends of older Americans.

- Describe rationales for public policy.

- Identify key historical long-term care (LTC) milestones and policies.

- Differentiate federal, state, and local LTC policies.

- Describe the role of Affordable Care Act (ACA) in strengthening LTC policies.

This chapter will discuss briefly key demographic trends and impacts on long-term care continuum and what long-term care is, and review the key historical milestones and major policies in the U.S., the rationales for government policies, and cost/quality-related public control mechanisms. In addition, the chapter will discuss how public perceptions have shaped and influenced development of long-term care policies in the United States.

Key Demographic Trends of Older Americans

Some key demographic trends that will influence the long-term care service industry include rapidly increased retirement age group, lower acuity level of aging population, longevity and healthier lifestyle, socioeconomic status, gender imbalance, culture and ethnicity, and same-sex marriage and the lesbian, gay, bisexual, transgender, and queer (LGBTQ+) communities.

Demographic Bulge

As aforementioned, the population of the United States is aging, rapidly. In 2011, the oldest baby boomers reached the retirement age, and in 2030, the youngest will join the group. The impacts of the increased retirement age population cannot be underestimated. California has the largest population of over 65-year-olds in the country, estimated at 4.4 million in 2011 (Administration on Aging, 2012). The age 65 to 74 population will grow at 300% of the overall rate of population growth over the next 50 years, and the age 75 years and older population will grow at 600% of the overall rate of population growth, making these the fastest-growing age groups in the state (California State Controller, 2014).

The dramatic increase in the older adult population will increase financial strains on government resources. Citizens aged 65 and older contribute proportionally less in taxes every year, with the share of federal income taxes paid by this group dropping from 14% in 2008 (U.S. Internal Revenue Service, 2008) to just 6% in 2012 (U.S. Internal Revenue Service, 2012). Despite their decreased contribution, the population over age 85 will accrue health expenses 3 times more than those who are between the ages of 65 and 74 (Davey, Takagi, & Wagner, 2013) due to the increased health challenges as one ages.

The combination of the increased size of the population of older Americans, their decreased contribution to government revenues and increased need for services, and the smaller size of the younger population all contribute to a situation in which the allocation of government resources will become an even greater challenge. This will have the hardest impact on the Social Security system, which will need to draw resources from a shrinking population of working-age Americans to fund benefits for a rising population of older Americans.

Lower Acuity Among the Aging

Balanced against the impact of the sheer number of older Americans is the potential that baby boomers will experience lower acuity levels as they age than earlier generations. A 2006 study by the Robert Wood Johnson Foundation (2014) estimated that overall acuity levels for baby boomers will remain lower than the preceding generation until this group begins to reach their 80s. These lower acuity levels may be the result of better living conditions during the baby boomers' lifetimes, healthier lifestyle choices, and advances in the quality and availability of medical care. One effect of lower acuity levels is that a larger proportion of this generation may have the opportunity to utilize lower levels of the long-term care continuum, and avoid using skilled nursing facilities (SNFs).

Longevity and Healthier Lifestyles

The longevity of older adults in the United States, generally defined as those older than 65 years of age, has changed in many ways since the 1900s. This segment of the population has tripled in percentage compared to the general population. In 2012, 13.7% of the population was over 65 years of age in comparison to 4.1% in the early 1900s (Administration on Aging, 2012). In addition, the actual number of older adults has increased due to advances in medical technology, healthier diets, and improvements in general lifestyle. Thus, from the 1900 to 2012, those 65 years and older increased from 3.1 million to 43.1 million (Administration on Aging, 2013). In addition, the life expectancy of Americans has increased by 20 years for women and 17 years for men. It is now anticipated that a baby born in 2011 will live 30 years longer than a baby born in 1900 as a result of medical advances (Administration on Aging, 2013).

Socioeconomic Status of Older Adults

The majority of older adults report that their primary income is from Social Security. Although 86% of older adults rely on Social Security for their major source of income, assets, private pensions, government pensions, and employment do provide some financial support (Administration on Aging, 2013). Studies have indicated that baby boomers are not as prepared for retirement as their parents. This is a result of poor financial planning, depressed market returns, and the opportunity to live to an older age. One in six older adults resides in poverty, equating to 9% to 15% in this age group. Poverty most greatly impacts older adults in African American communities (22% to 33%), followed by Asian Americans (11%), Latino Americans (22%), Native Americans (20% to 43%), and Euro-Americans (6%). A greater number of women than men experience poverty (U.S. Census Bureau, 2011).

Gender Imbalance

The baby boom generation started life with slightly more male births than female births, at a ratio of 50.3% male to 49.7% female. According to the 2009 Census, the percentage had reversed to 49.4% male to 50.6% female. However, female life expectancy averages 81 years, which is considerably longer than male life expectancy, which averages 76. This translates to a ratio of 45.1% males to 54.9% females when the baby boomers reach 80 (U.S. Census Bureau, 2009). Statistics also indicate that 28% of adults 65 years and older (8.4 million women; 3.5 million men) reside alone. It is interesting to note that 45% of women over the age of 75 years do live alone (Federal Interagency Forum on Aging Related Statistics, 2012).

By 2030, 62% of those age 85 years and older will be women (Administration on Aging, 2012). Due to the increase in availability of quality health care, it is anticipated that by 2040, there will be 127 women for every 100 men age 65 years or older. Data from the Administration on Aging (2012) indicate that for baby boomers, 7 out of 10 married women will outlive their husbands. Additionally, since women tend to live 7 years longer than men, the implications for social policy and services are great.

Diversity in Culture and Ethnicity

Cultural diversity in the United States has evolved. The number of individuals from non-Euro American backgrounds has increased from 5.7 million in 2000 (16.3% of older adults) to 8.5 million in 2011 (21% of older adults). This number is projected to increase to 20.2 million in 2030. Thus, 28% of the older population will be from a culturally diverse background (Administration on Aging, 2012). Data from the Administration on Aging (2013) related that in 2011 the older adult population consisted of 9% African American; 7% Hispanic/Latino; 4% Asian or Pacific Islander; 1% American Indian or Native Alaskan; and 0.6% of persons identifying as being of two or more races (*race* is the term used in the U.S. Census data collection and analysis). Cultural practices affect the residential options chosen by older adults (Administration on Aging, 2012). Therefore, it is important to be aware that cultural factors influence decisions made by families, groups, and communities.

Same-Sex Marriage and LGBTQ+ Gender Identity

The U.S. Census Bureau (2014) now includes partnership status in the census. This area was once ignored and negatively impacted services available for individuals in the LGBTQ+ communities. California is the home for the largest number *overall* of same-sex households, followed by the state of New York. Vermont, Florida, and New Mexico have the highest number of same-sex households among the United States' *older adult* population. Santa Rosa and San Francisco, California, and Santa Fe, New Mexico, have the largest *metropolitan* concentration of same-sex coupled older adults (U.S. Census Bureau, 2014).

Until 2013, same-sex couples were denied equal treatment given to legally married couples with respect to spousal benefits and power of attorney. This inequity impacted Social Security, veteran's benefits, family medical leave, and Medicare, and created severe inheritance tax consequences. In 2013, the United States Supreme Court found that Section 3 of the Defense of Marriage Act (DOMA) was unconstitutional and same-sex married couples were entitled to benefits given other legally married couples. However, this ruling impacted only couples living in states that allowed same-sex marriages. This has led to increased efforts to provide these benefits in the remaining states that do not yet recognize same-sex marriage.

Some regulatory issues involving same-sex marriage and LGBTQ+ lifestyle were addressed in the Affordable Care Act of 2010, which banned lifestyle-based discrimination in healthcare insurance and service delivery (Family Equality Council, 2014). However, changes to tax and Social Security survivor law, which will be required to ensure full equity for same-sex couples, still need to be enacted (Smith, Maechtlen, & Tyman, 2014). Federal and state laws governing SNFs will also require changes in order to capture residents' rights issues relating to these societal changes.

Impacts on Long-Term Care Continuum

The impacts of these demographic and societal changes on the long-term care continuum are starting to be felt. There has been an emphasis on community-based services due to resource constraints, longer life expectancy, and lower acuity. There has been a growth in facilities targeted to specific groups of the population. As a result there are community-based organizations and assisted living and SNFs that have catered to specific cultural, ethnic, social, or national groups ever since the advent of the concept of long-term care. This includes agencies and facilities run by religious groups, such as the Catholic or Jewish faiths, by particular nationalities, such as Armenians or Italians, by fraternal and social groups, such as the Masons or the Order of the Eagle, and by professional groups, such as the Motion Picture & Television Fund. In general, the décor, food, entertainment, and services offered are designed to meet the interests of the sponsoring group and the residents who choose to live in the facilities who may be affiliated in some fashion with the sponsoring group.

As new national groups prosper in America, they are beginning to create their own long-term care social services agencies and facilities. The 1990s saw the rise of Asian community long-term care facilities, including facilities that catered primarily to Koreans, Chinese, and Filipinos. There are efforts underway to create new facilities to serve members of Arab and Somali communities. As immigrants who arrive in the United States from other areas of the world thrive and age, it seems inevitable that this process will continue. At the assisted living level, there has been a growth in LGBTQ+ specific care facilities (Feather, 2013).

Long-Term Care and Public Policy

What Is Long-Term Care?

Long-term care (LTC) is a range of services and supports needed by persons with reduced functional capacity—physical or cognitive. This personal care need includes basic medical services, nursing care, prevention, or palliative care. However, most of them will not be a medical care service but assistance with basic personal tasks of everyday life. Health professionals often use ability to perform **activities of daily living** (ADLs) to measure functional status of a person. There are five categories of ADLs: (1) personal hygiene (i.e., ability to bathe (wash), shave, brush teeth), (2) dressing (i.e., ability to pick out appropriate clothes, put on, button, zip, tie), (3) self-feeding (i.e., ability to eat and drink), (4) functional mobility (i.e., ability to move freely within limitation, walking to and from, sitting, getting up), and (5) toileting (i.e., ability to get to and use facilities for urination and defecation, clean up properly). **Instrumental activities of daily living** (IADLs), on the other hand, are not necessarily those basic functions, but everyday tasks needed to live independently, such as shopping, housekeeping, accounting, food preparation/taking medications as prescribed, and telephone/transportation. With population aging and increased female labor-force participation, the need for care to maintain quality of life of the frail and disabled is growing. With increasing demand, decreasing supply, and limited financing mechanisms, there is a need to address access and financing challenges.

What Is Public Policy?

Public policy refers to actions or decisions taken by the government that are intended to solve problems and improve quality of life of its citizens. Long-term care policies address both users and providers of long-term care services: (a) consumers, such as elderly and physically or mentally impaired individuals, (b) provider organizations, such as nursing homes and assisted living facilities, (c) workers who provide long-term care services, both informal workers, such as family (friend) caregivers, and formal workers, such as nurses and nursing home administrators, and (d) other related suppliers, such as durable medical equipment suppliers. Even in a liberal society like in the United States, which prefers market solutions, there is a need for effective and efficient government regulation, financing, and supervision in the field of long-term care. Past and current public policy practices are intended to protect consumers, workers, and payers, to control costs, to ensure adequate supply, and to improve quality of care.

Rationales (Goals) for Public Policy

Americans now work longer and live healthier (Benz, Sedensky, Tompson, & Jennifer, 2013). However, there is an increasing demand for long-term care due to increased longevity and decreased fertility rates. Numerous shifts in long-term care services will occur in the next few decades due to the increasing number of elderly and disabled people, and there will be more emphasis on home and community-based services due to their desire to remain independent as long as possible. This desire will increase the needs of family caregivers, including family members, partners, and close friends. As the needs increase, the future availability of family caregivers is declining. The caregiver ratio will decline from seven caregivers per one frail elderly today to four in 2030, and continue to decline to 2.9 in 2050 (Redfoot, Feinberg, & Houser, 2013).

Given the lack of balance between needs and supply, long-term care is not characterized as a viable market or to be perfectly fit to the conditions of the idealized competitive economy. The market tends to fail due to **externalities**, any unintended costs or benefits resulting from any action that affects someone who did not fully consent to participate in voluntary exchange (Weimer & Vining, 2005). Other reasons for the market failures include **asymmetric information**, where there is a discrepancy in information received or shared between sellers (providers) and buyers (consumers). The discrepancy results in an inefficient market due to **adverse selection**, in which high-risk individuals will be more likely to buy insurance, or to **moral hazard**, where individuals who purchase the insurance will be more likely to utilize excessive services. In addition, the market, similar to the healthcare industry in general, is subject to individual preferences and it is a challenge to assess performance and quality objectively. Interventions are needed to alter *providers'* and *consumers'* behaviors and incentives.

Why Public Policies for LTC?

Government or public control mechanisms are intended to resolve the long-term care market failures by addressing problems and challenges as results of underlying causes. The rationales include:

- The target market is the most *highly vulnerable population*—frail and vulnerable elders and disabled people

- Long-term care is often *negatively perceived* in terms of cost and quality

- Resources are *limited*, both in financing and workforce

- *Non-viable* financing protection mechanism

Highly Vulnerable Population

Long-term care users include the elderly and nonelderly physically and/or mentally impaired population. The users can be categorized by age, conditions that caused incapacity, and place of residence (Kaye, Harrington, & LaPlante, 2010). In addition, long-term care needs vary depending on the users' circumstances—for example:

- Most children under the age of 18 incur impairment at birth or infancy. The impairment could be physical, intellectual/developmental, or both. Even though this group is a small of percentage of **long-term care services and supports** (LTSS) users, they require extensive care, which results in substantial costs.

- For working-age adults, age 18 to 44, the impairments include intellectual disabilities, paralysis and nervous system disorders, back problems, and mental disorders.

- For older adults, age 45 to 64, most of the impairment occurs at adulthood. It is mainly related to physical disabilities, but it could also be mental disabilities.

- For 65+, 50% of the physical impairment occurs after age 65, and is mainly caused by arthritis, heart disease, and diabetes.

- Cognitive impairment, such as **dementia**, is a complicating comorbidity that causes a need for LTC. Alzheimer's disease, which accounts for a majority (60% to 80%) of dementia cases, affects 1 of 9 (11%) Americans over 65 and 1 of 3 (32%) Americans over 85, and 82% of those with Alzheimer's disease are aged 75 or older (Alzheimer's Association, 2014).

These groups are highly vulnerable and some are not capable of exercising the autonomy to make critical decisions or protect themselves from risks to their health. According to a report of the federal Department of Health and Human Services (DHHS) Office of the Inspector General (OIG), in February 2014, about 22% of Medicare beneficiaries experienced adverse events during their SNF stays and an additional 11% of the beneficiaries experienced temporary harm events during their SNF stays. Most (59%) of those adverse events and temporary harm were clearly or likely preventable. Those incidents were mostly caused by substandard treatment, inadequate resident monitoring, and failure to provide or delay of necessary care. As a result, more than half of the residents who experienced temporary harm were hospitalized and Medicare spent $2.8 billion spent on hospital treatment for harm in SNFs in FY 2011 (Levinson, 2014). In another OIG report, in May 2011, about 22% of the atypical antipsychotic drugs in nursing homes claimed were not administered according to the CMS standards. Eighty-three percent of Medicare claims for atypical antipsychotic drugs from elderly nursing home residents were associated with off-label conditions, and 88% were administered to dementia patients, a condition specified in the FDA boxed warning (Levinson, 2011).

Negative Perceptions in Costs and Quality

Very few people plan ahead for long-term care. They may be overly optimistic about their health and the ability or willingness of family members to provide needed care. When people think about retirement, they envision more time with family and friends, traveling, pursuing new or long-neglected interests, and perhaps pursuing a new career or volunteering for an organization or cause. It is a lot less pleasant to think about and plan for loss of mobility and/or mental functioning, and how to find, select, arrange, and pay for the services one will need if the worst-case scenario becomes a reality.

According to the 2013 Naturally Occurring Retirement Communities (NORC) survey of Americans age 40 and older, 30% of them were reluctant to think about getting older at all and only 35% of them were very comfortable thinking about getting older. Being older, more educated, and healthier was associated with greater comfort in thinking about getting older. Some concerns of getting older include: losing independence, losing memory or other mental abilities, paying for care, moving to a nursing home, being a burden for families, and being alone without families or friends (Tompson et al., 2013).

The 2013 NORC survey also reported that about half of respondents agreed that just about everyone will require some LTC at some point of time, even though they are not seriously ill. However, only a few took action. For example, more than half (65%) of them reported of doing a little bit of planning or none at all and only 16% of them reported a great deal of planning. Specific actions included creating an advanced directive (most common), discussing preferences with families, setting aside money to pay for it, looking for information about aging issues or LTC, modifying their home to make it easier to live in, and moving to a community designed for an older population (Tompson et al., 2013).

Another problem is that there is a widespread misperception about costs. The 2013 NORC survey of Americans 40 years or older reported that people tend to underestimate nursing home costs and overestimate home healthcare aide costs. More than half (54%) of the respondents underestimated the costs for a nursing home, 14% overestimated the costs, and only 23% correctly estimated the costs. On the other hand, more than half (52%) overestimated the home healthcare aide costs, 14% underestimated the costs, and 30% correctly estimated the costs (Tompson et al., 2013). The fact is that long-term care services are costly, and will only become more expensive in future years. In 2014, according to the Genworth 2014 Cost of Care Survey (Genworth Financial, 2014), the national median rates for different types of LTC services were:

- $212 to $240 per day for semiprivate and private rooms in a nursing home
- $3,500 per month for a one-bedroom single-occupancy assisted living community unit
- $20 per hour for a home health aide, $19 for a homemaker
- $65 per day for adult day care services

The 2013 NORC survey also reported that only 27% of Americans 40 years or older were very confident that they will have the resources to pay for the care. The survey also reported that many people misunderstand the role of Medicare as a source of payment. Forty-four percent believe that Medicare will pay for the ongoing expenses for home healthcare aides, 37% believe that Medicare will pay for ongoing expenses for nursing home care, and 71% believe that Medicare will pay for any medical equipment and assistive device. Medicare pays only for medically necessary services for a limited time and pays only for medical equipment or assistive devices prescribed by a physician (Tompson et al., 2013).

Resources Are Limited—Unaffordable and Limited Supply

Not only is long-term care expensive, but also the costs vary across states. Even in the most affordable market (Utah), the median nursing home cost far exceeds median income everywhere (Houser, 2012). The 2014 LTC State Scorecard reported that the cost was *unaffordable for middle-income families in all states.* This condition did not improve nationally from the State Scorecard report in 2011, and even became less affordable in three

Table 1.1   Summary of National Findings[*]

	Nursing homes		Assisted living communities	Home care		Adult day services
	Semiprivate room	Private room		Home health aide	Homemaker	
Rate type	Daily		Monthly	Hourly		Daily
2012 average rate ($)	222	248	3,550	21	20	70
2011 average rate ($)	214	239	3,477	21	19	70
$ (% increase from 2011)	8 (3.7)	9 (3.8)	73 (2.1)	0 (0)	1 (5.3)	0 (0)
2012 median rate ($)	206	231	3,324	21	19	65
2012 highest average rate ($) Location	682 AK, statewide	687 AK, statewide	5,933 Washington, DC	32 MN, Rochester Area	28 MN, Rochester Area	141 VT, statewide
2012 lowest average rate ($) Location	131 TX, rest of state	147 OK, rest of state	2,355 AR, rest of state	13 LA, Shreveport Area	13 LA, Shreveport Area	26 AL, Montgomery Area
2012 annual rate ($)	81,030	90,520	42,600	21,840	20,800	18,200

[*]Costs are rounded to the nearest dollar.
Annual rates for home care are based on 4 hours per day, 5 days per week; annual rates for adult day services are based on 5 days per week.
Source: MetLife Mature Market Institute (2012).

states (see Table 1.1). In 2014, the average cost of nursing home care is 246% of the median annual household income, ranging from 171% for the most affordable states to 382% for the least affordable states (Reinhard et al., 2014).

Not only is it unaffordable, but also the LTC "system" has a limited supply of trained workers. An adequate workforce, both clinical and non-clinical, will be a significant determining factor to address the challenges of the increasing demand for personal care and home health aides. Currently, due to workforce shortages, many states allow people to hire their family members to provide services to Medicaid beneficiaries. As a result, and due to the economic downturn during this period, the numbers of home health aide supplies in 2010 to 2012 improved compared to the 2007 to 2009 period (see Figure 1.1). The turnover rate of nursing home staffs also declined during this period (see Figure 1.2) (Reinhard et al., 2014). However, as mentioned before, the caregiver ratio is predicted to significantly decline in the next 15 years (Redfoot et al., 2013).

State Performance: Home Health Aide Supply, 2010–2012 Compared to 2007–2009

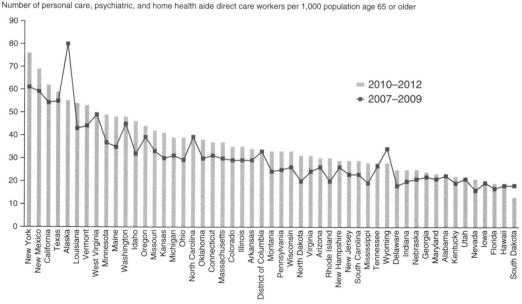

Number of personal care, psychiatric, and home health aide direct care workers per 1,000 population age 65 or older

Data: 2007–2012 American Community Survey Public Use Microdata, 2007–2012 U.S. Census Bureau Population Estimates.

Figure 1.1   State Performance: Home Health Aide Supply

Source: State long-term services and supports scorecard (2014).

State Performance: Nursing Home Staff Turnover, 2010 Compared to 2008

Ratio of employee terminations that occurred during the year, regardless of cause, to the average number of active employees during the same time period

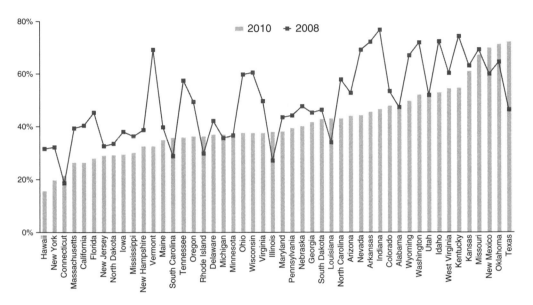

Note: Data not available for Alaska (2008–2010) and District of Columbia and Montana (2008), therefore, change in state performance cannot be shown.

Data: American Health Care Association, *Report of Findings: 2010 Nursing Facility Staffing Survey;* American Health Care Association, *Report of Findings: 2008 Nursing Facility Staff Vacancy, Retention and Turnover Survey.*

Figure 1.2   State Performance: Staff Turnover
Source: State long-term services and supports scorecard (2014).

Nonviable Financing Protection Mechanism, Both Public and Private Financing

The expenditures for long-term care impose significant burdens on families and states. Over $200 billion in annual spending on nursing care facilities, continuing care retirement communities (CCRCs), and home health accounts for more than 8% of our total health care spending annually. Of the $357 billion total long-term care spending in 2011, Medicaid paid 40% of the total (Kaiser Family Foundation, 2013). Even though Medicaid spending on LTC has been shifting toward community-based care, the expenses for long-term care services will increase sharply over the next decades (SCAN Foundation, 2012). Therefore, the pressure on federal/ state budgets and on personal budgets as well as on society is going to increase too. The growth of the elderly population and high healthcare costs will impose a significant additional burden on family/private financial resources and publicly financed programs. Changes and supports are needed to assure the well-being of the frailest.

Private financing, in the form of LTC insurance, may alleviate the burden. However, it is not a highly desired and profitable insurance product yet. Some insurance companies have left the market due to the enormous payouts. Only 4% of LTC expenditure was financed by private insurance (Brown, Goda, & McGarry, 2012). The barriers to expansion of this market include

> limited consumer rationality, the possibility that individuals may not value consumption as highly when institutionalized, as well as the availability of imperfect but cheaper substitutes for formal insurance, such as the public insurance provided by the means-tested public Medicaid program, financial transfers from children, or unpaid care provided by family members. (Brown & Finkelstein, 2009, pp. 3–4)

Other barriers include individual preferences and beliefs and undesirable features or distrust of the private market (Brown et al., 2012). Therefore, consumers will have fewer choices for private payment and will rely more on the government for intervention.

The previously referenced NORC survey (2013) of Americans over 40, in addition to revealing widespread misperception about costs and Medicare support, found that most respondents supported public policy options, such as tax breaks, government-administered long-term care programs, and a long-term care insurance individual mandate (Tompson et al., 2013). In summary, those who favor government interventions argue that public policy provides protection to consumers, particularly for those who are not capable of making well-informed decisions, and controls over costs.

Critiques of Public Policy

On the other hand, those who favor market solutions argue that the current system is not regulated effectively. They argue that many policies are uncoordinated and duplicative. Government interventions will also restrict innovation and benefits of having competition in market solutions. Policies could also produce unintended consequences that can be desirable or undesirable. For example, public policies intended to improve quality of care in nursing homes by providing higher reimbursement rates for better outcome measures exacerbate racial inequities in care (Konetzka & Werner, 2009). State tax subsidies for private long-term care insurance intended to increase private LTC insurance coverage and to reduce reliance on Medicaid funding for LTC produce unintended consequences, where the subsidies go to the high-income and asset-rich individuals, therefore produce no savings on Medicaid spending (Goda, 2011).

Key Historical Milestones and Major Long-Term Care Policies

Despite a variety of regulatory failures, long-term care is still a heavily regulated field. The principal policies (control mechanisms) regulate care providers and professionals/paraprofessionals working in the field. These control mechanisms are intended to improve quality of life of the society, safety, and health of its citizens by protecting consumers, workers, and payers. Public policies can be enacted in the form of acts or regulations. An act is a law that has been passed by some governing bodies, such as Congress or the president. A regulation is a more descriptive explanation of the way the legislation is actually implemented. One act can have numerous regulations. Both are imposed by a government unit—federal, state, or local government.

Federal Policies

The *Social Security Act of 1935* was a landmark piece of legislation that provided a monthly retirement benefit to people age 65. As the average life span of Americans increased and as society began moving from an agrarian orientation to a manufacturing orientation during the 20th century, there was a boom in homes for the elderly, particularly those associated with fraternal, faith-based organizations and other affinity groups. At the same time, large corporations began seeing the advantage of providing retirement programs, and a few states began providing old-age assistance programs. In 1935, with the effects of the Great Depression fresh in their minds, politicians enacted the Social Security Act, to federalize old-age pensions and get rid of the "poor farm" system that had become derelict and greatly overcrowded. The 1950 amendments to the Social Security Act mandated that any facility providing care for recipients of Social Security income had to be licensed by the state.

Following World War II, Congress passed the Hospital Survey and Construction Act of 1946 (also known as the *Hill-Burton Act*), which provided funding for the construction of hospitals and for state agencies to oversee its operation. This in turn provided the model for standards of design, regulation, and financing of healthcare institutions, as well as governmental agencies having jurisdiction over them. As this funding bill provided for construction of new facilities, many of the old hospital buildings were converted to nursing home use. Additionally, the burgeoning aged population and demand for long-term care nursing provided impetus for other structures, such as hotels and large houses, to be converted; a 1950 amendment to the Social Security Act provided for direct government payment to providers and stipulated that states must provide an authority to establish and maintain standards for such institutions (Institute of Medicine & Committee on Nursing Home Regulation, 1986).

In 1954 the Hill-Burton Act was amended to provide funding for the construction of nursing homes if they were part of a hospital. This amendment also provided a strong expectation of physical design based on what had been accepted practice for hospitals with regulatory oversight by the federal government. In 1959, the *National Housing Act* was amended to create a number of programs that enhanced the mortgages and provided low-interest loans through the Housing and Urban Development (HUD) Agency for construction of nursing homes, further increasing both the number of nursing homes and the federal government's involvement. However, all of these programs were aimed at financial aspects and not quality of care or consistency in nursing home environmental standards and safety (Institute of Medicine & Committee on Nursing Home Regulation, 1986).

Passed in 1965, the *Older Americans Act* (OAA) established the U.S. Administration on Aging (n.d.) within the Department of Health, Education and Welfare (today's Department of Health and Human Services) and state agencies on aging to organize, coordinate, and provide community-based services and opportunities for older Americans and their families. The act is intended to address social service needs of the aging population in order to maintain maximum independence in their homes and communities and to promote a continuum of care for the vulnerable elderly. The act also created authority for research, demonstration, and training projects in the field of aging. The 1973 amendment expanded the reach of the act by creating substate area agencies on aging. Currently the aging services network includes 56 state agencies on aging, 655 local area agencies on aging, 233 organizations serving tribal and Native Americans, and 2 organizations serving Native Hawaiians (Administration on Aging).

Some of the 2006 amendment provisions include the following:

- Authorize the assistant secretary for aging to be responsible for elderly abuse prevention and services, and to designate an office to be responsible for the administration of mental health services authorized under this act.

- Require the secretary of health and human services to establish an Interagency Coordinating Committee on Aging.

- The 2013 amendment reauthorized the Older Americans Act of 1965, proposed (not yet passed as of December 2015) in May 2013 to:

  - Include LGBTQ+, individuals with HIV and Alzheimer's disease, veterans, Holocaust survivors, among others, within the status of greatest social need caused by non-socioeconomic factors.

  - Require the director of the Office of Long-Term Care Ombudsman to collect, analyze, and report best practices for screening of elderly abuse.

  - Require the assistant secretary for aging to assist states with the development of Home Care Consumer Bill of Rights.

  - Require the Administration on Aging to work with Health Resources and Service Administration (HRSA) and secretary of labor to identify and address the workforce shortages in the field of aging.

Congress passed Title XVIII and Title XIX of the Social Security Act in 1965, creating *Medicare* and *Medicaid*, to provide insurance assistance to elderly and low-income individuals. As a result of this bill, the Center for Medicare and Medicaid Services (CMS) was created to oversee funding and regulate the quality of care and environment. In 1967, the Moss Amendments were passed, which put into place complete regulations requiring nursing homes receiving payments from Medicare and Medicaid to comply with building and life safety codes and quality of care standards. Since they are the largest source of payers, they have imposed detailed and stringent regulation to ensure quality. The regulation monitors the staffing levels, levels of coverage provided by each health professional, minimum amounts of care required to be received, and compliance in numerous specific procedures (preadmission screening, regular assessments of the functional status, internal quality assurance mechanisms, bill of rights implementation, and many others). They control costs and regulate eligibility and reimbursement rates. They also continue look at different ways to control costs, such as emphasizing home- and community-based services.

Medicaid is a joint state and federal program that helps low-income elderly to pay for long-term care services in nursing homes or at home. Medicaid does pay for custodial care in a SNF. In most states, Medicaid will also cover services to help the beneficiaries remain at home. Medicaid will pay for personal care needs; however, it will not pay for rent, mortgage, or food. To be eligible for Medicaid, a person needs to meet *general* requirements (e.g., citizenship or legal residency, be age 65 or older, have permanent disability determined by the Social Security Administration, be blind, be a pregnant woman, be a child or the parent of a child) and *financial* requirements (e.g., SSI recipients or with certain level of income). Eligibility rules and coverage of Medicaid vary from state to state (see Chapter 6 for Medicare and Medicaid coverage, eligibility, and reimbursement rates).

Containing the Nursing Home Reform Act, the *Omnibus Budget Reconciliation Act* (OBRA) of 1987 made significant changes in nursing home operations. On a continuing quest to address standards of care and to reduce federal reimbursements, OBRA established the Resident's Bill of Rights and provided a massive overhaul of federal regulations for both the care in and environment for nursing homes. The act intended to de-institutionalize the institution and change the care model from a traditional physical-only approach to a full-body approach, which includes physical, mental, and psychosocial aspects of each person. The Institute of Medicine's (IOM) report of 1986, entitled "Improving the Quality of Care in Nursing Homes," is widely acknowledged as the impetus of the *Nursing Home Reform Act* of 1987, in which a new set of standards applies to all nursing home facilities, not only for nursing home facilities that receive Medicaid and Medicare payments. The act leads to the development of the standardized Resident Assessment Instrument (RAI) for nursing home care management. The national minimum standard of care and rights of people who live in nursing facilities include: (a) resident rights, quality of life, and quality of care, (b) staffing and services, (c) resident assessment, (d) federal survey procedures, and (e) enforcement procedures.

There are three main contributions of the law for the nursing home operations. First, the OBRA 87 established new, higher, and much more resident-centered standards. The law established a number of rights, including freedom from abuse, mistreatment, and neglect and the ability to voice grievances without fear of discrimination or reprisal. The law also upgraded the staffing requirements and limited the use of physical restraints to very special circumstances. Second, the OBRA 87 introduced a range of enforcement sanctions. States were also required to conduct surveys without prior notice to the facilities, with the statewide interval not to exceed 1 year. Third, the OBRA 87 merged the Medicare and Medicaid survey and certification process into a single system.

The *Patient Self Determination Act* (PSDA) of 1990 required that all consumers have the right to understand the amount and type of care received in end-of-life situations, to create advance directives, and to hold providers accountable to their wishes. All healthcare providers, including nursing homes, home health agencies, hospice providers, and other healthcare institutions, are required to provide written information to patients concerning making decisions about medical care they received. The documentation includes the right to refuse or accept the treatment and procedures and the right to create advance directives at the time of admission. The act also requires providers not to condition provision of care or discriminate against an individual based on his decision about advance directives.

Another major federal policy affecting health care in general is the 1996 *Health Insurance Portability and Accountability Act* (HIPAA). Sections of HIPAA relatively more relevant to LTC include the administrative simplification sections that address the security and privacy of health data. The provision limits the release of patient protected health information without the written consent of the patient. The HIPAA also requires use of standard formats for processing claims and payments and standards for maintenance and transmissions of electronic health records and data. In addition, HIPAA ensures that the long-term care insurance policies that meet certain standards will receive favorable tax benefits.

Further federal quality-related regulation is a mandated use of *Minimum Data Set* (MDS). The MDS started in 1998 as a tool to assess nursing home residents. The MDS assesses the following: (a) cognitive patterns, (b) communication and hearing patterns, (c) vision patterns, (d) physical functioning and structural problems, (e) continence, (f) psychosocial well-being, (g) mood and behavior patterns, (h) activity-pursuit patterns, (i) disease diagnosis, (j) other health conditions, (k) oral/nutritional status, (l) skin condition, (m) medication use, and (n) treatment and procedures. Deficiencies will be reported based on comparison of those criteria with the standards. A similar assessment tool for home health care is called the *Outcomes and Assessment Information Set* (OASIS).

State and Local Government Policies

The designated state agencies provide oversight of Medicaid implementation. They may also impose additional regulations to ensure compliance with federal regulations. The main responsibility of state government in LTC regulation is in issuing licenses for healthcare providers. The local government agencies (both city and/or county government) ensure quality by regulating a variety of public health issues, including hygiene and sanitation, food handling (preparation and service), and many others. In addition, similar to any other business, LTC providers are obliged to comply with labor protection acts and regulations that address worker and public safety, environmental standards, and state and federal tax codes.

Several states have developed initiatives with Medicaid 1915(c) Home & Community-Based Service waivers to integrate assessment, information, care management, and other services to empower clients to choose the best settings and services for their needs. Such initiatives include the following program or services: Program of All-Inclusive Care for the Elderly (PACE), Cash and Counseling, Managed Long-Term Care Services and Supports (LTSS), such as Money Follows the Person (MFP), participant-directed services, and Balancing Incentive programs, and Testing Experience and Functional Assessment Tools (TEFT) "high-functioning" LTSS.

Significant growth in long-term care spending in 1970s led to the development of *Home- and Community-Based Services* (HCBS) or the *1915(c) waiver*, enacted in 1981 (Harrington, Ng, Kaye, & Newcomer, 2009). The waiver allows states to create flexible community-based services. The standard services include but are not limited to case management (i.e., supports and service coordination), homemaker, home health aide, personal care, adult day health services, rehabilitation (both day and residential), and respite care. The programs expanded rapidly; however, the nursing home expenses continued to grow as well.

Therefore, in the 1990s, a few states launched managed long-term care initiatives. The number of states that participate in *Managed Long-Term Care Services and Supports* (MLTSS) increased from 8 states in 2004 to 16 in 2012. By 2014, the number of states projected to have MLTSS is 26 (Saucier, Kasten, Burwell, & Gold, 2012). The MLTSS arrangements vary significantly across states. They are different in the type of enrollment (mandatory, voluntary, or both), type and size of MLTSS contractors (for-profit/nonprofit/public or quasi-public entities and local/national/mixed contractors), population groups (children, specific type of disabilities, older adults), level of care, capitation rates (comprehensive or partial services), whether they offer a consumer-directed option, whether they include Money Follows the Person through their MLTSS program, engaging members, relationship with Medicare, and quality measures (see Table 1.2).

Creating community/home-based LTC services is much more emotionally preferred, but it is also economically sound (Kaye, LaPlante, & Harrington, 2009; Kitchener, Ng, Miller, & Harrington, 2006). A review and synthesis study on cost-effectiveness of non-institutionalized LTC service programs suggested very positive outcomes and savings for home- and community-based services (Grabowski, 2006; Grabowski et al., 2010). Therefore, it is imperative to investigate factors that enable the transition. One study in Minnesota suggested that LTC facilities with more residents preferring community discharge, more Medicare days, higher nurse staffing levels, and higher occupancy have higher community discharge rates. In

Table 1.2 Population Groups Included in Existing MLTSS Programs, as of July 2012

State	Program	Children	Physical disability	Intellectual/developmental disability	65+
AZ	Long-Term Care System	V	V	V	V
CA	SCAN Connections at Home				V
DE	Diamond State Health Plan-Plus	V	v	V	V
FL	Long-Term Care Community Diversion				V
HI	QUEST Expanded Access	V	v	V	V
MA	Senior Care Options				V
MI	Managed Specialty Support & Services	V		V	
MN	Senior Health Options				V
MN	Senior Care Plus				V
NM	Coordination of Long-Term Services	V	v		V
NY	Managed Long-Term Care		V		V
NY	Medicaid Advantage Plus		v		V
NC	MH/DD/SAS Health Plan Waiver	V		V	
PA	Adult Community Autism Program			V	
TN	CHOICES	V	v		V
TX	Star+Plus	V	v		V
WA	Medicaid Integration Partnership		v	V	V
WI	Family Care Partnership		V	V	V
WI	Family Care		v	V	V

Source: Saucier et al. (2012).

addition, the rate is also higher when the facility is located within areas with higher home- and community-based services available to the community (Arling, Abrahamson, Cooke, Kane, & Lewis, 2011).

Several other new state consumer-directed strategies available in Medicaid include the following:

- State-plan optional personal care service benefit
- 1915(c) home and community-based services waiver
- 1915(j) state-plan "cash and counseling" authority
- 1915(i) state-plan home and community-based services

Important Policies Affecting LTC Professionals and Paraprofessionals

The *Americans with Disabilities Act* is a civil rights law established in 1990 to ensure fair treatment and to prohibit discrimination against individuals with disabilities in employment, state and local government services, public accommodations, commercial facilities, and transportation. Title I of the act prohibits discrimination against qualified individuals with disabilities in job application procedures, hiring, firing, advancement, compensation, job training, and other terms, conditions, and privileges of employment. It covers employers with 15 or more employees. Title II of the act protects qualified individuals with disabilities from discrimination in receiving services, programs, and activities provided by state and local government entities. Title III of the act prohibits discrimination in public accommodations and commercial facilities, and requires compliance with Americans with Disabilities Act (ADA) standards. Together with other federal laws, such as the **Civil Rights Act**, it ensures protection for consumers by guarantee of equal access and treatment for all. The act also ensures the protection of the rights of the disabled, including the ability to access public spaces and buildings.

The *Occupational Safety and Health Act* (OSHA) of 1970 is legislation to assure safe and healthful workplaces by setting and enforcing standards, and by providing training, outreach, education, and assistance. Many services delivered in nursing homes and residential care facilities involved occupational hazards, such as blood-borne pathogens and biological hazards, workplace violence, or ergonomic hazards due to resident lifting, transferring, and repetitive tasks. According to the Bureau Labor of Statistics, in 2010, nursing homes and personal care facilities had the highest lost workday rate due to injury and illness (LWDII) among private industries. The rate was 4.9 compared with 1.8 for private industries in general. Nursing aides, orderlies, and attendants had the highest rate of musculoskeletal disorders of all occupations. In 2010, the rate was 249 injuries per 10,000 workers compared with 34 per 10,000 workers for all occupation (Occupational Safety and Health Administration, n.d.). For more details on OSHA components, rules, citations, and penalties, see Chapter 5.

The *Department of Labor Wage and Hour Division* (WHD) was created with the enactment of the Fair Labor Standards Act (FLSA) in 1938. The division enforces the FLSA, government contracts labor standards statutes, the Migrant and Seasonal Agricultural Worker Protection Act (MSPA), the Employee Polygraph Protection Act (EPPA), and the Family and Medical Leave Act (FMLA).

The *Fair Labor Standards Act* (FLSA) determines the minimum wage, overtime pay, record keeping, and youth employment standards affecting workers in private sector and government. The federal minimum wage, effective as of July 24, 2009, is $7.25 per hour (as cited in http://www.dol .gov/whd/minimumwage.htm). States may also have minimum wage laws. Currently, there are only four states that have a minimum wage less than federal minimum wage. The rest of the states have either no minimum wage or a wage equal to or higher than the federal minimum wage. Employees are entitled to the higher minimum wage. The Patient Protection and Affordable Care Act of 2010 amended section 7 of the FLSA to require employers to provide reasonable break time for nursing mothers for 1 year after childbirth. Employers are also required to provide a place to express breast milk.

The *Family Medical Leave Act* (FMLA) of 1993 entitles eligible employees to take unpaid, job-protected leave for specified family and medical reasons. The employees are entitled to have 12 unpaid workweeks of leave in a 12-month period. The occasions include the birth of a child, to care for the newborn child, a child adoption, to care for core family members who have serious medical conditions that make the employee unable to perform essential duties of work, and any qualifying exigency due to active military duty of the employee's core family members. To take the leave, the employees have to give 30-day notice to their employer.

The *State Worker's Compensation Acts* were enacted by nine states in 1911. Currently, each of the 50 states has its own program. It varies in terms of who is allowed to provide coverage, the scope of coverage, levels of benefits, payment arrangement, and employer costs. Some states exempt mandatory coverage for special categories of workers, such as certain agricultural workers, charity or religious organization employees, or household workers. Employers with a fewer number of employees are exempted from mandatory coverage as well (Sengupta & Reno, 2007).

The *Equal Employment Opportunity Commission* (EEOC) enforces federal laws that make it illegal to discriminate against job applicants or employees based on the person's race, color, religion, sex, national origin, age, disability, or genetic information. The laws enforced by EEOC include:

- Title VII of the Civil Rights Act of 1964: It is illegal to discriminate against people based on race, color, religion, national origin, and sex.

- The Pregnancy Discrimination Act (PDA): This act amended Title VII to make it illegal to discriminate against a woman due to her pregnancy, childbirth, or medical condition related to pregnancy or childbirth. The law also makes it illegal to retaliate against a person who complains or participates in an employment discrimination investigation.

- The Equal Pay Act (EPA) of 1963: This act makes it illegal to pay different wages to men and women if they perform equal work in the same workplace.

- The Age Discrimination in Employment Act (ADEA) of 1967: This act prohibits discrimination against people who are 40 or older.

- Title I of the Americans with Disabilities Act (ADA) of 1990: This act prohibits discrimination against a qualified person with a disability in both the private sector and government. The law also requires employers to accommodate a person's physical or mental limitations.

- Section 102 and 103 of the Civil Rights Act of 1991: This law amended Title VII and ADA to permit jury trials and compensatory and punitive damage awards in intentional discrimination cases.

- Section 501 and 505 of the Rehabilitation Act of 1973: This law prohibits discrimination against a qualified person with a disability in the federal government.

- The Genetic Information Nondiscrimination Act (GINA) of 2008: This act makes it illegal to discriminate against a person due to genetic information. Except for Title I of this act—use of genetic information in health insurance—the provisions are enforced by the Department of Labor's Employee Benefits Security Administration (EBSA), with the Department of Health and Human Services' Office of Civil Rights enforcing Section 105 of Title I GINA.

Examples of State-Specific Laws

California Assembly Bill (AB) No. 663 amends Section 1562.3 and 1569.616 of the Health and Safety Code, and amends Section 9719 of the Welfare and Institutions Code, relating to care facilities in California. The existing law requires administrators of an adult residential care facility or an administrator of a residential care facility for elderly to have training in business operations and the psychosocial needs of facility residents. The law also requires the Office of the State Long-Term Care Ombudsman to sponsor training of ombudsmen, which needs to be completed prior to certification as an ombudsman. This bill would require the administrator and ombudsman training to include training in cultural competency and sensitivity in issues related to aging in the (LGBT) community.

The *Residential Care Facilities for the Elderly* (RCFE) Reform Act of 2014 proposed 12 bills to address some problems reported during investigation of 7,000 assisted living facilities in California. On July 24, 2014, the California governor signed **AB 1572** (one of the bills of the RCFE Reform Act), which requires facilities to allow residents to create or maintain resident councils.

The *California Partnership for Long-Term Care* (Partnership) is an innovative program launched in 1994 by the California Department of Health Care Services together with a few selected private insurance companies dedicated to educating Californians about planning for their future long-term care needs. The partnership just launched www.RUReadyCA .org as an independent source that provides information on high-quality long-term care insurance policies.

The Patient Protection and Affordable Care Act (PPACA) and LTC

Several LTC-related provisions in the ACA were created to address two main issues: costs and quality. Efforts to contain costs include expanding supports of Medicaid HCBS options. The most prominent LTC-related provision in the ACA is the CLASS Act (it is currently suspended). The CLASS Act was created to address the most imperative problem of LTC—financing. The act intended to create a government-run LTC insurance program within the parameters of the enrollment, eligibility, premium, coverage level, and administration. However, the act was repealed due to its inability to show evidence of solvency over a 75-year period (a statutory mandate) (Gleckman, 2011). Without the CLASS Act, the *Affordable Care Act* provisions mostly consisted of several programs and supports in helping people to receive long-term care service and supports in their home or the community. The law continues supports for the existing mechanisms/programs and creates new alternatives and financial incentives for states to provide home- and community-based services and supports (Reinhard, Kassner, & Houser, 2011). The supports include:

- The *State Balancing Incentive Payments* program, authorizing grants to states to increase access to non-institutional long-term care service and supports, which started October 1, 2011. The program offers a targeted increase in the Federal Medical Assistance Percentage (FMAP) tied to the percentage of a state's noninstitutional LTSS spending.

- The *Home and Community-Based Services (HCBS) State Plan Option*, which expands HCBS to more individuals and ensures the quality of services provided.

- *Community First Choice* provides enhanced federal funding to states that elect to provide person-centered home and community-based attendant services and supports to increase individuals with disabilities' ability to live in the community.

- *Money Follows the Person* (MFP) provides individuals with LTSS that enables them to move out of institutions and into their homes or other community-based settings. Forty-four states, including Washington, DC, participate in the MFP demonstration, part of the 2005 Deficit Reduction Act (DRA). The funding allows states to offer help to Medicaid beneficiaries transitioning from institution settings to community-based settings. Under the ACA, Medicaid beneficiaries who reside in LTC institutions for 90 consecutive days are eligible to participate (instead of 6 months to 2 years) and the funding is going to be extended until September 2016 (a total of $2.25 billion will be allocated for 2012 to 2016 or $450 million each fiscal year [FY]). Any unused funds awarded in 2016 can be utilized until 2020.

- Demonstration grants for *Testing Experience and Functional Assessment Tools* (TEFT) in LTSS test quality measurement tools and demonstrate e-health in Medicaid LTSS.

Efforts to improve quality include provisions affecting LTC workers both in institutions (nursing home) or communities (personal attendant and family caregivers). There are a few demonstration projects and grants to support training of LTC-related professionals and paraprofessionals. The ACA also includes several provisions to ensure and improve quality of nursing home care and to prevent elderly abuse and neglect. The provisions include disclosure of more detailed information, implementation of compliance and ethics programs, improvement of the Nursing Home Compare website, and adoption of standardized complaint forms. Also there are several national demonstration projects on culture change and the enhanced use of information technology and pay-for-performance in nursing homes.

Summary

In the next few decades, the graying of the baby boomers, increased longevity, lower fertility rates due to labor-force participation, and some other demographic trends will change the future of long-term care in the United States. With current policy directions, there will be major changes ahead. Increasing demand for any interventions or strategies to support independent living will become more and more popular. As the demand for long-term care service and supports continues to grow, it is important to seek alternatives for those increasing needs. Particularly with limited available resources, both labor and capital resources, it is imperative to create innovative ways to tackle the challenges. Public and private control mechanisms were created to control escalating costs and ensure adequate access and quality of care. Current policies that emphasize sociodemographic and culturally sensitive home- and community-based services need to be continued and supported. Quality measures need to be refined. Resources need to be properly allocated and redistributed.

Key Terms

The following terms are important to the chapter. Some of the terms may also be found in other chapters, but they may be used in different contexts.

Act: A law that has been passed by a legislative body

Activities of daily living: Routine activities of everyday life that individuals must perform in order to survive comfortably (ex. dressing, bathing, toileting)

Adverse selection: Unintended consequences due to imbalanced shared information in which individuals with higher risks of using services are more likely to purchase insurance

Asymmetric information: Imbalanced shared information

Custodial care: Help with activities of daily living, such as help to bathe, walk, shop, eat, and dress

Dementia: A wide range of symptoms associated with a decline in memory or other thinking skills that reduce a person's ability to perform everyday activities

Externalities: Unintended costs or benefits of certain actions/conditions

Instrumental activities of daily living: Skills needed to maintain independence (ex. preparing meals, homecare, paying bills and banking, shopping, managing medications)

Long-term care services and supports (LTSS): Any task that helps older adults and people with disabilities accomplish everyday tasks

Moral hazard: Unintended consequences due to imbalanced shared information that results in excessive use of services by individuals who purchase insurance

Public policy: Actions taken or decisions made by the government that are intended to solve problems and improve the quality of life of its citizens

Regulation: A law that describes how an act is implemented

Review Questions

1. Why should government regulate long-term care providers and practitioners?

2. What are the potential contributions and impacts of ACA on LTC?

3. Your state is concerned about increasing Medicaid spending on long-term care services and supports, and long-term care insurance is not growing as expected. What are some of the policy alternatives that could be used to increase the long-term care insurance rate?

4. What are the best alternatives besides expanding home- or community-based services?

Case Study

Public policies comprise authoritative decisions to address public issues and problems. Most public policies are intended to maximize benefits of the society. However, they often produce unintended consequences. The complexity of the issues and variability of the causes create unthinkable and unpredictable consequences. The graying of the baby boomers and lack of adequate and sufficient protection mechanisms need immediate attention. Using the U.S. demographic projections and the current existing financing mechanisms for long-term care, do the following:

•   Assess the need for government involvement in creating major policy changes.

- Discuss several alternatives to government intervention.

- Discuss the pros and cons (barriers and unintended consequences) of each alternative.

- Decide whether we should keep market involvement to allow flexibility and innovation in solving problems.

References

Administration on Aging. (n.d.). *Older Americans Act*. Retrieved from http://www.aoa.gov/AoA_programs/OAA/

Administration on Aging. (2012). *Aging statistics*. Retrieved from http://www.aoa.acl.gov/Aging_Statistics/index.aspx

Administration on Aging. (2013). *A profile of older Americans: 2013*. Retrieved from http://www.aoa.gov/Aging_Statistics/Profile/

Alzheimer's Association. (2014). *2014 Alzheimer's disease: Facts and figures.* Retrieved from http://www.alz.org/downloads/Facts_Figures_2014.pdf

Arling, G., Abrahamson, K. A., Cooke, V., Kane, R. L., & Lewis, T. (2011). Facility and market factors affecting transitions from nursing home to community. *Medical Care, 49*(9), 790–796.

Benz, J., Sedensky, M., Tompson, T., & Jennifer, A. (2013). *Working longer: Older Americans' attitudes on work and retirement*. Retrieved from http://www.apnorc.org/PDFs/Working%20Longer/AP-NORC%20Center_Working%20Longer%20Report-FINAL.pdf

Brown, J. R., & Finkelstein, A. (2009). The private market for long-term care insurance in the U.S.: A review of the evidence. *The Journal of Risk and Insurance, 76*(1), 5–29. doi:10.1111/j.1539-6975.2009.01286.x

Brown, J. R., Goda, G. S., & McGarry, K. (2012). Long-term care insurance demand limited by beliefs about needs, concerns about insurers, and care available from family. *Health Affairs, 31*(6), 1294–1302. doi:10.1377/hlthaff.2011.1307

California State Controller. (2014). *California's population*. Retrieved from www.sco.ca.gov/state_finances_101_california_population.html

Davey, A., Takagi, E., & Wagner, D. (2013). A national profile of caregivers for the oldest-old. *Journal of Comparative Family Studies, 45*(4), 434–490.

Family Equality Council. (2014). *The Affordable Care Act and families with parents who are LGBT: Everything you need to know*. Retrieved from www.familyequality.org/get_informed/advocacy/know_your_rights/affordable_care_act_guide

Feather, J. (2013). Making communities LGBT aging friendly. *Huffington Post*. Retrieved from www.lgbtagingcenter.org/newsevents/newsArticle.cfm?n=45

Federal Interagency Forum on Aging Related Statistics. (2012). *Federal agency on aging statistics: Older Americans 2012—Key indications of well-being*. Retrieved from www.agingstats.gov/agingstatsdotnet/Main_Site/Data/2012_Documents/Docs/EntireChartbook.pdf

Genworth Financial. (2014). *Cost of care survey: Home care providers, adult day health care facilities, assisted living facilities and nursing homes.* Retrieved from https://www.genworth.com/dam/Americas/US/PDFs/Consumer/corporate/130568_032514_CostofCare_FINAL_nonsecure.pdf

Gleckman, H. (2011). Requiem for the CLASS Act. *Health Affairs, 30*(12), 2231–2234.

Goda, G. S. (2011). The impact of state tax subsidies for private long-term care insurance on coverage and Medicaid expenditures. *Journal of Public Economics, 95*(7), 744–757.

Grabowski, D. C. (2006). The cost-effectiveness of noninstitutional long-term care services: Review and synthesis of the most recent evidence. *Medical Care Research and Review, 63*(1), 3–28.

Grabowski, D. C., Cadigan, R. O., Miller, E. A., Stevenson, D. G., Clark, M., & Mor, V. (2010). Supporting home- and community-based care: Views of long-term care specialists. *Medical Care Research and Review, 67*(4 suppl), 82S–101S.

Harrington, C., Ng, T., Kaye, H. S., & Newcomer, R. J. (2009). Medicaid home and community based services: Proposed policies to improve access, costs and quality. *Public Policy & Aging Report, 19*(2), 13–18.

Houser, A. (2012). *A new way of looking at private pay affordability of long-term services and supports.* Washington, DC: AARP Public Policy Institute.

Institute of Medicine & Committee on Nursing Home Regulation. (1986). Appendix A: History of federal nursing home regulation. In *Improving the quality of care in nursing homes* (pp. 238–253). Washington, DC: National Academies Press.

Kaiser Family Foundation. (2013). A short look at long-term care for seniors. *JAMA, 310*(8), 786–787. doi:10.1001/jama.2013.17676

Kaye, H. S., Harrington, C., & LaPlante, M. P. (2010). Long-term care: Who gets it, who provides it, who pays, and how much? *Health Affairs, 29*(1), 11–21.

Kaye, H. S., LaPlante, M. P., & Harrington, C. (2009). Do noninstitutional long-term care services reduce Medicaid spending? *Health Affairs, 28*(1), 262–272.

Kitchener, M., Ng, T., Miller, N., & Harrington, C. (2006). Institutional and community-based long-term care: A comparative estimate of public costs. *Journal of Health & Social Policy, 22*(2), 31–50.

Konetzka, R. T., & Werner, R. M. (2009). Review: Disparities in long-term care building equity into market-based reforms. *Medical Care Research and Review, 66*(5), 491–521.

Levinson, D. R. (2011). *Medicare atypical antipsychotic drug claims for elderly nursing home residents.* Retrieved from http://oig.hhs.gov/oei/reports/oei-07-08-00150.pdf

Levinson, D. R. (2014). *Adverse events in skilled nursing facilities: National incidence among medicare beneficiaries.* Retrieved from http://oig.hhs.gov/oei/reports/oei-06-11-00370.pdf

MetLife Mature Market Institute. (2012). *Market survey of long-term care costs: The 2012 MetLife market survey of nursing home, assisted living, adult day services, and home care costs.* New York, NY: Author.

Occupational Safety and Health Administration. (n.d.). *Nursing homes and personal care facilities.* Retrieved from https://www.osha.gov/SLTC/nursinghome/

Redfoot, D., Feinberg, L., & Houser, A. (2013). *The aging of the baby boom and the growing care gap: A look at future declines in the availability of family caregivers.* Retrieved from http://www.aarp.org/content/dam/aarp/research/public_policy_institute/ltc/2013/baby-boom-and-the-growing-care-gap-insight-AARP-ppi-ltc.pdf

Reinhard, S. C., Kassner, E., & Houser, A. (2011). How the Affordable Care Act can help move states toward a high performing system of long-term services and supports. *Health Affairs, 30*(3), 447–453.

Reinhard, S. C., Kassner, E., Houser, A., Ujvari, K., Mollica, R., & Hendrickson, L. (2014). *Raising expectations: A state scorecard on long-term services and supports for older adults, people with physical disabilities, and family caregivers.* Retrieved from http://assets.aarp.org/rgcenter/ppi/ltc/ltss_scorecard.pdf

Robert Wood Johnson Foundation. (2014). *Long-term care: What are the issues?* Retrieved from www.rwjf.org/en/research-publications/find-rwjf-research/2014/02/long-term-care--what-are-the-issues-.html

Saucier, P., Kasten, J., Burwell, B., & Gold, L. (2012). *The growth of managed long-term services and supports (MLTSS) programs: A 2012 update.* Retrieved from http://www.medicaid.gov/medicaid-chip-program-information/by-topics/delivery-systems/downloads/mltssp_white_paper_combined.pdf

SCAN Foundation. (2012). *Growing demand for long-term care in the U.S. (updated).* Retrieved from http://www.thescanfoundation.org/growing-demand-long-term-care

Sengupta, I., & Reno, V. (2007). Recent trends in workers' compensation. *Social Security Bulletin, 67*, No. 1, 2007.

Smith, C., Maechtlen, L., & Tyman, A. (2014). *President Obama expands LGBT non-discrimination protections with executive order.* Retrieved from www.laborandemploymentlawcounsel.com/2014/07/president-obama-expands-lgbt-non-discrimination-protections-with-executive-order/

State long-term services and supports scorecard. (2014). Retrieved from http://www.longtermscorecard.org/

Tompson, T., Benz, J., Agiesta, J., Junius, D., Nguyen, K., & Lowell, K. (2013). *Long-term care: Perceptions, experiences, and attitudes among americans 40 or older.* Retrieved from http://www.apnorc.org/PDFs/Long%20Term%20Care/AP_NORC_Long%20Term%20Care%20Perception_FINAL%20REPORT.pdf

U.S. Census Bureau. (2009). *Selected characteristics of baby boomers 42 to 60 years old in 2006.* Retrieved from www.census.gov/population/age/publications/files/2006babyboomers.pdf

U.S. Census Bureau. (2011) *The older population: 2010*. Retrieved from http://www
.census.gov/prod/cen2010/briefs/c2010br-09.pdf

U.S. Census Bureau. (2014). *Same sex couples*. Retrieved from www.census.gov/
hhes/samesex

U.S. Internal Revenue Service. (2008). *Tax year 2008, Table 3.7—All returns: Tax
liability, tax credits, and tax payments for tax year 2008*. Retrieved from www
.irs.gov/pub/irs-soi/12in37ag.xls

U.S. Internal Revenue Service. (2012). *Tax year 2012, Table 3.7—All returns: Tax
liability, tax credits, and tax payments for tax year 2012*. Retrieved from www
.irs.gov/pub/irs-soi/12in37ag.xls

Weimer, D. L., & Vining, A. R. (2005). *Policy analysis: Concepts and practice*. New
York: NY: Routledge.

CHAPTER 2

LONG-TERM CARE CONTINUUM

Marian Last
Jean Schuldberg
Kenneth Merchant

The dramatic growth in the older adult population in the United States has contributed to rapid changes in the field of long-term care. Each day, 10,000 **baby boomers** (those born between 1946 and 1964) are reaching the age of 65 years (West, Cole, Goodkind, & He, 2014). Long-term care refers to the continuum of care services available to people who need minimal assistance in coping with ongoing conditions while residing either at home or in a long-term care facility. Factors that impact the type of services needed and appropriate residential environment include medical conditions, mental health status, social factors, and challenges resulting from physical disability.

The U.S. Department of Health Services, Administration for Community Living (ACL) (2013) reports that an average of 3.5% of the older adults aged 65 or above reside in an institutional setting at one given time. The 3.5% is an average of all older adults 65 years and older. It is important to note that this number increases with age. For example, only 1% of adults age 65 to 74 reside in institutional settings, while for those 75 to 84 years of age, the percentage increases to 3%. This number then increases dramatically to 10% of older adults who are 85 years of age and older residing in institutional settings (ACL, 2013).

The Long-Term Care Continuum Defined

The long-term care continuum consists of a wide range of services, all directed to caring for people with long-term

LEARNING OBJECTIVES

- Identify the major components in the long-term care continuum.

- Describe the benefits and challenges of aging in place, as compared to receiving care in an institutional setting.

- Describe some of the caregiver services that are available to support aging in place.

- Identify the characteristics of skilled nursing facilities and how they differ from non-institutional healthcare settings.

- Discuss the professions of the key staff who provide services within the long-term care continuum.

- Discuss the requirements to become a healthcare administrator, in either skilled nursing or assisted living.

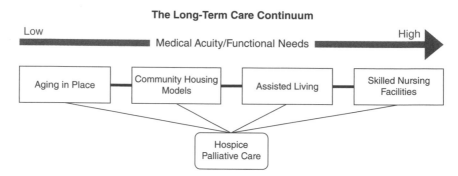

Figure 2.1   The Long-Term Care Continuum
Source: Merchant (2014b).

health issues. It can be as simple as family members providing assistance to elderly relatives who are otherwise independent and aging in place in their own home. Or, it can be as challenging as providing 24-hour nursing care to individuals with complex medical conditions, who require advanced technological interventions in order to survive. Figure 2.1 depicts the long-term care continuum.

Activities of Daily Living (ADLs) and Instrumental Activities of Daily Living (IADLs)

Activities of daily living (ADLs) are the routine activities of everyday life that individuals must attend to in order to survive comfortably. ADLs include toileting, eating, bathing, ambulating (walking) and transferring, and dressing. Instrumental activities of daily living (IADLs) focus on skills needed to maintain independence, such as preparing meals, homecare, paying bills and banking, shopping, managing medications, monitoring basic health indicators, such as temperature and blood pressure, and attending to in-home medical treatments, such as oxygen. Many individuals require increasing assistance with ADLs and IADLs as they grow older, or as a result of disabilities.

In some cases, community-based agencies can provide resources for people to age in place independently. Nonprofit organizations and local government agencies can offer a variety of services to help people sustain independent lifestyles, ranging from assisting with ADLs and IADLs to providing subsidized housing. These services may be provided to the individual at limited cost, with either a fixed or a sliding scale fee.

The categories of long-term care are organized in a sequence from lowest acuity level to highest acuity level: aging in place, assisted living, skilled nursing, and acute care. These levels will be addressed in detail later in this chapter, with an overview of the continuum of care, beginning with the private home environment, followed by community home environments, community support programs, and transitional housing from home community to formalized care facilities, and skilled nursing facilities (SNFs).

It is a truism that aging in place (in one's home) is the preferred long-term care solution. It is also the preference of the U.S. federal government, as codified in the 2006 amendments to the Older Americans Act (OAA) of 1965 (Administration on Aging, 2006a). This chapter will pay particular attention to the different levels of care that will not be addressed elsewhere in this book.

Medical Acuity

An individual's place on the continuum is generally determined based on a combination of his medical and mental capacity (functional living skills), activities of daily living, instrumental activities of daily living, and financial and familial considerations. **Medical acuity** can be defined as the measurement of the intensity of nursing care required by an individual (American Sentinel University, 2014). The goal of the care provider is to "attain or maintain the highest practicable physical, mental, and psychosocial well-being possible" (U.S. Dept. of Health and Human Services, 2014b, p. 58) at the lowest level of care possible on the long-term care continuum.

The Long-Term Care Continuum

Aging in Place

Aging in place refers to individuals growing older within their home environment, surrounded by a familiar network of family and friends, sometimes utilizing community-based services. This option is often the preferred level of care for individuals, offering the greatest level of independence, and causes the fewest disruptions to one's lifestyle. The ACL of the federal government officially supports aging in place as the recommended course of action for individuals because of its potential impact on quality of life, and because it costs the government less in services in the long run (U.S. Department of Housing and Urban Development, 2013a).

Choosing an Appropriate Service

Planning is advisable to best prepare consumers for a future informed decision regarding needed services. Before services become absolutely essential, it is advisable that an extensive search of community service options be facilitated and contact be made with the respective agency or agencies. This allows time to assess eligibility requirements and documents needed to process an application. Agency staff also must identify community-based services that are paired to the mental and physical capabilities of the individual. Many agencies utilize a uniform, universal, comprehensive assessment and/or intake form for gathering vital information on the client. Additional assessment tools may be used to assess activities of daily living (ADL) and instrumental activities of daily living (IADL). The changes in a person's ability to perform ADLs and IADLs often impact the need for transitioning into a higher level of care.

Quality of Life Factors

Quality of life relies on a continuum of care from formal networks requiring payment for services (lawyers and home health aides) and informal networks (friends, family, and neighbors), holistic management, assessment of an individual's medical, physical, and psychosocial care that maintain independent lifestyles. In Figure 2.2, the Diminished Capacity Chart (Last, 2014) illustrates the path of interventions to follow as the ADLs and IADLs of the client become compromised.

Care Managers and Case Managers

The terms **care manager** and **case manager** are frequently used synonymously, referring to the same skill set and type of services provided to clients and their families. Thus, when this chapter discusses care managers, the education and duties are reflective of case managers.

A care manager has completed a formal education with a focus on providing advocacy for clients and their families. The **geriatric care manager**'s role is to assist individuals and families to assess and choose appropriate services from the options available from community programs and agencies. Geriatric care managers include those who have received degrees in human services that include nursing, gerontology, psychology, and social work. Specific professionals, who are versed in mental health and gerontology, may also assist clients to reside in the least restrictive residential environment. These include licensed marriage family therapists (LMFTs), licensed clinical social workers (LCSWs), and licensed professional counselors (LPCs).

Care managers' duties may vary, but overall they include completing an initial, in-depth assessment with clients to evaluate their goals and in turn secure resources to help meet these goals. Care managers "assists clients in attaining their maximum functional potential" (National Association of

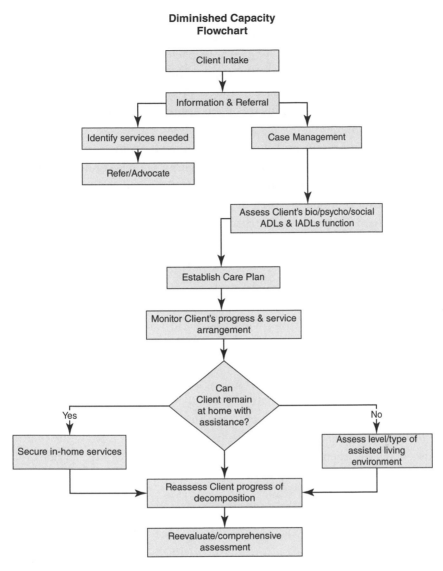

Diminished Capacity Flowchart

- Client Intake
- Information & Referral
  - Identify services needed
    - Refer/Advocate
  - Case Management
    - Assess Client's bio/psycho/social ADLs & IADLs function
    - Establish Care Plan
    - Monitor Client's progress & service arrangement
    - Can Client remain at home with assistance?
      - Yes → Secure in-home services
      - No → Assess level/type of assisted living environment
    - Reassess Client progress of decomposition
    - Reevaluate/comprehensive assessment

Figure 2.2 Diminished Capacity Flowchart
Source: Last (2014).

Professional Geriatric Care Managers, 2014, p. 2). Thus, "the goal of care management is to achieve an optimal level of wellness and improve coordination of care while providing cost effective, non-duplicative services" (Health Care Administration, 2008).

To provide services, care managers complete routine home visits. A thorough assessment is utilized to evaluate ADLs and IADLs, safety concerns, needed home modifications, and challenges that may occur due to poor nutrition, medication management, mental status, mental health, and social needs. The frequent contact with a client allows the care manager to evaluate and modify care plans due to changes in physical or mental health or social situation. A team approach is frequently utilized, with care managers collaborating with hospital and SNF discharge planners and home health agencies. A care manager may refer the client to various community services, and thus this team approach is designed to minimize hospital readmission.

The Older Americans Act provides funding for some care management services administered through state and county agencies or nonprofit organizations (Administration on Aging, 2006a). Private-pay care management services are becoming an integral part of elder care, and the people who provide them are termed geriatric care consultants.

Documents Relevant to Securing Services

It is important for individuals to keep copies of their own medical records. Consumers are entitled to request such documentation from their respective healthcare providers as mandated under the *Health Insurance Portability and Accountability Act* (HIPAA) of 1996. A document following HIPAA guidelines is commonly utilized as the standard reference by professionals provided to the consumer before rendering services and offering any health care. Updated financial and legal records, such as bank statements, pension benefits, and durable powers of attorney, should be executed while the client's cognitive functions are intact. Such information also helps the client qualify for public benefits and various services relevant to maintaining his care. Documents should be maintained in various formats (digital and hardcopies) and secured in safe places, such as a safety deposit box at the bank or a fireproof safe at home.

The Private Home Environment: Aging in Place

Informal Supports

Informal supports are unpaid family or friends providing caregiving within the home. The Administration on Aging (2012) related that 85% of all older adults will need some in-home caregiving services during their lifetime. Unpaid (family and/or friends) caregivers provide 84% of care; 30% of these caregivers are over 65 years old. Studies affirm that more than three-fourths of caregivers feel the need for increased help related to their duties. The majority of these caregivers receive no formal instruction or training on how to perform these tasks (American Association of Retired Persons [AARP], 2011b).

Davey, Takagi, and Wagner (2013) studied older adults with some form of disability. In their study, almost 58% of respondents described themselves as experiencing "poor health." Over one-third lived alone, approximately 45% resided with a spouse, and 22% lived with a child. The majority of the caregivers did not receive additional assistance, and those who worked in urban regions related greater stress than those in rural areas. The researchers suggested that informal supports from community and family would have reduced the tension for caregivers employed in less populated areas.

Private-Duty Aide

A **private-duty aide** provides a variety of services that includes medical and custodial care. Medical services are provided by **registered nurses (RN)** or **licensed vocational nurses (LVN)** in any environment, such as a personal home, acute hospital, skilled nursing, or assisted living facility. The services of aides, nurses, and medication technicians may be covered under a long-term care policy, Medicare, Medicaid, health maintenance organization (HMO), preferred provider organization (PPO), or private pay. Additionally, private-duty non-medical (custodial) nursing care services can be provided by **home health aides**. Home health aides are caregivers who provide assistance to individuals in their homes with their ADLs and can be certified or non-certified, depending on the state. The activities within this category consist of personal or companion care and housekeeping services and may be covered under a long-term care policy or by in-home supportive services funded by a state or a county, or private pay.

Home Care

Homemaker or chores services are typically not medical in nature. **Home care** eases the burdens of housework, shopping, laundry, ironing, and cooking. Personal care attendants or assistants may support an individual in performing daily living activities (ADLs and IADLs), such as eating, dressing, bathing, toileting, and transferring, and those activities that generally are instrumental to routine functioning that facilitates independent living.

Home Health Care

With a medical emphasis, **home health care** services include skilled nursing care, such as the care of a catheter, physical therapy, occupational therapy, speech therapy, and respiratory therapy. Services of this nature must be prescribed by a physician and involve ongoing medical supervision. Home health agencies employ a myriad of professionals, such as registered and licensed vocational nurses, physical and occupational therapists, and social workers. Services may be covered by Medicare, private plans, cash, or long-term care insurance.

Home Modifications

Home modifications are adaptations to the home environment to alleviate specific barriers that may impede the ability to remain in the home. According to the AARP (2009) 80% of older adults are homeowners. This number is projected to reach 89% in 2030. Of this group, 82% have expressed a wish to live in their home for as long as possible. A survey by AARP indicated 2,260 adults ages 45 to 65 echoed the desire to remain at home, but showed an awareness of the need for structural modification. For example, 91% of respondents expressed the importance of having a bedroom on the main floor (AARP, 2011a). With baby boomers aging in place, there will be an increase in the need for home modification.

Most homes today are not modified to meet the needs of those over the age of 65. Physical hazards include stairs, slippery floors, limited access to bathing facilities, cabinets and counter access, and obstacles preventing appliance use. To mitigate these obstacles, home modifications can make a physical environment more user-friendly. The modifications may include special consideration for the ingress and egress of doorways and rooms. Safety features might include the addition of grab bars, ramps, fire and carbon monoxide alarms, medication prompt systems, and home tele-health monitors.

Szanton et al. (2011) performed a pilot study of older adults averaging 78 years of age. The goal of the study was to evaluate the participants' needs for a safe and supportive living environment that would allow aging in place in their own homes. The participants in this study were primarily from African American communities. Forty-four percent of the participants experienced difficulties with three or more ADLs. Nursing and occupational therapy were provided to participants, along with minor to moderate home repairs. Modifications ranged from fixing loose floor tiles and providing grab bars to replacing defective gas stoves. The average cost of these basic modifications was $1,285. Results showed that these modifications improved daily functions, such as ambulation, and increased the participants' sense of well-being and ability to continue to reside in their home.

Houses in need of repairs to ensure a safe and sanitary environment may qualify for subsidies if income guidelines are met. Additionally, the U.S. Department of Health and Human Services (n.d.) funds the Low-Income Home Energy Assistance Program (LIHEAP) and the Weatherization Assistance Program (WAP). In the United States it is becoming more common for communities to assist with subsidizing home modifications through federal and state programs. Eligibility requires that the owner occupy the home and meet the low-income requirements applicable to the state where he resides. With several locations throughout Southern California, nonprofit organizations, such Rebuild America (n.d.), provide home modification.

Federal Housing Programs

The U.S. Department of Housing and Urban Development (HUD) facilitates the Section 8 housing program that provides vouchers that are portable that augment rent for income-eligible recipients. Up to 66% of the rent for income-eligible recipients can be covered. This means that arrangements with an existing landlord can occur that will require the property to be certified as safe, sanitary, and secure for occupancy. One and two bedrooms are available and must meet the requirements mandated under the Americans with Disabilities Act (ADA). Senior congregate housing, funded under HUD, does not provide on-site ancillary health or social services (U.S. Department of Housing and Urban Development, 2013c).

Section 202, Supportive Housing for the Elderly, directs independent living resources toward individuals at least 62 years of age with very low incomes. Standardized units feature one bedroom, private bath, kitchen, and other amenities (special ramps, flooring, and grab bars) that facilitate a safer environment for individuals with compromised physical abilities. Section 202 requires provisions for ancillary supportive services on-site, including meals, information, and assistance, and essential transportation to life-sustaining activities. Both Section 8 and Section 202 have a limited number of slots available each year for eligible individuals (U.S. Department of Housing and Urban Development, 2013b).

Shared Housing Programs

In **shared housing** programs, people live together in a home or an apartment with shared common areas. Private sleeping quarters are usually available. People move into shared housing for various reasons, such as reduced housing costs, help with chores, support for household responsibilities, or feeling safer with others at home.

Congregate Housing

Congregate housing refers to complexes with separate apartments (including kitchens) that provide some housekeeping services and some shared meals. These facilities may be subsidized under Section 202 of the federal housing programs administered by the U.S. Department of Housing and Urban Development (HUD).

Veterans Affairs Supportive Housing (VASH)

Since 2008, the Department of Housing and Urban Development, through the Veteran's Administration, has issued an average of 10,000 housing vouchers to veterans and their families who are at risk of becoming homeless. A case manager is assigned to assist families in securing housing and monitor the progress to help veterans maintain sustainable housing and employment (U.S. Department of Veterans Affairs, 2014).

Community Resident Environments

Continuing Care Retirement Community (CCRC)

A **continuing care retirement community** (CCRC) is a residential model that offers a range of housing options (normally independent living through nursing home care) and varying levels of medical and personal services. A CCRC is designed to meet residents' needs in a familiar setting as they grow older while they are healthy.

Some CCRCs are licensed to provide care at both the skilled nursing and the assisted living levels. Individuals typically pay the cost of their care in a CCRC, though they may receive public assistance once they transition into receiving skilled nursing care. Caregivers at CCRC facilities are typically a blend of the assisted living and the SNF models. CCRCs have a non-medical support staff and medical staff, comparable to assisted living facilities and skill nursing respectively.

A CCRC resident signs a long-term contract that outlines housing, personal care, housekeeping, yard maintenance, and nursing obligations. An entry fee, in addition to a monthly service charge, is also specified. These costs may change according to the medical or personal care services required. Fees vary depending on whether the person owns or rents the living space, its size and location, the type of service plan choice, and the current risk for needing intensive long-term care.

Active Living Communities

Active living communities promote independent living, allowing older adults to age in place with support to perform home and personal care. An example of this is the Village Model of a community, such as Beacon Hill, located in Boston, Massachusetts, which is one of the fastest-growing concepts in the United States. The types of support can range from assistance with home repairs and house cleaning to assistance with ADLs, transportation, and recreational activities. This innovative approach to "aging in place" provides a community to support the older adult. To maintain the "village," participants pay an annual fee, ranging from $50 to several thousands of dollars, to a community volunteer, an agency, or an independent provider.

Some villages are formally constructed and consist of single-family units, townhomes, or duplexes constructed for adults aged 55 years and above; these may contain properties to purchase and/or rent. Some communities are as comprehensive as providing gated complexes that feature meals in a restaurant-type setting, recreation, aquatic centers, angulating walkways, and lush golf courses. Floor plans incorporate state-of-the-art kitchens, bathrooms with Jacuzzi bathtubs, and expansive patio areas and gardens. Other common attributes may include recreational activities, college-level classes, fitness centers, computer labs, medical clinics, theaters, and libraries. Leisure World of Seal Beach and Laguna Woods Village are among some of the more long-standing communities, established in the 1960s by Ross Cortese, a developer and builder (Laguna Woods Village, n.d.).

Naturally Occurring Retirement Community

A **naturally occurring retirement community (NORC)** is a community that was not originally designed to serve as a senior community, but that evolved into one over time (SeniorHomes.com, 2014). The Older Americans Act of 2006 (Title IV, Section 422) defines a NORC as a community where "40 percent of the heads of households are older individuals" or "a critical mass of older individuals exist," but that is "not an institutional care or assisted living setting" (Administration on Aging, 2006b).

NORCs do not conform to a set pattern. They range from unorganized communities of seniors who have aged in place to organized communities that allow only senior residents, who live in private residences and receive assistance with ADLs.

Community Support Programs

Adult Social Day Care

Adult social day care programs throughout the United States all have the same goals, but may provide varying types of care. Programs operate daily throughout the week. Community-based social day care programs engage adults with mild memory loss over the age of 18. Supervised individual and group activities take place in structured environments that facilitate interaction among peers and staff. Activities vary depending on whether they are privately or publicly funded. Services under this program category are not covered under Medicare; however, costs may be reimbursed through a long-term care policy. Otherwise individuals pay privately for this service.

The focus of adult social day care is on preventing or delaying institutionalization. These programs provide a social model that may include meals and group and individual activities that have a physical component as well as ones that enhance socialization. Adult social day care provides not only the older adult with opportunities for supervised care and social interaction but also the caregivers with another form of respite. Knowing that one's loved one is in a safe environment allows the caregiver to have much needed time away from caregiving responsibilities (Administration on Aging, 2012).

Adult Day Health Care

Adult day health care differs from social day care in that there is more of a healthcare emphasis, targeting adults and older adults with defined medical, mental health, and/or physical disabilities that put them at risk of being prematurely institutionalized. Services include supervised activities, nursing care, personal care, social services, physician/psychiatric oversight, rehabilitative care, meals, and transportation. The costs for services may be covered under Medicare and/or long-term care insurance.

Hospice and Palliative Medicine

The Medicare Hospice Benefit was enacted in 1982 and was made a permanent part of Medicare in 1986 (Centers for Medicare and Medicaid Services, 2014). To receive care covered by an insurance or Medicare, an individual must be diagnosed by a physician of having 6 or fewer months to live. **Hospice** is a program that provides services in a variety of locations. As the American Cancer Society (2014) relates, the idea of quality of life, versus quantity, is paramount. The idea of hospice is that death is neither hastened nor postponed, but that during the time between life and death, compassionate care with pain management is provided. This most frequently occurs within a home, but may also be provided within an institution, such as a SNF.

A hospice team consists of doctors, nurses, social workers, spiritual advisors, personal and home care aides, physical therapists, and volunteers, all working together to provide comprehensive care. Hospice services are provided to not only those diagnosed with cancer but also individuals with end-stage renal disease, congestive heart failure (CHF), and other conditions. As stated by Dame Cicely Saunders, the founder of the hospice movement in 1948, "You matter because of who you are. You matter to the last moment of your life, and we will do all we can, not only to help you die peacefully, but also to live until you die" (American Cancer Society, 2014, para.1).

When discussing hospice, it is important to include **palliative care**. Palliative care is a term that was previously used in reference to only those who received hospice services. It is a specialty and is offered in conjunction with curative therapies or end-of-life care, with specific emphasis on meticulous symptom management and maximizing functional status.

Intergenerational Caregivers

Intergenerational caregivers may consist of children, grandchildren, parents, or others of a generation other than the client's. Piercy's (2007) study on intergenerational caregivers reported that they have a strong commitment to caring for their elders. This dedication also "had moral and religious bases that extended beyond notions of duty or obligation" (p. 385). Current support within the community varies, depending on geographic location and the economic status of the family.

Respite Care Programs

Respite refers to short-term, temporary care provided to people with cognitive or physical disabilities to allow family members relief from the responsibilities of caregiving. Respite may involve overnight or daytime care. Research on caregiver fatigue, frequently termed "burnout," indicates that respite care is imperative to proactively avoid the challenges that may occur for the older adult and/or caregiver. This includes negative impacts on the caregiver's health and mental health and an increase in potential neglect and/or abuse of the older adult (AARP, 2011b). Longer-duration respite care is generally provided in an assisted living or nursing community setting. Each facility has its own respite policies (Area Agency on Aging and Disabilities of Southwest Washington, n.d.) and costs vary. Long-term care insurance may cover the respite expense.

Congregate and Home-Delivered Meal Programs

Proper nutrition is critical to the maintenance of good health. Many people who are aging in place need assistance with meal preparation. Congregate meals are available to low-income and socially isolated individuals over the age of 60 years and their respective spouse, regardless of age, through designated agencies. Congregate meals are typically offered Monday through Friday at community or neighborhood centers. Menu patterns are created under the supervision of registered dietitians, who comply with recommended daily allowance (RDA) guidelines, in addition to reducing sodium and saturated fat levels. While these programs are free of charge for qualified individuals, donations are accepted.

Meals on Wheels (www.mowaa.org) (sometimes referred to as home-delivered meals) is typically organized and staffed by volunteers, who prepare and deliver nutritionally supportive meals. There is usually a payment required from the recipient, but much of the cost of the program is borne by community donations and government assistance programs. A benefit of home-delivered meals is that clients are monitored by program staff or volunteers, who can identify areas of concern or changes in condition.

Other Community-Based Programs Organizations That Provide Assistance

The following programs serve as a one-stop shop, providing clients information about a magnitude of community resources and helping them to access vital services.

Area Agency on Aging

The **Area Agency on Aging** (AAA), created by federal law in 1974, falls under the umbrella of the ACL through each state's Administration on Aging. The focus is to form countywide networks designed to fund and coordinate programs for dependent adults over the age of 18 and individuals 60 years and older. AAAs link individuals to community-based services that will allow them to remain in their homes. The nature of information disseminated includes, but is not limited to, care management, information and assistance, family caregiving services, meals, legal services, housing, and public benefits. The National Association of Area Agency on Aging (N4A) serves as the umbrella organization in promoting standardized methods in the delivery of services.

Multipurpose Senior Citizen Centers (MSCC)

Numbering 10,000 nationwide and more than 700 in the State of California (California Commission on Aging, 2010), multipurpose senior centers offer a convenient, one-stop entry for both active and at-risk individuals needing a variety of programs and services. Senior centers help to minimize the confusion by advocating on behalf of the adult and family as well as promoting interagency cooperation.

Offering a variety of on-site services, senior centers also integrate at-risk older persons through participation in recreation, care management, nutrition, health and wellness, and adult education programs. Their strong community orientation further ensures lasting client relationships by promoting aging in place. Therefore, centers serve as conduits in enabling transitions from assisted living back home. Under one roof, both non-medical and medical services for older adults are marshaled to provide comprehensive, multidisciplinary programs that meet the many diversified needs of their particular communities.

Program for All-Inclusive Care for the Elderly (PACE)

PACE is a federal program through which clients qualify for placement in a SNF but may be able to receive services in their own homes or at adult day healthcare programs. Recipients must be dually eligible for Medicare/Medicaid in order to participate in the program; they are eligible with their Medicare/Medicaid coverage and use the PACE provider network for their care and assistance. Applications are available through each state's Medicaid office. In addition to the income guidelines under Medicare/MediCal, PACE recipients are aged 55 or older, with compromised ADL and/or IADLs, and meet the standards for nursing home placement.

The novelty of the PACE program is that services are all-encompassing, including prescription drugs, home health, and personal care. Another unique feature is that clients can qualify for adult day healthcare services outside the home in active environments that stimulate cognitive function (Li, Phillips, & Weber, 2012; On Lok Lifeways, 2014).

Cash Assistance Program for Immigrants (CAPI) is a state-funded program, offering cash assistance to certain aged, blind, and disabled legal non-citizens ineligible for Supplemental Social Security Income or State Supplemental Payment (SSI/SSP) due to their immigration status. Clients may also qualify for other public benefit programs, such as Medi-Cal, In-Home Supportive Services (IHSS), and/or Food Stamps benefits.

Applications can be submitted through the designated Department of Social Services in the respective counties of residence.

In-Home Supportive Services (IHSS)

In-home supportive services (IHSS) are a public benefit program that provides basic assistance at clients' residences. Examples of personal care include feeding, bathing, transferring, and assistance with laundry, shopping, and other functions that enable independence. A formula is used to rate the client's ADLs and IADLs, determining time allotted for attendant care. For instance, clients may be awarded 20 minutes to consume a meal, 5 minutes for toilet functions, and so forth (formulas are subject to change).

Health Information Counseling and Advocacy Program (HICAP)

The **Health Information Counseling and Advocacy Program (HICAP)** is a federally funded program that assists Medicare recipients with individualized counseling to maximize their health insurance coverage vis-à-vis supplemental Medicare gap insurance plans, prescription drug, and long-term care insurance. Advocacy services are provided by a professional staff and volunteers; they may assist clients in filing Medicare appeals. HICAP volunteers also help individuals assess appropriate Medicare supplement policies and the impact of the Affordable Care Act on their insurance status.

Adult Protective Services

Adult protective services (APS) are provided in each state to address financial, physical, or mental abuse, and/or neglect. Most APS programs provide services to not only older adults 65 years of age and older, but also to adults adult 18 years and older who are disabled. Each state has specific laws regarding **mandated reporters,** those individuals who must report to APS concerns of neglect, exploitation, and/or abuse. Mandated reporters include healthcare workers and administrators, and social service workers (National Center on Elder Abuse, n.d.).

Transportation Services

Other forms of community assistance include specialized senior transportation programs offered by local mass transit districts for older adults and the disabled. It is common practice to provide older adults with discounted fares, and in many cases they are provided free tickets or vouchers.

Access Services is a federally mandated curb-to-curb transit program under Article 42 U.S.C. /12143, Alternative Mode of Flexible Passenger

Transportation, available to clients with compromised functional limitations and, if applicable, their caregivers. Riders must meet certain requirements and participate in a face-to-face interview in order to determine eligibility for this highly specialized service. Many senior centers transport participants to their facilities, bolstering attendance at nutrition and recreation programs, as well as community and adult education.

Utility and Public Service Workers Programs

Some jurisdictions have mail carrier alert programs that monitor the homes of at-risk individuals to insure that mail is picked up on a daily basis. Participants must register with the local post office and provide information of a designated person to be contacted in case of any suspicious activity.

Equipment to Assist With Independence: Assisted Technology Programs

Visual impairments. Within communities, there are often agencies that offer low-vision products and computer accessories to assist individuals who are visually impaired. The National Federation of the Blind (NFB), based in Maryland, maintains state affiliations and local chapters throughout the United States that link clients to the products that best suit their needs. These may include assistive magnifying devices, such as screen readers, digital materials, and large-print books.

Devices to increase physical mobility. Independent living centers are located on a regional basis to facilitate access to adaptive equipment, making homes more functionally livable for clients who have difficulty ambulating. A caseworker conducts a home assessment to determine client eligibility and home readiness.

Audio impairment. Telephone companies provide special equipment that increases the phone volume as well as special flashing lights installed throughout the house to alert the client that the phone is ringing.

Emergency response/call systems. Medical alert monitoring systems involve connecting equipment to a telephone line that is activated by a wireless signal device (either in the form of a wristband or a necklace) worn by the client. The signal has a 700-foot radius so that the clients can easily roam around their homes and yards freely and in the event of feeling ill or falling can activate a 911 response by pressing a button, alerting the system to seek help. There is usually a one-time-only equipment setup fee and monthly service fee that may range from $40 to $90 a month. Once the apparatus has been installed, trained personnel can talk to the clients through a speaker system and activate 911 networks on their behalf as well as connect with clients every day to make sure they are well.

A number of groups offer services to assist individuals to age in place. Pharmacy services can offer home delivery of prescriptions that are paid for by Medicare or secondary healthcare insurance programs. Additionally, experts may be available to examine an individual's home to identify potential issues that might cause problems. This would include rugs that may represent tripping hazards or doorways that need to be widened to accommodate walkers or wheelchairs or adding grab bars in the bathroom to assist with balance. While Medicare does not offer any assistance in modifying homes for aging in place, there is an assistance program for veterans through the Veterans Health Administration, and some states are conducting pilot programs that allow the use of Medicaid money for this purpose (Paying for Senior Care, 2014).

Healthcare providers can provide a wide range of medical services that are performed in the home, typically paid for through Medicare or a long-term care insurance policy. Services include visits by therapists and nurses, a variety of assistive medical devices, including hospital beds, walkers, and critical supplies, such as oxygen tanks or concentrators. Healthcare providers can also provide access to experts in the hospital, on an outpatient or a clinic basis. In addition to seeing a family physician or internal medicine specialist, this can include physical therapy, dialysis or infusion therapy, and consultation with registered dietitians, who can design therapeutic diets to meet special nutritional or physiological needs. Medicare will provide these services for most eligible individuals.

Transitional Housing From Home Community to Formalized Home Care Facilities

There is a sharp dividing line between the home- and community-based care models at the lower end of the long-term care continuum and the institutional care models at the high end of the continuum. Facilities operate under stricter, more obtrusive regulatory constraints.

Financial and familial considerations can play a critical role in determining what level of care on the long-term care continuum is practical for an individual. Individuals with adequate financial resources or long-term care insurance policies can afford to spend more for required assistance. Individuals with strong family or community support structures may be able to remain in a home environment longer.

Board and Care and Adult Care Homes

Board and care and adult care homes are forms of assisted living communities, which are often converted residential homes. Residents receive meals and assistance with their activities of daily living, but are otherwise independent. Individuals in board and care and adult care homes typically pay for their lodging, and pay either a fixed amount or a share of costs to cover the cost of care staff and food. Facility administrators will generally be required to be licensed as assisted living administrators.

Intermediate Care Facilities (ICF)

Intermediate care facilities provide health-related services beyond basic custodial care, but not at the depth of a SNF or an acute care hospital. Throughout the United States, immediate care facilities have been primarily designed for individuals who experience intellectual and developmental disabilities. For older adults, this type of facility provides care for those who experience chronic health challenges that need medical monitoring on a regular basis, and who may respond well to rehabilitation therapy resulting in returning to their home environment. An ICF may provide physical and occupational therapy, recreational activities, and other support services.

Assisted Living Facilities

Assisted living facilities are residential settings that provide services for older adults who do not require 24-hour medical care, but require some assistance from others with their activities of daily living. Assisted living may also be referred to as residential care facilities for the elderly (RCFE). Typically, assisted living facilities are organized using a social model. Services can range from limited on-call assistance to assisting with the full range of activities of daily living. The cost of assisted living facilities is significantly higher than aging in place within one's home, borne exclusively by the individual receiving care.

Caregivers in assisted living facilities are not required to have any formal training, or to hold government or industry certifications. Facility administrators at this level are required to be certified as assisted living administrators. Assisted living facility staff also includes dietary services personnel to operate the kitchen, housekeeping services, laundry and maintenance staff, and administrative staff.

Twenty-Four-Hour Nursing Care

As an individual's acuity increases, the level of medical care they require increases, which may involve 24-hour nursing care. Twenty-four-hour nursing care is routinely offered only at **SNFs**, **subacute facilities**, and **acute care**

hospitals. These facilities have licensed nurses on-site at all times. Acute care hospitals will have physicians available on-site, while skilled nursing and subacute facilities will have them on call. While a SNF will operate three staff shifts (day, evening, and night), they are required to have at least one RN on-site on each shift.

Skilled Nursing Facilities

Skilled nursing care is long-term care that takes place in skilled nursing facilities (commonly abbreviated as SNF, which is pronounced "sniff"). SNFs are institutional healthcare settings where individuals live in the facility and receive 24-hour nursing care and assistance with their activities of daily living. Residents in SNFs generally fall into two categories, short-term or long-term stay.

A **short-term stay** in an SNF is one that lasts less than 14 days (National Association of Boards of Nursing Home Examiners [NAB], 2014). This category of care applies to individuals requiring assistance while they undergo recovery or rehabilitation from medical events, such as illness or surgery. The goal is to transition the individual back to his home once his recovery or rehabilitation is completed. Short-term stay may be funded by Medicare, private insurance, or the resident's self-pay.

A **long-term stay** in an SNF lasts 14 or more days (NAB, 2014). Most residents receiving care require assistance for chronic conditions, such as permanent disability, or infirmities associated with advanced age. Care for long-term stay is paid by Medicare (for up to 100 days), state Medicaid programs, long-term care insurance, or self-pay by the resident. The majority of individuals receiving this level of care receive public financial assistance, typically through Medicaid. Figure 2.3 provides an organizational chart of SNFs.

Subacute care facilities are for individuals who do not require acute care (hospitalization), but need more intensive skilled nursing care than what is provided in a SNF. Their condition could include injuries, an acute illness, or the worsening of a chronic or progressive disease. The services provided by the facility may include the care of a wound or tracheotomy, intravenous medication management or tube feeding, and intensive rehabilitation (California Department of Health Care Services, 2014). Subacute care may be provided in a section of a SNF or a hospital, or an entire facility that provides this comprehensive medical care.

Acute Care Facilities

Acute care is short-term medical care that provides intensive treatment for an urgent medical condition. This can include an acute illness or

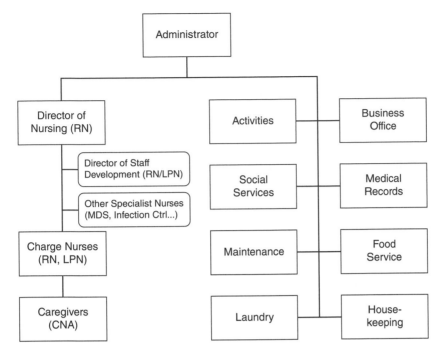

Figure 2.3   SNF Organizational Chart
Source: Merchant (2014a).

injury and/or recovery from surgery. This brief care is provided in a hospital setting by specialized medical personnel who have access to highly technical medical equipment.

The Workforce in Care Facilities

The professionals who work in long-term care play a critical role for those individuals requiring long-term care. In this section we examine the tasks they perform and where they are found within the continuum of care.

Administrators

Administrators in SNFs

At every level of the long-term continuum of care, the top position within a healthcare organization is the **administrator**. Healthcare provider organizations are businesses, performing many functions beyond providing health care. These include services such as dietary, housekeeping, maintenance, medical records, human resources, and finance. The role of the administrator is to manage all of these, including healthcare services, ensuring compliance with government laws and regulations.

Administrators in SNFs do not need to be healthcare professionals but are subject to federal and state regulations. Each state has set its own standards for becoming a nursing home administrator (NHA). However, every state subscribes to a standard national nursing home administrator exam managed by a nonprofit organization, the National Association of Long-Term Care Administrator Boards (NAB). The purpose of the licensing examination is to "protect the public by ensuring that entry-level nursing home administrators have mastered a specific body of knowledge and can demonstrate the skills and abilities essential to competent practice within the profession" (NALCAB, 2015, p. 4).

Administrators in Assisted Living

The field of assisted living/residential care for the elderly is not regulated at the federal level, and laws vary considerably from state to state. The duties of an assisted living administrator mirror those of the skilled nursing home administrator, being responsible for every aspect of the operation and management of the facility (Assisted Living Federation of America, 2014; California Health & Safety Code, Section 1520-1526.8). The primary differences derive from having lower levels of government regulation, not receiving government funding, and having less responsibility for medically licensed personnel and services (Mollica, 2009).

Physicians

The Family Doctor

The family doctor, licensed at the state level, is trained to diagnose and treat a wide range of medical conditions. However, when the care required exceeds the family doctor's ability, they serve as "gatekeepers" for advanced medical care, making referrals to medical specialty services when necessary. In the United States, the family practice specialty replaced the general practice physician (or general practitioner) starting in 1969 (American Board of Family Medicine, 2014).

Physicians in Skilled Nursing

In SNFs, residents continue to be under the care and orders of their family doctor. However, SNFs will also have on-call physicians on staff, commonly referred to as medical directors. The medical director is available either on-site or on-call to provide medical orders or prescriptions for residents in the event of sudden changes in their condition or emergencies. In addition, some SNFs may have nurse practitioners or physician's assistants (PAs) on staff. These two professions, working in conjunction with medical directors, have the ability to evaluate changes in conditions and emergencies, and issue or modify prescriptions for some medications.

Nurses

Nurses play a critical role in the delivery of health care, by serving as the interface between physicians, medical specialists, and patients.

Nurses are divided into two major categories, registered nurses (RN) and licensed practical nurses (LPN), also called licensed vocational nurses (LVN) (American Nursing Association, 2014). The differences between these categories differ between the states, and will be addressed in detail later in this section.

Governing Bodies and Scope of Practice

Nurses are licensed at the state level, with each state governing what services nurses can and cannot perform. Each state maintains a Board of Nursing that serves to interpret the state's scope of practice, while enforcing discipline and professional standards among the licensed nurses in its jurisdiction (National Council of State Boards of Nursing, 2014a). In all but three states there is a single state nursing board for both categories of nursing. The exceptions are California, Louisiana, and West Virginia. Each has a separate board for each category (National Council of State Boards of Nursing, 2014b). At the national level there are only general laws pertaining to nursing, with the exception of programs such as the armed forces and the Veterans Health Administration. In each case, these are governed by their specific scope of practice documents.

Registered Nurses (RN)

Registered nursing is the higher of the two nursing licensure categories. In most states, RN training programs are required to include a defined program of nursing course work, and are tied to attaining a college degree. The additional requirements to earn an associate's degree make a typical associate degree RN (ADN) program take approximately 2 years, and a bachelor of science RN (BSN) program take between 3 and 4 years.

Director of Nursing

The **director of nursing** (DON) is an RN who supervises the medical care of all patients in a healthcare setting. In acute care the DON typically reports to the medical director and the chief physician, and is responsible for managing the nursing staff. In skilled nursing, the DON reports directly to the facility administrator, and frequently serves as the second in command for the facility. The position includes responsibility for ensuring that the facility is in compliance with state and federal regulations in all areas.

Licensed Practical Nurses (LPN) and Licensed Vocational Nurses (LVN)

Licensed practical nurses (LPN) and **licensed vocational nurses (LVN)** provide basic medical care, have a lower educational requirement, and are required to work under the supervision of a RN. Licensed vocational nurse (LVN) is an alternative designation for LPN and is used primarily in California. LPNs can be employed in the acute care hospital settings, performing bedside patient care. There are a number of specialized roles in SNFs that can be performed by either an RN or an LPN as well as the director of staff development.

Director of Staff Development (DSD)

All SNFs are mandated by federal law to have one nurse, the **director of staff development (DSD)**. The DSD is assigned to monitor and document the continuing education training of the direct patient care staff. This nurse also serves as a trainer and serves as the instructor if a facility offers the nursing assistant pre-certification training program on its premises.

Licensed Versus Certified Healthcare Personnel

Physicians and nurses are classified as licensed healthcare professionals under U.S. law, and acknowledged by the jurisdiction that licenses them. A licensed healthcare professional has the authority to conduct any medical procedure or activity within his scope of practice without having to work under another medical professional's supervision.

Certified healthcare professionals are also acknowledged by government agencies, and must meet the minimum requirements to practice in their field, which includes completing a program of education and possibly a licensure examination. However, certified professionals have scopes of practice more limited than those of licensed professionals, restricted to a specific type of healthcare workplace. They are required to work under the supervision of a licensed healthcare professional.

Unlicensed Assistive Personnel

There are four primary categories of unlicensed assistive personnel within the long-term care continuum. Two of these, certified nursing assistants and home health aides, are subject to government certification and regulation. The medical assistants may be certified in some states, and have nationally recognized industry certifications. The fourth group is a general category of workers who provide patient/resident care services, but work in environments that are not subject to government regulation.

Certified Nursing Assistants

Certified nursing assistants are entry-level caregivers with specialized training, and are authorized to work in SNFs regulated by both federal and state law.

The job category of certified nursing assistant (CNA) was developed in California in the 1970s to improve the quality of care in nursing homes. California law established a formal training and certification process for CNAs. When Congress passed OBRA, which established national standards for SNFs, they adopted the California concept and standards for certified nursing assistants. Federal law sets a minimum standard for training CNAs, delegating responsibility to the states for establishing training, testing, and certification programs.

Within SNFs, CNAs serve as direct caregivers, working within their scope of practice and under the supervision of nurses. They assist residents with their ADLs, as well as recording medical data for the residents' charts.

Medical Assistants

Medical assistants are entry-level caregivers who have specialized training, and who are authorized to work in acute care hospitals and medical clinics. Medical assistants are not governed by federal law. Ten states, Arizona, California, Florida, Illinois, Maryland, New Jersey, Ohio, South Dakota, Virginia, and Washington, have defined the medical assistant's scope of practice (American Association of Medical Assistants, 2014). There is also a recognized certification for medical assistants through the American Association of Medical Assistants.

Therapeutic Specialists

Therapeutic specialist services are offered in the acute care and skilled nursing settings. These generally seek to improve the quality of life of residents, and involve collaboration between physicians, nurses, and direct caregivers as described ahead.

Physical Therapy Staff

The goal of physical therapy is to improve quality of life by helping residents to maintain their mobility, flexibility, and motor functions. Professional therapy staff will typically include physical therapists, who help residents improve their movement and manage their pain; occupational therapists, who treat ill or disabled residents through the therapeutic use of everyday activities; and speech pathologists, who treat swallowing disorders and work to diagnose, prevent, and treat communication disorders (Bureau of Labor Statistics, 2014).

Registered Dietitians (RD)

Registered dietitians work with acute care and SNFs to plan and provide nutritious meals for all residents. They also develop therapeutic meals for residents who have special nutritional needs or who have physical difficulty in swallowing.

Social and Quality of Life Specialties

Social Services (SS) Staff

Social service designees are "entry-level social work assistants" (Houston Chronicle, 2010) who work in SNFs. They serve as representatives and advocates for residents and may include individuals with undergraduate degrees in social work. The National Association of Social Workers (NASW) (2003) developed standards for social work services in long-term care facilities. These standards address the social worker's role in long-term care settings that focuses on "the social and emotional impact of physical or mental illness or disability, the preservation and enhancement of physical and social functioning, the promotion of the conditions essential to ensure maximum benefits from long-term healthcare services, the prevention of physical and mental illness and increased disability, and the promotion and maintenance of physical and mental health and an optimal quality of life" (NASW, 2003, p. 9). **Social workers** are defined by NASW as having, at a minimum, a bachelor's degree in social work from a program accredited by the Council on Social Work Education (CSWE).

Long-Term Care Ombudsman Program

Each state is mandated by federal law to have a **Long-Term Care Ombuds-man Program** that is administered by the state's Administration on Aging. The program is designed to provide advocates in resolving any complaints from residents in skilled nursing and other residential facilities. Advocates are trained to work closely with administrators in long-term care facilities and other mandated reporters to promote quality of life, and to ensure that a resident's rights to privacy, care, information and expression, and safety are sustained (National Consumer Voice, 2013).

Activities Staff

Activities staff are non-medical personnel who provide recreational, educational, and social activities that stimulate and enrich the lives of residents. Staff is required to be certified by the state in which they operate. These requirements vary from state to state (Education Portal, 2014), with the lowest level being completion of a 20-hour certification course, and the highest being a requirement that facilities use an occupational therapist, which requires a master's degree (U.S. Department of Labor, 2014).

Summary

The population of Americans aged 65 to 85 is growing rapidly. The needs of the baby boomer population will be different from their parents as a result of cultural diversity and the vast number of older adults. The demand for innovative long-term healthcare services can be expected to increase. The goal is to provide services to allow elders to age in place, within the comfort of their community and support systems.

Long-term care is provided in a variety of levels by differing types of licensed and professional service providers and informal caregivers. These providers can be characterized as part of the long-term care continuum that brings different levels of care into the home to placing an individual into a facility. The appropriate type of care to be provided may be dictated by an individual's acuity.

With the focus on aging in place in the private home environment, it is important to be knowledgeable of alternatives, including community home environments and community support programs, to maintain maximum independence. For a small percentage of older adults, it may be necessary to transition to a formalized home care faculty, such as a board and care. SNFs offer short- and long-term stays, providing a level of medical care not available within the home environment. Long-term care service providers and facilities are staffed by a variety of social service medical and non-medical professionals. Within each level of care, key professional staff provide services to enhance physical, emotional, and social well-being.

Key Terms

Active living community: Community living allowing older adults to age in place with support with home and personal care.

Activities of daily living (ADLs): Routine activities of everyday life that individuals must perform in order to survive comfortably.

Acute care: Short-term medical care that provides intensive treatment for an urgent medical condition.

Acute care facilities: Hospitals that provide short-term, intensive medical treatment for urgent medical conditions.

Administrator: The senior manager of a healthcare facility.

Adult day health care: Provides day care with a healthcare emphasis, targeting dependent and older adults with defined medical, mental health, and/or physical disabilities that put them at risk of being prematurely institutionalized.

Adult social day care: Provides day care for individuals with the goal of preventing or delaying institutionalization.

Aging in place: Individuals growing older within their home environment.

Area Agency on Aging (AAA): Created by federal law in 1974 to link individuals to community-based services.

Assisted living facility: Residential settings for older adults who do not require 24-hour medical care, but require some assistance with their ADLs.

Baby boomers: Generation consisting of people born between 1946 and 1964.

Care manager: Assists individuals and families to assess and choose appropriate services from options available from community programs and agencies. Frequently used synonymously as "case manager," referring to the same skill set and type of services provided to clients and their families.

Case manager: Assists individuals and families to assess and choose appropriate services from options available from community programs and agencies. Frequently used synonymously as "care manager," referring to the same skill set and type of services provided to clients and their families.

Community-based home programs: Governmental, nonprofit, or private organizations that provide services at the local level.

Congregate housing: Housing complexes with separate apartments (including kitchens) that provide some housekeeping services and some shared meals.

Continuing care retirement community (CCRC): Residential housing model with a range of housing options (i.e., independent living through nursing home care) and varying levels of medical and personal services within a single facility or complex.

Director of nursing (DON): A registered nurse (RN) who supervises the medical care of all patients in a healthcare setting.

Director of staff development (DSD): A nurse assigned to monitor and document the continuing education training of the direct patient care staff in an SNF.

Family doctor: Physician with whom an individual interacts at the start of every interaction with the healthcare system.

Geriatric care managers: Care managers who specialize in geriatrics, who serve as advocates for older adults and their families.

Health Information Counseling and Advocacy Program (HICAP): Federally funded program that assists Medicare recipients with individualized counseling to maximize their health insurance coverage.

Health Insurance Patient and Accountability Act (HIPAA): Federal law governing the privacy of healthcare records.

Home care: Assistance with functions needed in home.

Home health aide: Caregivers who provide assistance to individuals in their homes with their ADLs.

Home health care: Health care provided in the home environment, receiving assistance with medical needs and ADLs from trained professionals.

Home modifications: Adaptations to home environment to alleviate specific barriers that may impede ability to remain in the home.

Hospice: A program that provides specialized medical support for individuals at the end of life.

In-home supportive services (IHSS): Government-funded program that provides non-certified home health aides to assist individuals with ADLs in a home setting.

Informal supports: Unpaid family or friends providing caregiving within the home.

Instrumental activities of daily living (IADL): Skills needed to maintain independence.

Intergenerational caregivers: Caregivers who consist of children, grandchildren, parents, or others of a generation other than the client's.

Intermediate care facility: A facility that provides health-related care and services above the level of custodial care, but not at the level of a SNF or a hospital.

Licensed practical nurses (LPN): Nurses who provide basic medical care. LPNs have a lower educational requirement than RNs; they are required to work under the supervision of a RN.

Licensed vocational nurse (LVN): An alternative designation for LPN.

Long-term care continuum (LCC): The range of services available to care for people with long-term health issues, from aging in place to 24-hour nursing care in a hospital.

Long-term Care Ombudsman Program: A federally funded program placing advocates in long-term care facilities to help resolve resident complaints and ensure client/patient rights are enforced.

Long-term stay: Admission to an SNF that lasts 14 or more days.

Mandated Reporter: Individuals who are required by state law to report abuse, neglect, and/or exploitation of older adults to Adult Protective Services or the Long-Term Care Ombudsman Program.

Medicaid: Federal medical assistance program for low-income individuals.

Medical acuity: Measurement of the intensity of nursing care required by an individual.

Medical assistants: Entry-level caregivers who are authorized to work in acute care hospitals and medical clinics.

Medicare: Federal medical insurance program for the elderly and disabled.

Naturally occurring retirement community (NORC): Community that was not originally designed to serve as a senior community, but which evolves into one over time.

Nursing assistants: Entry-level caregivers who have specialized training and are authorized to work in SNFs.

Nursing home administrator: The senior manager in an SNF licensed by the each state.

Palliative care: Care offered in conjunction with curative therapies or hospice care with specific emphasis on meticulous symptom management and maximizing functional status.

Private-duty aide: Provides in-home services that include medical and custodial care.

Program of All-Inclusive Care for the Elderly (PACE): A federal program through which clients qualify for placement in a SNF, but are able to receive services in their own homes or at adult day healthcare programs.

Registered nurses (RN): A nurse who has earned an associate's, bachelor's, or master's degree in nursing and has passed a national license exam.

Respite: Short-term, temporary care that allows family members relief from the responsibilities of caregiving.

Scope of practice: The care and services a healthcare professional is legally permitted to perform.

Shared housing: Groups live together in a home or an apartment with a shared common area.

Short-term stay: Admission to an SNF for less than 14 days.

Skilled nursing facility (SNF): An institutional healthcare setting where individuals live in the facility, receive 24-hour nursing care, and receive assistance with their ADLs.

Social worker: Social service provider who has the minimum of a bachelor's degree in social work from a program accredited by the Council on Social Work Education.

Subacute care facilities: Facilities that provide care for those who do not require hospital acute care, but need more intensive skilled nursing care than what is provided in a SNF.

Therapeutic specialist: Interdisciplinary specialists (ex. physical therapy and dietitians) who work collaboratively with physicians, nurses, and direct caregivers to meet the needs of a patient.

24-hour nursing care: Level of health care that provides around-the-clock monitoring and care service.

Review Questions

1. What are the elements of the long-term care continuum?

2. What three services might allow an individual to receive support to remain in the community environment?

3. What is the role of the case manager?

4. Explain factors that may impact an individual requiring care in a SNF.

5. What is the role of the family doctor in managing health care for people receiving care? In a SNF?

6. Who sets the standards for becoming a SNF administrator?

Case Studies

Case Study #1: Community Care

Ms. M., age 85, has resided in her current home for the past 25 years. Her husband of 60 years died 2 months ago. Ms. M.'s only child, a daughter, lives in another state, and it takes her all day by air to visit her mother. Ms. M. relates she has a "good" relationship with her daughter, talking with her on the phone every Sunday; her daughter visits her once a year.

Two days ago, Ms. M. was released after a 24-hour stay in the hospital, following an angioplasty procedure. Soon after returning to her home, she fell and was found lying on her living room floor for several hours until a neighbor came over to visit. She seemed to be somewhat disoriented and refused to go to the hospital. Ms. M. told her neighbor that she was afraid she would be not allowed to come back home if she returned to the hospital.

Ms. M's neighbor noticed that Ms. M. was wearing the same clothes she had worn two days ago, and Meals on Wheels containers were piled on the kitchen countertop. Ms. M. was agreeable to have her neighbor call her family doctor, and he referred her to a home health agency. The nurse, following an assessment, implemented physical therapy, weekly nursing visits, a nurse's aide to assist with personal care, and a referral to a care manager to secure meals and home care services.

1. As a case manager, to what additional services and community resource would you refer Ms. M. to assist her to continue to reside in her home?

2. What level of care might Ms. M. need if she fell again in her home and became increasingly confused?

Case Study #2: Skilled Nursing

Mrs. Jones was born in 1944, at the start of the baby boom generation. She married, had children, and had a career as a teacher. Mrs. Jones retired in 2008, at age 65. Between 2008 and 2011, Mrs. Jones and her husband aged in place, living in their home. In 2010, Mrs. Jones suffered a stroke, but was able to continue living at home with the aid of her children and an in-home supportive services worker, who helped her with her activities of daily living. In addition, Mrs. Jones and her husband started receiving hot meals delivered by Meals on Wheels.

In 2011, Mrs. Jones's husband died and she was unable to continue to maintain her quality of life living on her own. She sold her family home and moved into an assisted living facility.

In 2013, she fell and broke her hip. Mrs. Jones was hospitalized, where she received hip replacement surgery. Following her hospitalization, she was placed in a SNF on a short-term stay basis for rehabilitation. Mrs. Jones then returned to her assisted living facility. In 2014, it became clear to Mrs. Jones that she needed more care and assistance than she could receive at her assisted living facility. She then had herself admitted to a SNF.

1. Identify three community resources that could have assisted Mrs. Jones and her husband in preparing their home for aging in place, and for providing support after her stroke.

2. Identify two alternative approaches Mrs. Jones could have taken rather than moving into an assisted living facility after her husband's death.

3. What services would a SNF provide for Mrs. Jones that she would not receive in a formalized home care facility?

References

Administration for Community Living. (2013). *A profile of older Americans: 2013.* Retrieved from http://www.aoa.gov/Aging_Statistics/Profile/

Administration on Aging. (2006a). *Older Americans Act and aging network.* Retrieved from http://www.aoa.gov/AoA_Programs/OAA/introduction.aspx

Administration on Aging. (2006b). *Older Americans Act of 1965, as amended in 2006.* Retrieved from www.aoa.gov/AOA_programs/OAA/oaa_full.asp

Administration on Aging. (2012). *Aging statistics.* Retrieved from http://www.aoa.gov/Aging_Statistics/index.aspx

American Association of Medical Assistants. (2014). *State scope of practice laws.* Retrieved from http://www.aama-ntl.org/employers/state-scope-of-practice-laws

American Association of Retired Persons. (2009). *Universal design home modification devices.* Retrieved from www.aarp.org/universalhome/

American Association of Retired Persons. (2011a). *2011 housing survey.* Retrieved from www.aarp.org/home-family/livable-communities/info-10-2012/boomers-housing-livable-communities.html

American Association of Retired Persons. (2011b). *Becoming disabled after age 65: The expected lifetime costs of independent living.* Retrieved from www.aarp.org/home-garden/livable-communities/info-2005/2005_08_costs.html

American Board of Family Medicine. (2014). *About ABFM.* Retrieved from www.theabfm.org/about/index.aspx

American Cancer Society. (2014). *Choosing hospice care.* Retrieved from http://www.cancer.org/treatment/nearingtheendoflife/nearingtheendoflife/nearing-the-end-of-life-hospice

American Nursing Association. (2014). *What is nursing?* Retrieved from www.nursingworld.org/EspeciallyForYou/What-is-Nursing

American Sentinel University. (2014, February 5). Using patient acuity to determine nurse staffing: Health care on call. *Healthcare desk of American Sentinel University.* Retrieved from www.americansentinel.edu/blog/2014/02/05/using-patient-acuity-to-determine-nurse-staffing/

Area Agency on Aging and Disabilities of Southwest Washington. (n.d.). *Senior housing options definitions.* Retrieved from www.helpingelders.org/wpcontent/uploads/downloads/2013/01/2012-senior-housing-definitions.pdf

Assisted Living Federation of America. (2014). *Assisted living regulations and licensing.* Retrieved from www.alfa.org/alfa/State_Regulations_and_Licensing_Informat.asp

Bureau of Labor Statistics. (2014). *Occupational outlook handbook entries for physical therapist, occupational therapist and speech pathologist.* Retrieved from www.bls.gov/ooh/healthcare/

California Commission on Aging. (2010). *Senior center initiative: Final report, 2010.* Retrieved from http://www.ccoa.ca.gov/2008-2010%20Senior%20Center%20Initiative.htm

California Department of Health Care Services. (2014). *Subacute care.* Retrieved from http://www.dhcs.ca.gov/provgovpart/Pages/SubacuteCare.aspx

California Health & Safety Code, Section 1520-1526.8, *Residential care for the Elderly Administrator Practice Act.* Retrieved from www.leginfo.ca.gov/cgi-bin/displaycode?section=hsc&group=01001-02000&file=1520-1526.8

Centers for Medicare and Medicaid Services. (2014). Quality of care. *Medicaid State Operations Manual* (SOM), Appendix PP, F-309, 42 CFR 483.25. Retrieved from https://www.cms.gov/

Davey, A., Takagi, E., & Wagner, D. (2013). A national profile of caregivers for the oldest-old. *Journal of Comparative Family Studies, 45*(4), 434–490.

Education Portal. (2014). *Become a nursing home activity director: Step-by-step career guide.* Retrieved from portal.com/articles/Become_a_Nursing_Home_Activity_Director_Step-by-Step_Career_Guide.html

Health Care Administration. (2008). *Care management: The office of quality and care management.* Retrieved from http://www.hca.wa.gov/medicaid/healthyoptions/documents/ccm_finalopdef.pdf

Houston Chronicle. (2010). *Job description of a social service designee.* Retrieved from http://work.chron.com/job-description-social-service-designee-19253.html

Laguna Woods Village. (n.d.). *Laguna Woods Village.* Retrieved from http://www.lagunawoodsvillage.com/

Last, M. (2014). *Diminished capacity flowchart.* Unpublished manuscript.

Li, G. K., Phillips, C., & Weber, K. (2012). *On Lok: A successful approach to aging at home.* Retrieved from http://pacepartners.net/wp-content/uploads/2012/04/GLi-OnLok-ASuccessfulApproachtoAgingatHome.pdf

Merchant, K. (2014a). *Skilled nursing facility organizational chart.* Unpublished manuscript.

Merchant, K. (2014b). *The long-term care continuum.* Unpublished manuscript.

Mollica, R. L. (2009). *State Medicaid reimbursement policies and practices in assisted living.* American Health Care Association. Retrieved from www.ahcancal.org/ncal/resources/documents/medicaidassistedlivingreport.pdf

National Association of Boards of Nursing Home Examiners. (2014). *NAB study guide: How to prepare for the nursing home administrators examination* (5th ed.). Washington, DC: Author.

National Association of Long-Term Care Administrator Boards. (2015). *Nursing home administrators licensing examination: Information for candidates.* Washington, DC: Author.

National Association of Professional Geriatric Care Managers. (2014). *About care management.* Retrieved from www.caremanager.org/

National Association of Social Workers. (2003). *NASW standards for social work services in long-term care facilities.* Retrieved from www.socialworkers.org/practice/standards/naswlongtermstandards.pdf

National Center on Elder Abuse. (n.d.). *Adult protective services.* Retrieved from http://www.ncea.aoa.gov/Stop_Abuse/Partners/APS/index.aspx

National Consumer Voice. (2013). *The national long-term care ombudsman resource center.* Retrieved from http://ltcombudsman.org/about/about-ombudsman

National Council of State Boards of Nursing. (2014a). *About the NCLEX.* Retrieved from www.ncsbn.org/nclex.htm

National Council of State Boards of Nursing. (2014b). *Member boards.* Retrieved from www.ncsbn.org/521.htm

On Lok Lifeways. (2014). *How PACE works.* Retrieved from www.onlok.org/HowPACEWorks.aspx

Paying for Senior Care. (2014). *Making and paying for home modifications to enable aging in place.* Retrieved from www.payingforseniorcare.com/home-modifications/how-to-pay-for-home-mods.html#title5

Piercy, K. (2007). Characteristics of strong commitments to intergenerational family care of older adults. *Journal of Gerontology, 62B*(6), 381–387.

Rebuild America. (n.d.). *Rebuilding together.* Retrieved from http://rebuildingtogether.org/whoweare/

SeniorHomes.com. (2014). *Naturally occurring retirement communities.* Retrieved from www.seniorhomes.com/p/naturally-occurring-retirement-communities

Szanton, S., Thorpe, R., Boyd, C., Tanner, E., Leff, B., Agree, E., . . . Gitlin, L. (2011). Community aging in place, advancing better living for elders: A bio-behavioral-environmental intervention to improve function and health-related quality of life in disabled older adults. *The American Geriatrics Society, 59*, 2314–2320.

U.S. Department of Health and Human Services. (n.d.). *Office of Community Services: Low income home energy assistance program (LIHEAP).* Retrieved from www.acf.hhs.gov/programs/ocs/programs/liheap

U.S. Department of Housing and Urban Development. (2013a). *Aging in place: Facilitating choice and independence.* Retrieved from www.huduser.org/portal/periodicals/em/fall13/highlight1.html

U.S. Department of Housing and Urban Development. (2013b). *Section 202.* Retrieved from www.huduser.org/portal/publications/sec_202_1.pdf

U.S. Department of Housing and Urban Development. (2013c). *Section 8 assistance for public housing.* Retrieved from http://portal.hud.gov/hudportal/HUD?src=/programdescription/phrr

U.S. Department of Labor. (2014). *Occupational therapist.* Retrieved from www.onetonline.org/link/summary/29-1122.00

U.S. Department of Veterans Affairs. (2014). *Homeless veterans update.* Retrieved from www.va.gov/homeless/hud-vash.asp

West, L. A., Cole, S., Goodkind, D., & He, W. (2014). *65+ in the United States: 2010.* Retrieved from www.census.gov/

CHAPTER 3

RESIDENT ADVOCATES, DIVERSITY, AND RESIDENT-CENTERED CARE

Ann Wyatt

The push for nursing home regulation and practice improvement over the past 30 years has been entirely toward individualized care. In essence, this means that regardless of role—administrator, nursing assistant, housekeeper, family member, volunteer—that individual must act as an advocate on behalf of people needing long-term care.

In the early 1980s there was a move on the part of the Reagan administration to largely eliminate federal standards for nursing home care. However, Congress, in response to widespread consumer objections, determined that before such drastic action could be taken, a study should be conducted to review the history and effectiveness of nursing home regulation along with ways to improve it. This led to the establishment of the Institute of Medicine's Committee on Nursing Home Regulation. Their report, "Improving the Quality of Care in Nursing Homes," issued in 1986, laid the groundwork for the Omnibus Budget Reconciliation Act of 1987 (**OBRA '87**, often referred to as the Nursing Home Reform Act [NHRA]), as well as the foundation for nursing home quality improvement.

Long-term care providers, researchers, consumers, regulators, and medical professionals were members of the committee, and were also represented through testimony regarding their views on nursing home quality and regulation at public meetings. Extensive interviews and surveys were conducted, as well as case studies of nursing home regulation in several states. Existing research was

LEARNING OBJECTIVES

- Be able to articulate how and why quality of care and quality of life are inextricably connected in long-term care, and the responsibility administrators have for achieving this integration.

- Understand how the long-term care regulatory system (OBRA) is based on the individualized needs of residents, and the role of staff in advocating for these needs.

- Understand how community groups and volunteers support residential care facilities to more effectively respond to the diverse needs of residents, and the role of administrators in promoting these relationships.

- Understand the different ways that emerging models of care attempt to address the underlying principles of OBRA.

- Understand the importance of knowledge and competence about state-of-the-art dementia care among leadership and staff, and the organizational adaptations necessary to promote effective dementia care.

reviewed, and several papers were commissioned. Among its conclusions, the committee acknowledged that although regulations alone cannot guarantee high-quality care, a stronger federal regulatory role was essential.

Specifically, the committee recommended that regulations be promulgated to create a system to obtain standardized data on residents, because high-quality care requires "careful assessment of each resident's functional, medical, mental, and psychosocial status upon admission, and reassessment periodically thereafter" (Committee on Nursing Home Regulation, 1986, p. 74). This action was necessary to reorient the regulatory system from a structural and facility-oriented approach to a resident-centered and outcome-oriented approach. Both good care and good regulatory oversight need to be tied to the resident's experience of care. This, combined with the committee's finding that quality of care is inextricably linked to quality of life, formed the foundation for individualized care that is the heart of OBRA.

Hearing directly from residents is an essential component of providing effective care, and OBRA sets the expectation that everyone who works in a long-term care setting has a role to play in finding and affirming the voice of the resident. *Advocacy* is defined as the provision of "active support," which is what is required to translate the resident's voice into care that meets his clinical, physical, and psychosocial needs. Over time, OBRA has demonstrated the link between quality of care and quality of life. Whether someone needs short-term rehabilitation to recover from a hip fracture or long-term support because of a stroke or other chronic illness, research and experience consistently point to individualized care as essential to high quality.

Where Does Quality Start?

Quality starts with each person who works in long-term care. Every job in the organization has the potential for affecting residents positively or negatively. Leadership has a huge impact on quality of care and quality of life, but too often care in these communities tends toward the compartmentalized and hierarchical, which leads to service delivery fragmentation and less than optimum care. Classic performance theory teaches that most problems occur in the handoff from one department or function to another, and this is frequently exactly what happens in long-term care. To avoid this, an approach to problem solving is needed that (a) puts the resident at the center, and (b) sets the expectation that the various disciplines will succeed only to the degree that they work collaboratively.

This means that organizations need to address the needs of the whole person, not just the part that is sick. The opportunity for retaining decisions for one's life is essential for a resident's social and emotional health, as Rosalie Kane, and many other researchers have documented. Such autonomy extends from decisions about medical treatment to the myriad of small activities that make up a day, such as when to get up, what to wear, what to eat, which activity to attend (if any), and which book to read. In a communal setting, a resident will not have unlimited options for such decisions because they are living in community with others, but the best are those that maximize these options to the fullest possible extent. Regardless of whether a person can move easily about the building or must stay in bed, it is in the activities of everyday life where autonomy and comfort make a big difference. While every member of staff has an impact on quality of care and quality of life, it is the leadership of the building that sets the benchmark for individualized, **person-centered care**.

Nursing

In long-term care, certified nursing assistants (CNAs) are central to the provision of individualized care. As part of the Institution of Medicine's (IOM) 1986 study, the National Citizens' Coalition for Nursing Home Reform conducted research to ascertain the consumer's perspective on quality. The study, funded by the Robert Wood Johnson Foundation, the Retirement Research Foundation, Health Care Financing Administration (HCFA) (now CMS), and American Association of Retired Persons (AARP), surveyed 455 residents of 107 nursing homes. Residents ranged in age from mid-20s to 102, and had spent an average of 4 years in a nursing home. The majority of homes were proprietary, while one-third were nonprofits.

In the study residents indicated that staff were the most important factor in achieving good care. All levels of staff were included in these statements, although CNAs and nurses were mentioned most frequently. Personal characteristics and attitudes of the staff were as important to them as the help they received in meeting care needs. Residents were well aware that good staff morale, good pay, good supervision, and administrative support were essential in achieving quality care.

J. Neil Henderson, PhD, who spent more than a year as a nurse's aide in an Oklahoma nursing home, describes the critical link between quality care and individualized care as follows:

> When I began working as a nurse aide, the first striking discovery I made was that every aide had memorized a large array of each resident's personal habits that made services more personal and time-efficient. Knowledge of and attention to seemingly minor details is of extreme importance, such as the placement of a juice glass on the left

side of [the] breakfast tray to make the glass more visible and accessible for one resident, ensuring two packages of sugar for another resident, three for another, no napkin for still another resident because of being prone to eating paper. Mastering the details is critical to proper job performance....Only lengthy, daily contact and a commitment to provide quality care can make such a feat possible. More importantly, this same intimate knowledge of patients enables the nurse aide to observe behavioral changes that may be indicative of impending medical consequences. Actual hands-on contact with patients, such as feeding, bathing, clothing, and changing diapers and bed linens, provides the nurse aide with a vital set of information. (Henderson, 1987, pp. 8–10)

Consistent, dedicated staff are a hallmark of all person-centered models of care. A 1996 study found that low turnover of staff was associated with the opportunity for aides to contribute suggestions and concerns about resident care. As a study conducted by Banaszak-Holl and Hines (1996) attests, even lower turnover of staff occurred in situations where aides were included in resident care planning meetings; consistent staffing and staff engagement work better for residents, as well as for staff. *Advancing Excellence* has developed a very useful tool for facilities to determine just how much consistency they provide. The tool specifies that all caregivers assigned to a resident over 1 month be identified; unfortunately, it is not uncommon to discover that as many as 20 to 30 different nursing assistants care for a single resident. Carrying out an individual plan of care is virtually impossible with this number of staff. Consistent assignments and thoughtful organizing of replacement staff can make a significant positive difference.

This tool is an example of the technical support being offered by *The Advancing Excellence in America's Nursing Homes Campaign*, which is an initiative of the Advancing Excellence in Long-Term Care Collaborative. More than 60% of the nation's nursing homes have signed on to the campaign, which provides assistance to homes for improving their clinical and organizational outcomes, and establishes and provides support to local area networks that are formed to provide collaboration opportunities.

Nurses also have a huge influence over the resident's experience of care, by acting as role models in resident and family interactions, in how they assess priorities, and in their interactions with CNAs. An important role for management is supporting nursing staff, through supervision, education, and organizational policies and procedures, to ensure their competence and confidence in promoting individualized care.

Housekeeping

Although CNAs are responsible for the majority of hands-on care, house-keepers spend large chunks of uninterrupted time with residents. As J. Neil Henderson (1995) has also noted,

> The potential for housekeepers to engage in meaningful interaction with patients is naturally enhanced by their job performance demands.... Demonstration of job fulfillment for housekeepers involves a lengthy stay of about 20 minutes in patient rooms. This indirectly conveys a message of thoroughness of cleaning, and provides a social field for engaging patient-housekeeping interactions. (pp. 48–49)

Such encounters provide an opportunity for the resident to have a one-on-one connection, someone who listens, someone to speak with about everyday things, someone who does not necessarily make you feel like a "patient." This means it is not unusual for housekeepers to forge relationships with residents and sometimes learn things that can be helpful. It is essential that housekeepers be considered part of the care team. In one home, a housekeeper regularly leads a men's group for residents, and in the dementia neighborhood where he works, he has been offering lollipops to residents for years. At another home, a housekeeper stopped by almost every day to converse with a resident at lunchtime, specifically to provide company and encourage her to eat.

Therapeutic Recreation

For many years, the emphasis on recreation has tended to be on large-group activities in the hopes of reaching as many residents as possible. While these events can bring a great deal of pleasure to residents, the goal of assisting residents to find meaningful engagement on a day-to-day basis is a much more individualized process, requiring input from recreation staff, other departments, family members, friends, and volunteers.

Several years ago, Anita Schacher, then administrator at Clatsop Care Center in Astoria, Oregon, gave a workshop on activities at a LeadingAge conference, and started by asking participants to list 10 ways they most liked to spend their free time. There were at least 50 people in the room, and no one listed more than two or three large-group activities. In most cases, people listed activities such as reading the paper while drinking coffee, taking a walk, praying, listening to the radio or watching television, reading a magazine or book, talking on the phone to a family member, having coffee with a friend, knitting, playing games on the computer, listening to music, and listening to ballgames. These activities are the habits, preferences, and comforts of a lifetime, and what makes them meaningful is that they are personal: specific newspapers, books, radio stations, and television programs, particular music, close friends, and family members. Schacher then went on to describe how understanding the importance of these kinds of moments led her and her staff to reframe the activities program at Clatsop Care Center (see Case Study #1).

The importance of knowing each resident is underscored in an article entitled "Large Parties Are Not for Everyone," in which Dr. Judah Ronch reminds us that there can be a tendency to focus on thinking and memory, but ignore personality, and specifically the fact that there are people "who tend to find large groups to be tiring or even stressful." He based his comments on *Quiet: the Power of Introverts in a World That Can't Stop Talking*, by Susan Cain (2013). He goes on to note,

> What struck me was how we—as a field, especially in the congregate setting—see these preferences as risk factors for depression and/or isolation and not as ways for introverts to be at their best. Any strengths-based approach to care has to re-orient typical institutional evaluations of these behaviors and understand their value as positive and adaptive to an environment that too often sees extrovert behavior as normality and any deviation as pathological. (Ronch, 2012)

Individualized activities are also effective for those who come for shorter-term stays. Rehabilitation is often demanding, and people needing facility-based care usually come after suffering trauma and/or serious illness. This is a time when retaining a sense of personal identity can be very important, and part of the rehabilitation process itself.

Volunteers

One of the most effective ways for organizations to widen and normalize the world of those who reside there is to actively promote wide-ranging roles for volunteers and community members. Nursing homes benefit from strong community connections because isolation creates barriers, stigma, and fear. Organizations that welcome and encourage community involvement gain positive interaction that benefits residents, families, and staff alike. A remarkable example of what can be accomplished by engaging with volunteers is the work social worker and one-time volunteer Dan Cohen has done to bring personalized music to nursing home residents through use of the iPod. As a nursing home volunteer he tried out using iPods with only a few residents in one home, and was so successful that the nonprofit he established, Music and Memory, Inc., now assists hundreds of nursing homes across the country to establish personalized music programs.

Years ago, a home in New York developed a novel approach to resident birthdays: A group of community residents put together a committee who bought and delivered flowers and a card for each of the facility's 200 residents' birthdays. A local block association took on the task of raising the money (through bake sales and other events) to pay for these flowers and cards. This activity brought much joy to the residents and life into the community.

Involving staff in volunteer activities is another way to enrich the life of a home. Another home encourages staff from various departments to commit to volunteering on a regular basis. For example, a trio of staff from finance and human resources performs ballroom dancing, and other staff members formed a Latin music group called Parranda.

Dietary

Mealtimes are an extremely important part of every resident's day, and dietary is an area where small things can make a big difference. While dietary preferences are routinely assessed at admission, the real challenge comes when trying to incorporate specific favorite foods into meal plans. A lovely example of this is a facility where the dietary worker prepares waffles on the unit at breakfast once a month for whoever wants them. Other facilities have taken a more careful look at snacks, and have determined that peanut butter and jelly sandwiches are a particular favorite and should always be an available option. Being able to choose among alternates is desirable, but not very satisfying if those alternatives rarely include something the resident particularly enjoys. Both the American Diabetes Association (2008) and the Academy of Nutrition and Dietetics recognize that in nursing homes there is rarely a need for restrictive diets, which are often not very appealing and can result in residents not getting enough nourishment. Family members can play a role here by bringing in favorite foods. Whether a resident prefers to eat alone in their room or in a dining area, everything possible should be done to make the dining experience itself as pleasant as possible.

Social Work

Social workers have traditionally been seen as primary advocates in long-term care, the person most likely to speak up on behalf of residents. Their role as advocate should continue, but what OBRA makes clear is that advocacy is a shared responsibility among disciplines. The psychosocial histories that social workers develop help staff to get to know the resident, by conveying the life the resident has lived, what is important to him, what provides comfort, and what his priorities are in terms of care and treatment. These histories should not be filed away in the chart; they should be actively incorporated into care plans. Social workers bring a unique focus to care with a strengths-based approach, and are also instrumental in working with families and residents to address concerns and facilitate desirable outcomes.

Other Disciplines and Departments

Everyone working in a facility has the potential for affecting quality either positively or negatively: Staff from Admissions, Finance, Human Resources, Laundry, Maintenance, Medical Records, Medicine, Rehabilitation, Security, and Staff Development all have a role to play. Wherever possible, it is desirable to include staff (at all levels) from these departments in quality improvement projects. They often have invaluable information to contribute, and they also benefit from relating to other departments in the process of organizational problem solving. Such collaboration also helps all staff remain in touch with the overall mission and purpose of the organization.

A physician who doesn't call families back, a front desk receptionist who is less than welcoming, or someone in the business office who is short with a resident regarding access to his allowance chips away at the very foundation: an atmosphere where staff support one another to honor the dignity of the people in their care.

Quality Assurance and Performance Improvement

An effective performance improvement program provides a perfect opportunity to engage all levels of staff across the disciplines, as well as residents and family members. This is in keeping with classic improvement models, which stress the importance of including those closest to the problem in improvement efforts. While nursing homes have tended to focus their improvement projects on clinical areas, a broader source for improvement ideas is preferable. Someone in the dietary department may have an idea about how to make meals more enjoyable, a resident council may have suggestions about how to improve the activities program, or a family member may offer a way to lessen the stress at the time of move-in. Ideas for change can also come from family and staff satisfaction questionnaires, Department of Health surveys, and letters of complaint.

For example, one facility decided to look for ways to reduce the amount of noise throughout the building, a concern that had been noted by residents, families, and staff members. Included on the workgroup were staff members from nursing, a beautician, a family member, and someone from finance. One of the more irritating sources of noise identified was the ice machine on each floor. After some research, they identified a quieter model, and the finance person was able to include noise as an element in the ongoing purchase criteria.

It is not always feasible (scheduling can be very challenging) to include a resident or a family member, or, for example, someone from the night shift, in an actual improvement workgroup. However, it is absolutely essential that their perspective be sought, and incorporated into the workgroup's efforts, if the area of concern has any impact on them.

Resident Councils

Federal law gives residents the right to meet as a council. A resident council is an organized and independent group of nursing home residents who meet at times of their choosing to discuss issues of concern to them. Homes are required to provide space for councils to meet, and councils typically request that a member of the home's staff act as a liaison between them and administration. Councils provide an opportunity for improved communication, help to identify problems early, when they may be easier to correct, and promote a sense of community among residents. They provide residents with the opportunity to raise both systemic and individual concerns in an atmosphere where residents feel supported by each other. Councils have the right to meet privately, or to invite members of the staff, relatives, friends, or members of community organizations to attend meetings. There is variety from one home to the next in size, structure, and amount of participation by residents.

Establishing a process for tracking resident concerns is an important part of quality improvement for an organization. Too often resident council issues are seen in isolation from the rest of the organization, and integrating them into the QI program in the organization will assist in sustaining resolutions. Those homes that take their resident councils seriously, and make an authentic effort to be responsive, are greatly the better for it.

Family and Friends

Family and friends have a huge role to play in advocating for residents, but too often the partnership of families is not actively sought, or sometimes avoided altogether, and a gap is created, which is frustrating to everyone. The best time to engage families is at the moment of admission, when the stage is often set for the days and months ahead. It is usually a very emotional time for families and residents alike, and therefore all the more important to find ways of making families feel welcome.

One home recently realized they often give mixed messages to family members. For example, family members on one floor who wanted to bring a glass of water to their relative were told by the nurse they were not allowed to use the ice machine, while on another floor another nurse made a point of showing the ice machine to the family on their first visit, and invited them to help themselves whenever they needed ice. In this tiny example, it is possible to see the seeds of partnership, or its opposite.

INTERACT (http://www.interact2.net/)is a quality improvement program designed for staff to assist them in improving the early identification, assessment, documentation, and communication about acute changes in the status of residents. The goal is to reduce the need for hospitalizations. Some homes have decided to extend the idea to families by educating them about INTERACT and inviting them to tell staff when they see changes in their relative. This changes the dynamic from "the family is complaining" to "thank you for telling us."

Active engagement with families in the care planning process is essential. Soon after a resident was admitted to a dementia unit in one home, the staff talked with his wife about his resistance to care and learned that he had a previous stay in another facility and a brief stay in a psychiatric facility. The resident's wife relayed that at home her husband was accustomed to staying up until about 4 A.M., having a snack, going to bed, and sleeping until about noon. Staff adjusted the resident's care plan to reflect this long-time habit, and the resistance to care almost completely disappeared. As his wife described it, "I have my husband back."

In addition to making families comfortable on the unit, comfortable with asking questions and raising concerns, and truly welcome at care plan meetings (does the home make it a priority to accommodate family members when scheduling these meetings?), there are many ways of engaging families:

- Encouraging participation in quality improvement projects.
- Welcoming participation at mealtimes.
- Welcoming participation in activities.
- Making them aware of activity options available on the unit, such as checkerboards, puzzles, and playing cards.
- Inviting assistance in personalizing the resident's living space.
- Forming family councils. A family council is made up of family members and friends of residents, who come together to discuss areas of mutual concern. As with resident councils, family members may choose to meet with or without the presence of staff. Their concerns should be tracked as part of an organization's quality improvement process.

National Nursing Home Ombudsman Program

In 1972, the **Nursing Home Ombudsman Program** was first created as a public health demonstration project in seven states. The demonstration was deemed successful, and in 1974 it was moved to the Administration on Aging (AoA). States initially had the option of developing a program; however, in 1978, Congress passed an amendment requiring each state to develop one. There are programs in all 50 states and in Puerto Rico, the District of Columbia, and Guam, funded under Titles III and VII of the Older Americans Act, along with other federal, state, and local sources (e.g., the United Way, or a local foundation). Each state program operates somewhat differently, although most are housed in their State Units on Aging. Local programs are often housed in local Area Agencies on Aging. While the programs include paid staff, the majority of ombudsmen are volunteers.

Currently there are thousands of local ombudsmen in almost 600 regional (local) programs. All ombudsmen, paid or volunteer, are required to complete a training program, and each local program submits statistical reports to their state agencies, which are then submitted to AoA. Local programs (operating under state supervision) develop their own protocols, depending on the needs and resources available in that community.

AoA also funds the National Long-Term Care Ombudsman Resource Center, operated by the National Consumer Voice for Quality Long-Term Care, in conjunction with the National Association of States Agencies on Aging United for Aging and Disabilities (NASUAD), to provide training and technical assistance to state and local ombudsmen. The Resource Center and NASUAD work closely with the National Association of State Long-Term Care Ombudsman Programs (NASOP) and the National Association of Local Long-Term Care Ombudsmen Programs (NALLTOP) in providing this training and technical assistance.

Ombudsmen have many roles, including: (a) resolution of complaints by or for residents; (b) education of residents and the public about residents' rights and good care practices, (c) promotion of community involvement through volunteer opportunities, (d) promotion of citizen organizations, family councils, and resident councils, and (e) systemic advocacy—that is, commenting on proposed legislative and regulatory changes and monitoring changes once made. Their most important role, however, is as an advocate on behalf of residents. Nursing homes are incredibly busy places, with most staff working at a very fast pace. It can be easy for staff to forget that for the average resident or family member, nursing homes can be confusing and overwhelming. Residents don't always know who they should talk to about a particular problem, or they may fear that they will anger someone (a staff member or another resident) if they raise a complaint. By definition, most residents are frail and often ill, thus making them even more vulnerable. This is precisely why the Ombudsman Program was developed, to ensure that residents could count on having someone to speak up on their behalf when needed.

Nursing homes are required by the Older Americans Act to provide access for ombudsmen to individual residents, to groups of residents, and to resident records. While much of their time is taken up with talking directly to residents and staff, it is sometimes necessary to see charts as well. While most of the time they do so after obtaining the permission of the resident (or the resident's representative), there are occasions when this is not possible. For example, if a resident wants his concerns kept confidential, and the ombudsman needs to review the record, the ombudsman may look at two or three records to protect the specific identity of a resident. Some residents may be unable to give consent, and may not have a representative. HIPAA does not apply to access by ombudsmen. Resident consent is required prior to any ombudsman viewing records except in special circumstances which require the approval of the state long-term care ombudsman (e.g. someone who lacks capacity and has no family) (see Case Study #3).

Advocacy Organizations

The leading consumer organization working for nursing home quality is the National Consumer Voice for Quality Long-Term Care (**The Consumer Voice**), originally known as the National Citizens' Coalition for Nursing Home Reform (NCCNHR), founded in 1975. The organization's founder, Elma Holder, was heading Ralph Nader's Long-Term Care Action Project of the Gray Panthers when she organized a group of advocates to attend a nursing home industry conference in Washington, DC. These advocates represented 12 citizen action groups from all over the country. The organization now has more than 200 member groups, in addition to a growing list of individual members. Many member groups are composed of resident and family members, and residents and family groups are often represented on the board. Federal and state legislative and regulatory matters, adequacy of staffing, overuse of antipsychotics, and homes with a history of especially poor care have all been areas of concern.

The Consumer Voice has continued to play an active role in seeking out the concerns of residents, and in providing them with information on issues of importance (e.g., residents' rights, staffing, person-centered care, and falls prevention). In recent years, they have hosted a series of free national conference calls for residents, to support them in becoming empowered advocates for quality care and quality of life, both for themselves and for their peers who lack the capacity to self-advocate (L. Smetanka, personal communication, January 25, 2014).

In 1995, it was NCCNHR that brought together several providers to their annual meeting to share with consumers the efforts they were making to change the culture of their homes. In 1997, these same providers were among the founders of the **Pioneer Network**, discussed later.

For her work in bringing the voice of the consumer to the national stage, and for her leadership in the development and adoption of OBRA, Ms. Holder was named by AARP as a "Champion of Aging," one of the 10 most influential people in aging over the last century.

The National Disability Rights Network was established as a non-profit membership organization to represent the interests of the federally mandated network of Protection and Advocacy Systems (P&A) and Client Assistance Programs (CAP). This network provides a variety of advocacy services to people with disabilities—in particular, training and technical assistance on behalf of residents wishing to move out of nursing homes and back into the community.

Diversity

Diversity in nursing homes is rich and quite complex. In addition to the values, beliefs, practices, and customs that attach to cultural differences, there are differences in religious affiliation, language, gender, sexual orientation, age, political orientation, socioeconomic status, and marital, geographical, and occupational history. There are also differences in disability (physical and mental), diagnoses, medical complexity, and length of time in the facility.

There is also significant diversity among those who work in nursing homes. It is common for homes to have staff from dozens of different countries of origin, with great variety in language and culture. Such variety offers opportunity and interest to the long-term care environment; however, sometimes these differences can make communication more complicated, not only between staff and residents but also among staff. It is important for leadership to recognize that barriers may arise, so that conflicts and misunderstandings can be promptly and appropriately addressed.

There is always diversity in lifestyle, certainly among residents, but also among staff, regardless of their background or circumstances, which leads to different ways of coping with the kind of adversity that illness brings. Sharing a room with a stranger can be extremely challenging. There is also the ever-present tension between the needs of individuals and the requirements of institutions, which inevitably brings a tension of its own. Finally,

> when thinking about cultural knowledge, it is critical to remember the concept of intra-cultural variation—there is more variation within cultural groups than across cultural groups . . . . No individual is a stereotype of one's culture of origin, but rather a unique blend of the diversity found within each culture, a unique accumulation of life, and the process of acculturation to other cultures. (Campinha-Bacote, 2003)

These considerations of diversity underscore the need for individualized, person-centered care. As Campinha-Bacote (2003) further points out, "Cultural values give an individual a sense of direction as well as meaning to life." By recognizing and supporting the individuality of residents, providers are far better able to help residents build on their strengths.

One of the greatest challenges providers face is helping residents and staff appreciate and value the differences they encounter with one another. Leadership must acknowledge that diversity is not only present and deserving of attention but also something to be valued and even celebrated. Many years ago the commentator John Hockenberry said that diversity is thought of as resolved by bringing "one of each" to the table (a man, a woman, someone black, someone Asian)—essentially, a problem to be fixed. Instead, he says, diversity is the richness of life around all of us, and in our differences, we are complete (J. Hockenberry, personal communication, March 17, 1997).

Organizational policies and staff education should ensure that they promote, rather than detract from, the acceptance and welcoming of diversity. As an example, most facilities have residents who identify as lesbian, gay, bisexual, transgender, and queer (LGBTQ+) yet many facilities are either unaware or deliberately ignore this fact, too often leaving the person anxious about his status in the facility and fearful of how he may be treated by others. While a person's sexual orientation and gender are only two aspects of his overall identity and life experience, treating everyone equally, regardless of sexual orientation or gender identity, often results in treating everyone as heterosexual. Doing this glosses over challenges LGBTQ+ elders may have faced, including discrimination, physical and emotional stress, and violence. Active and visible steps to demonstrate organizational acceptance are important. The National Resource Center on LGBT Aging (2012) is the country's first and only technical assistance resource center aimed at improving the quality of services and supports offered to lesbian, gay, bisexual, and transgender older adults, and they have published a useful resource, "Inclusive Services for LGBT Older Adults: A Practical Guide to Creating Welcoming Agencies."

It is important to create ongoing monitoring mechanisms for residents, visitors, and staff to report biased behavior of any kind. This process should be presented to residents and staff and also posted in high-traffic areas. Complaints should be addressed promptly.

One resource for information and guidance regarding diversity is the U.S. Department of Health & Human Services (DHHS) Office of Minority Health (OMH) (n.d.), which released national standards for culturally and linguistically appropriate services in 2000, is an ongoing source for information, and links to a wide variety of other resources.

Changing the Culture: Person-Centered, Person-Directed Care

In the early 1990s, several providers around the country began exploring new approaches to providing care. These explorations largely coincided with the gradual implementation of OBRA, as well as shifts toward the more complex needs of many of those needing long-term care. They arose from dissatisfaction about the quality of care being offered, as well as the recognition that the quality of life for most residents left much to be desired. The term **culture change** arose when the people involved in these efforts recognized that in order to achieve the improvements they hoped for, they would need to "change the culture" of their care environments.

There are several examples of culture change homes described ahead, and new models continue to evolve. What they have in common is a focus on the resident, with approaches that integrate quality of care with quality of life.

Mount St. Vincent

One of the earliest new models was developed by Mount St. Vincent Nursing Home in Seattle, where staff felt compelled to seek change when an audit of their traditional nursing units found that residents were being cared for an average of only 4% of their waking days: "Residents were mostly isolated and barely interacting with anyone, spending most of their time waiting, either to be gotten up, fed, put to bed, or taken somewhere." As their administrator described the situation, "Staff were doing exactly what they have been trained and were expected to do . . . We had a committed and hard-working staff forced to use an antiquated and stupid system" (Mount St. Vincent, 1994, p. 13).

Their changes started with the recognition that relationships between nursing assistants and residents are at the heart of both individualized care and a sense of community. Staffing patterns were reorganized to reduce the ratio between CNAs and residents, making it possible for CNAs to spend more time with each resident. Nursing units were redesigned to better promote the frequency and quality of resident and staff interaction. Instead of the traditional 40-bed units with few private rooms, the new design features only 20 residents per unit, occupying private bedrooms, with a central common area for the kitchen, dining area, and living room. Breakfasts are prepared individually, and other meals are served family style. There is no nursing station, but rather small work areas incorporated into the common area to encourage more interaction among residents and staff. For variety there is a cafeteria in the building open to residents, staff, and visitors, and a small restaurant-like dining area, with waitress service, where residents may entertain guests. There are also child day care programs located in different parts of the building, open to staff and to the wider community. Charlene Boyd and Robert Ogden originated this change effort at Mount St. Vincent, and Charlene Boyd is still actively involved.

The Live Oak Regenerative Community

Barry Barkan and his wife and partner, Debora Barkan, established the Live Oak Institute in 1981, to develop and spread their "regenerative" community approach. They developed their approach in the former Live Oak Living Center, a combined skilled nursing and assisted living home, where they focused on the challenge of engaging and keeping volunteers and staff members active in providing meaningful activities for all residents, with particular emphasis on the most isolated residents. Their goal was to transform homes from institutions to person-centered communities.

While the Barkans no longer operate the Living Center, their experience there was the basis for what has evolved into their current focus, the development of *The Pleasure of Your Company*, a comprehensive system that helps nursing homes bring meaning and relationship to residents who are most at risk for social isolation. In 2010 the Hulda and Maurice Rothschild Foundation funded the institute so that the program could become widely available to homes throughout the country.

The Eden Alternative

One of the most well-known of the early change efforts is the Eden Alternative, pioneered by Dr. William Thomas. In response to the malaise Dr. Thomas observed, which he believed was the result of loneliness, helplessness, and boredom, he developed a model based on creating a "holistic environment" (with birds, cats, dogs, plants, child care, gardens, and visiting school children) in which residents were able to give as well as receive care and feel valued. Thomas eliminated restraints, encouraged residents to give lessons in their own areas of expertise, and trained workers for holistic care. Nursing assistants worked together to develop their own schedules, and staff attendance improved, with fewer staff calling in sick. The facility experienced a statistically significant reduction in mortality, illness, and drug use. Contact with the local community increased, and an on-site child care facility was established.

Now there are more than 200 Eden homes, in the United States, Canada, Europe, and Australia. Eden today considers itself a philosophy that can be applied in any organizational or physical model, across the entire continuum of care, rather than a specific programmatic approach to or model for transformation.

Wellspring

The Wellspring approach was launched in 1994, when a core group of 11 independent nonprofit homes throughout eastern Wisconsin formed an alliance to network and share performance improvement practices. The goals focused on improved outcomes for residents, aligned with more educational support for staff. They did not promote any particular structural design; rather, they focused on the improvement model as an approach that could be applied in any setting.

Training programs were developed in specific practice areas, with homes in the alliance sending members of their staff for shared training. Findings from a 2002 evaluation by Stone and others and funded by the Commonwealth Fund found Wellspring homes had fewer residents who were bedfast, lower restraint usage, more preventive skin care, fewer psychoactive medications, less resident incontinence, fewer tube feedings, and more individualized diets (Stone et al., 2002). Most significantly, these outcomes were accomplished with the same staffing levels as non-Wellspring facilities. Over time, most Wellspring Alliances dissolved, as individual organizations became more experienced and more effective in their own internal quality improvement programs. In 2012 Wellspring was acquired by the Eden Alternative.

The Green House

The **Green House** model evolved from Dr. Thomas's experience with the Eden Alternative. The first Green House was opened in 2003, and currently there are hundreds in operation or in development in most states. The goal is to create an environment that provides the experiences and comforts of being at home. Each home is designed for 10 to 12 residents including private rooms (with private bathrooms) opening to the central communal area, which offers a family-like atmosphere. In this model, empowerment happens when residents (referred to as elders) feel comfortable about expressing their needs and preferences to staff, and when staff are able to respond to these requests (e.g., bringing someone a glass of milk and a cookie, or skipping lunch, or helping someone to bed earlier than usual) because they are confident they understand the resident well enough to make those kinds of decisions without having to check in with anyone else. Shahbazim is the term used to describe the CNAs who provide personalized care, meal preparation, light housekeeping, and laundry. The Shahbazim partners with nurses and other clinical team members to oversee care in the home. Green Houses are licensed and provide the same level of care as other skilled nursing settings.

More recently, the first urban Green House, the Leonard Florence Center for Living, was opened in Boston. Earlier efforts were developed in communities where land was much more readily available; the challenge in an urban environment was to reconfigure and structure the concept of a multi-unit home with much less available land, while preserving a smaller home dynamic. The solution was a single building with five resident floors. There is a first floor with some dining and other amenities. Each of the higher floors has two separate houses, and each house is home to 10 residents. Each house has a distinct doorbell and mailbox.

Another feature of this first urban Green House is that some of the houses serve younger and also specialized populations. Three of the houses are for people with subacute needs (with therapy areas located in each of them). Two are specialized residences, one for people with ALS and one for people with multiple sclerosis (MS). These two houses are fitted with state-of-the-art assistive technology, to maximize independence for the people living there. For example, there are lifts attached to the ceiling, and buttons that residents can use to open doors or turn lights on or off.

The Household Model

In this model, between 14 and 20 residents reside in the home, and each home has its own kitchen, dining room, and living room. The first household opened at Northern Pines (now Bigfork Valley) in Bigfork, Minnesota. Residents get up when they choose, bathe when and how they choose, go to bed when they choose, and eat what and when they choose. Each household has decision-making autonomy—regardless of how many households are part of the larger facility—and each is consistently staffed. Traditional departments like nursing and dietary have been eliminated, and the focus is on integrating care within the household. One of the earliest and most prominent examples of the **household model** is the Meadowlark Hills Retirement Community in Kansas, where the CEO was Steve Shields, who is now very active in helping to spread the model to other settings. There is now an Association of Households International (AHHI), which promotes the household model.

Planetree

Since its founding in 1978 by a patient who had experienced a difficult and lengthy hospital stay, Planetree has worked with hospitals and ambulatory care settings around the world who have implemented the Planetree philosophy. A nonprofit organization that provides education, training, and resources in a collaborative community to healthcare organizations, Planetree facilitates the creation of person-centered care in healing environments.

Beginning in 2002, Planetree began to translate its designation criteria and implementation process to continuing care environments and post-acute settings.

Advocacy and Dementia Care

As models for person-centered care have evolved, all based on knowing the needs of residents, the question is often asked, do these models work for people with dementia: How can people with dementia know or state their needs and preferences (and implicitly, would it make any difference)? Experts in the field of dementia care have long endorsed the principle that, for people with dementia, behavior is communication. As Case Study #2 powerfully illustrates, people with dementia, even in the most advanced stages, do indeed communicate their needs, and it does make a difference.

The Pioneer Network

The Pioneer Network is a national, nonprofit organization founded in 1997 by a group of national leaders in the field of long-term care and aging. Their vision was to move away from the traditional, institutional, provider-driven models to consumer-driven approaches that focus on flexibility and self-determination for residents. The organization has many strategic partnerships, including provider organizations and foundations, and sponsors a wide variety of educational, research, and advocacy efforts. Their annual conference is attended by hundreds of people, and focuses on practice improvements and change strategies. There are over 65 state and local culture change coalitions around the country, all charged with advancing person-centered, person-directed care. The Pioneer Network website contains links to a wide variety of organizations, research, and resources that focus on culture change.

The Role of Philanthropy

Philanthropies have played a significant role in the quest for quality. The Robert Wood Johnson Foundation has been very actively involved in promoting the Green House model, most recently by funding several academic research departments to conduct evaluations in Green House settings. The Hulda B. & Maurice L. Rothschild Foundation has worked on person-centered care issues for many years, most recently by sponsoring a series of regulatory task forces, which have helped/are working to shape the Life Safety Code, the International Building Code (IBC), Health Facilities Guidelines, dining standards, lighting, and acoustics, all in an effort to permit more comfortable environments for residents. The Retirement Research Foundation funded the Pioneer Network to promote the use of the MDS resident preference data as a way of enabling long-term care culture change. The Commonwealth Fund has funded many research projects, such as an evaluation of the Wellspring model.

The Language of Culture Change

Karen Schoeneman, formerly senior policy analyst in the Division of Nursing Homes in the CMS, has written about the impact language can have on how we think about people. Schoeneman (n.d.) relates that in 1972, when she first started working in long-term care at a state school or hospital, people were referred to as "inmates" and "retarded," and categorized as "moron," "idiot," "imbecile," and "mongoloid." As she says, these words were not intended as insults, just as diagnoses. Today, these words have very negative connotations.

In the culture change movement, the term "feeders" is an example of a word that is unintentionally demeaning, and under this movement it has been changed to "person who needs assistance with dining." Similarly, "wheelchair-bound" has been replaced by "person who uses a wheelchair." While these changes may seem insignificant, what they convey is the difference between being defined by the disability (wheelchair-bound or a feeder) and a person who, in addition to other qualities, needs mobility assistance or dining assistance. People living in nursing homes are often referred to by their diagnosis (a diabetic, a quad, a CVA). The culture change movement teaches the concept of "a person who 'has' (diabetes, quadriplegia, a CVA)," not "is" a diabetic, a quad, or a CVA.

Among those engaged in culture change efforts, many have come to prefer "person-directed" rather than "person-centered." While this shift may also seem small, it represents the perspective that the person is active in care planning and care delivery, rather than the more passive "recipient" of person-centered care.

Institutional language creates perceptions, and those perceptions affect how one receives care, and also leads to generalizations and the perpetuation of stereotypes about aging that affect not only how care is delivered but also how the profession is viewed by others.

Summary

The goal of a nursing home never changes: to provide the best possible care for the people who live there, and to nourish the spirit of residents and staff alike. At the same time, nursing homes are places that change every day: Residents and workers (in all their variety) come and go, staff learn better ways to deliver care, equipment is modernized, and new regulations are introduced. Adapting to change and continuously learning new and more effective ways of working—as individuals, as teams, and as organizations—result in care that is both more effective and more compassionate, and in a work environment that is more satisfying.

As Sallie Tisdale (1987) states in her book, *Harvest Moon: Portrait of a Nursing Home*, "Ordinary, even familial things happen here, though often unwitnessed. Wounds are healed, muscles strengthened, faces washed, and hands held. Each small movement is tiny in its fruition, huge in its absence" (p. xii).

To fill that absence, everyone has a part to play in advocating for the resident's voice.

Key Terms

The Consumer Voice (originally, the National Citizens' Coalition for Nursing Home Reform): A nonprofit organization made up of consumer groups and individual consumers, founded in 1975, and focused on improving care in nursing homes. It played a leadership role in the development and passage of OBRA '87.

Culture change: A term used to describe the effort of many providers and consumers to improve care by changing the culture of nursing homes.

Green House: A model of care, first developed by Dr. William Thomas and colleagues, which focuses on the creation of small homes (licensed as SNFs) designed for 10 to 12 residents with an environment that provides the comforts and experiences of home.

Household model: In this model, households are designed to be to between 14 and 20 residents, also with an environment intended to provide the comforts and experience of home.

Nursing Home Ombudsman Program: The Older Americans Act requires that all 50 states (and Puerto Rico, the District of Columbia, and Guam) have a long-term care ombudsman program, whose purpose is to address complaints by or for residents, advocate on their behalf, educate residents and the public about resident rights and good care practices, and promote the development of citizen organizations, family councils, and resident councils.

OBRA '87: Also known as the Nursing Home Reform Law of 1987, OBRA '87 was the first major revision of federal standards for nursing home care since Medicare and Medicaid were in enacted in 1965. OBRA '87 is the basis for current nursing home regulations.

Person-centered, or person-directed, care: A term that is intended to convey that the person's needs and preferences should direct care planning and care delivery.

Pioneer Network: A national, nonprofit organization founded in 1997 by leaders in long-term care and aging who wanted to move away from the traditional, more institutional models of nursing home care to consumer-driven approaches that emphasize flexibility and self-determination for residents. They hold an annual conference, which is attended by hundreds of people from all over the country, and which focuses on both practice improvements and change strategies.

Review Questions

1. What are the different ways diversity manifests itself in long-term care settings?

2. Why is advocacy an important role for staff?

3. How are quality of care and quality of life linked in long-term care?

4. Why does the language we use in long-term care matter?

5. What has been the overall thrust of emerging models of care in residential care settings?

6.   How can volunteers improve care?

7.   How can advocates from outside the facility—such as ombudsmen and advocacy groups—improve care?

Case Studies

Case Study #1

Typical activities at Clatsop Care were parties with entertainment, bingo, church services, exercise classes, ice cream socials, and theme parties. They began to realize that most of these were focused on entertaining rather than engaging residents. To supplement the work of the activities department, they formed the "Nightingales," a work group (which included the administrator, the cook, and a housekeeper) charged with finding ways of engaging residents in activities that were personally meaningful. They knew they could not proceed without actively listening to residents, and without engaging and soliciting staff support. They conducted "learning circles" with both residents and staff, listening, observing, and experimenting with different ideas as they went along.

Early on, they realized that while past history can be extremely helpful for some residents in identifying pleasurable activities, this was not always the case. For example, someone who was once an accomplished pianist no longer enjoyed playing because she was frustrated that she could not play at the level she once did. On the other hand, someone else who had always enjoyed music started a singing group. Another resident who loved houseplants was provided with a greenhouse space. Yet another resident was given space outside the home for growing tomatoes—she had lived and worked on the family vegetable farm.

Not everything involved a specific activity. On a hunch, after a donation of clothing came in that included a bright red sheer nightgown, the administrator brought it up to a resident who had had a stroke, and had been unwilling to participate in any activities. The resident became quite animated, the home secured some additional gowns, and the resident began getting out of bed, had her hair done, and began to be more engaged.

Another change came when, instead of monthly birthday parties, they started recognizing resident's birthdays individually, on the day, with singing and a small gift at lunch. They also started to focus more on smaller group activities; for example, instead of playing trivia with 20 residents, they would break the residents into groups of 5 or so, dividing according to ability, to increase the likelihood of resident engagement. Even more visits from children, and from pets, were encouraged.

The most common response, when residents were asked what they would like, was "get out of here," and so what had been monthly trips evolved to two trips a week, usually an outing to a destination of interest for one trip (a fish hatchery, the beach, the Coast Guard station), with a second trip for lunch or dinner out. This didn't mean every resident went out every week; it meant that those who were able got to count on going out regularly, and had something to look forward to.

Staff was another source of many activities: A housekeeper who was a member of the American Legion suggested residents go to the Legion for bingo, which residents now do at least quarterly. A custodian who brews beer has given demonstrations and provides samples. A cook who likes crafts started a group that makes handmade cards, which residents can keep, or sell at the front desk. Staff members of various ethnicities have provided a meal, dance, or song specific to their country.

It became evident that expansion of individual and small group activities could not occur without additional support. A part-time volunteer coordinator was hired, and volunteer hours increased from 40 to 400 hours per month. This was due partially to having the new position, and to the effectiveness of the person they hired, but it was also due to the fact that the home's approach to so much individualization of activities meant a much richer, more interesting, and more appealing set of activities for volunteers to relate to with residents. This increase in volunteers also allowed staff to focus more of their time on residents with dementia, and other residents who need more individualized attention.

While they would be the first to acknowledge that their efforts to find meaningful, more individualized engagement for residents are not always easy and not always successful, there is no question that they have improved the quality of life as well as the quality of care for the great majority of residents, and have had an extremely positive impact on staff and family members as well (A. Schacher, personal communication, January 2014).

Study questions: (1) Why does leisure time matter for people living in long-term care? (2) Why is engagement, as well as entertainment, important?

Case Study #2

In the late 1990s, staff at Beatitudes Campus made the determination that the care they were providing to residents on their dementia unit was not acceptable. Residents were frequently in distress, calling out, moaning, and sometimes rejecting care when offered assistance. There was a lot of staff turnover: It was not a place where people liked to work. Starting with the premise that behavior is communication, staff determined they would try to understand what the person with dementia was trying to communicate, to see if they couldn't make them more comfortable than they appeared to be. They gradually determined that most of the discomfort they were observing could be traced to unmet needs: hunger, pain, loneliness, over- or understimulation, sleep deprivation, the need for toileting, being too hot or too cold, or boredom.

Gradually they made a number of organizational changes to address these concerns. Staff on the neighborhood held weekly meetings to pin down exactly what and when the distress occurred, and also what brought the resident comfort/pleasure. They spent as much time as they needed, until they felt they were meeting the resident's needs, although at any point things could and often did change, at which point they would reassess. All disciplines were involved in these meetings.

Early on, they decided to see what they could do about that time at the end of the day when so many residents seemed especially agitated or upset (the time of the day commonly associated with "sundowning," a term used to describe the agitation, pacing, irritability, and disorientation that many people with Alzheimer's experience during the late afternoon, evening, or night). The staff saw that many residents looked tired and frazzled and wondered if they would be more comfortable if they were to lie down and rest. Much of the time, these rest periods were not necessarily convenient for the staff, and it was challenging at first; however, the team decided if someone looked tired, no matter when that occurred (even mealtimes or during an activity), they would help him to rest either in a comfortable chair or on the bed (some prefer a chair or the couch, some may only lay on top of their bed, with a throw, while others prefer to change and get back into bed—the decision is based on the resident's comfort). As residents started to sleep when they were tired and wake when they were rested, the change was obvious. Residents were much happier. The nurses didn't give PRN medication for agitation any longer and felt comfortable asking the physicians to begin tapering medications. Another positive outcome was that there were fewer falls—staff realized that many falls (especially in the evening) came about because residents were tired.

Staff also observed the overall neighborhood environment. What was seen and heard was appalling. The general chaos at shift change was compounded by the common room television and general noise on the unit. Watching the residents respond to the din was enlightening. Sometimes people covered their ears or tried to get away from it. Some just looked scared and bewildered. It became clear to the staff that they needed to stop talking so loudly and slow down, and they worked successfully toward a "silent" shift change. The television was moved. The milieu became quiet, and everyone responded positively to the change in the environment. Being confused and unable to make sense out of the environment can be extremely tiring for the person with Alzheimer's, and overstimulation only makes this worse.

Once the changes were in place, residents didn't call out, become angry or upset, or try to leave. Families and friends increased their visits in the afternoon and evening.

Weight loss is another area where the staff at Beatitudes have been very successful. Knowing what people with dementia like to eat is even more important than knowing what they don't like to eat: Restricting food options can increase the risk of weight loss. Beatitudes eliminated special diets and now makes snack foods available 24 hours a day. They are offered every hour or so around the clock and are usually finger foods, offered in small portions, geared to what staff can see that residents truly enjoy: peanut butter sandwiches, fruit slices, chocolate, lollipops, and ice cream. Every afternoon, the smell of cookies baking can be found on the unit. The need for supplements has been eliminated, and weight loss is now rare.

Better identification and treatment of pain have been a hugely significant factor as well. Pain is more common for people with dementia than is commonly understood, because they are often not able to tell us about it due to their confusion and lack of insight. Once again, by focusing on behavior as communication, it became clear that calling out, moaning, or striking out at caregivers during care occurred because the person was in pain. If non-pharmacological solutions are not effective, then analgesics and other pain medications are explored—these often prove effective, treating the very real pain and thus preventing or minimizing the distressed behavior.

Finally, staff observed that large-group activities left most residents unengaged, and many of them restless and even distressed by the confusion they experienced from all the stimulation. Activities have been redefined to include all interactions between staff (all departments) and residents, and now, regardless of whether the interaction involves helping someone to dress, to toilet, or a walk down the hallway, a few moments of sitting side by side, or sharing a piece of chocolate, all staff look for opportunities to make a meaningful connection with residents, starting with knowing as much about what makes the person comfortable and what brings him pleasure as possible. Large-group activities have been replaced almost entirely by one-on-one and small group activities.

Significantly, now there is almost no staff turnover and there is a waiting list for those who want to work on the unit. Staff at Beatitudes now train others all over the country in their Comfort Matters approach (T. Alonzo, personal communication, January 2014).

Study questions: (1) Why is it important to understand that people with dementia have specialized needs? (2) Why is comfort an important concept to understand in the long-term care setting?

Case Study #3

A local ombudsman in Virginia was contacted by a resident's family member because the facility where his aunt, Mrs. Jones, was a resident had informed him that she would be discharged because her "behaviors" were posing a threat to other residents and staff. Specifically, staff complained that she tried to hit staff when personal care was provided and that she seemed generally restless but unwilling to engage in the activities offered to her. The ombudsman talked with the resident and the nephew as well as staff to learn more about the concerning behaviors and whether there were particular situations that seemed to trigger the resident's lashing out at others. The nephew explained that the resident had lived on her own for many years out in the country, managing a small farm and handling many tasks that many of her neighbors considered "man's work." She primarily kept to herself, was fiercely independent, and also had a very significant hearing loss. In observing staff approaching the resident in the nursing home, the ombudsman could see that the staff did not seem to be aware that the resident was sometimes startled when approached or touched from behind or even from the side, and that this is when the resident would tend to strike out. It became clear to the ombudsman that staff had not considered how this might impact a resident who could not hear or who also had a certain degree of discomfort when strangers provided personal care. The ombudsman followed up with the staff regarding the need to make sure they were fully aware of care/assessment issues identified in the MDS and that they received training in how to approach residents with hearing or visual impairments. The resident's history also pointed up the need to consider "less traditional" options for activities, including those that might interest a resident like Mrs. Jones (e.g., tabletop gardening), who preferred a more solitary endeavor that got her hands into the dirt. Since the hearing impairment had not gotten adequate attention to this point, at the next care planning meeting staff explored possibilities for offering the resident the opportunity to have her hearing evaluated to assess the potential for improved hearing through assistive devices. Once the ombudsman and staff understood how to better approach and advocate for the resident, the nursing facility no longer had an interest in discharging the resident (J. Latimer, personal communication, January 2014).

Study questions: (1) Why is an outside, fresh perspective on a dilemma sometimes helpful? (2) What can get in the way of staff being thorough when investigating a resident's perspective?

References

Academy of Nutrition and Dietetics. (2005). Position of the American Dietetic Association: Liberalization of the diet prescription improves quality of life for older adults in long-term care. *Journal of the Academy of Nutrition and Dietetics, 105*(12), 1955–1965.

Advancing Excellence. Retrieved from https://www.nhqualitycampaign.org/goalDetail.aspx?g=ca

American Diabetes Association. (2008). Nutrition recommendations and interventions for diabetes: A position statement of the American Diabetes Association. *Diabetes Care, 31*(Suppl 1), 561–578.

Banaszak-Holl, J., & Hines, M. A. (1996). Factors associated with nursing home staff turnover. *The Gerontologist, 36*(4), 512–517.

Cain, S. (2013). *Quiet: The power of introverts in a world that can't stop talking.* New York, NY: Broadway Books.

Campinha-Bacote, J. (2003, January 31). Many faces: Addressing diversity in health care. *Online Journal of Issues in Nursing, 8*(1), Manuscript 2. Retrieved from http://www.nursingworld.org/MainMenuCategories/ANAMarketplace/ANA Periodicals/OJIN/TableofContents/Volume82003/No1Jan2003/Addressing DiversityinHealthCare.aspx

Committee on Nursing Home Regulation, Institute of Medicine. (1986). *Improving the quality of care in nursing homes.* Washington, DC: National Academy Press.

Henderson, J. N. (1987, April). When a professor turns nurse aide. *Provider,* pp. 8–12.

Henderson, J. N. (1995). The culture of care in a nursing home: Effects of a medicalized model of long-term care. In J. N. Henderson & M. D. Vesperi (Eds.), *The culture of long-term care* (pp. 37–54). Westport, CT: Bergin & Garvey.

Kane, R., & Caplan, A. (1990). *Everyday Ethics: Resolving Dilemmas in Nursing Home Life.* New York, NY: Springer.

Mount St. Vincent, Providence. (1994). *An alternative to nursing homes: Impacting resident functional and health decline.* Sisters of Providence.

National Citizens' Coalition for Nursing Home Reform. (1985). *A consumer perspective on quality care: The residents' point of view.* Washington, DC: Author.

National Resource Center on LGBT Aging. (2012, March). *Inclusive services for LGBT older adults: A practical guide to creating welcoming agencies.* Retrieved from www.lgbtagingcenter/resources

Office of Minority Health. (n.d.). *Think cultural health: Advancing health equity at every point of contact.* Retrieved from https://www.thinkculturalhealth.hhs.gov/GUIs/GUI&uscore;TCHRegister.asp?mode=new&clas=yes

Ronch, J. (2012, December 11). Large parties are not for everyone. Retrieved from http://www.ltlmagazine.com/blogs/judah-ronch/large-parties-are-not-everyone

Schoeneman, K. (n.d.) Language. Retrieved from http://www.pioneernetwork.net/CultureChange/Language/

Stone, R. I., Reinhard, S. C., Bowers, B., Zimmerman D., Phillips, C. D., Hawes, C., . . . Jacobson, N.(2002) Evaluation of the Wellspring model for improving nursing home quality. Retrieved from http://www.commonwealthfund.org/Publications/Fund-Reports/2002/Aug/Evaluation-of-the-Wellspring-Model-for-Improving-Nursing-Home-Quality.aspx

Tisdale, S. (1987). *Harvest moon: Portrait of a nursing home.* New York, NY: Henry Holt.

Acknowledgments

To Elma Holder, Barbara Frank, and a multitude of colleagues and friends at NCCNHR (now Consumer Voice), it is impossible to convey the debt we all owe you, for all you have brought to quality care, to me personally, for bringing us OBRA, and for every minute of your passionate and never-ending commitment to improving nursing home care. My endless appreciation, and love, to the residents, staff, and board at Village Nursing Home during my years there, where it all began, especially George Karelitsky, Judy Levin, Paul Rounsaville, and the memory of Lenore Zola, Tom Spicuzza, Bob Lott, and Nick Rango.

To the residents and my colleagues at Isabella Geriatric Center and Cobble Hill Health Center, I can only say thank you for inviting me in, and letting me stay, to learn and grow alongside you all these years.

Special thanks to Dan Cohen at Music and Memory, Sara Joffe at PHInational, and to Anita Schacher, formerly at Clatsop Care Center, for all the ways you have enlarged my life, and for all you do and have done to enhance the lives of people who live in nursing homes.

My thanks to Jim Kinsey for his contribution of the section on Planetree. Finally, my deep gratitude to the staff at Beatitudes Campus, Phoenix, Arizona, especially Tena Alonzo, Carol Long, Karen Mitchell, and Maribeth Gallagher at Hospice of the Valley, for all that I have been privileged to learn from you about palliative care for people with advanced dementia. To Jed Levine and the staff at the Alzheimer's Association, NYC Chapter, and to our partner colleagues Karen Harper, Deirdre Downes, Kris Kuhn, and Rob Herel—working with you has been an extraordinary privilege, and I am enormously grateful.

CHAPTER 4

PHYSICAL ENVIRONMENT OF LONG-TERM CARE

Andrew Alden
Jeffrey Anderzhon
Sarah Moser

Is **long-term care** an environment for work, rehabilitation, and healing, or a living environment? The answer is "yes, it is." Long-term care settings for older adults are a unique combination of functions, containing layers of public and private spaces.

The activities that take place in a building, and the people who live, work, and socialize there, can be supported or hindered by the design of the **physical environment**. The physical environment is the external, tangible surroundings in which a person exists. A typical problem that long-term care environments face today is a mismatch between what the physical environment offers and what is needed by those who live and work there.

History of Long-Term Care Design in the United States

In this chapter we will look at the highlights and most influential events that have brought this care profession to its current state. The first step in understanding the existing physical environment of long-term care is to understand its origins and links with hospitals.

Origins of the Acute Care Hospital and Aged Care

In the 13th century, monks established infirmaries for the care and treatment of the sick and injured. Medical

LEARNING OBJECTIVES

- Identify the historical origins of long-term care from an operational, policy, and physical environment perspective and the impact on contemporary environments.

- Grasp the link between a resident-centered model of care and the trend toward smaller non-institutional settings with an emphasis on a residentially scaled built environment.

- Understand the connection between the contemporary resident-centered model of care and associated aspects of both the physical environment and operations.

- Recognize the changes that are occurring in long-term care operations, programming, and physical environments in direct contrast to a traditional institutional model of care.

- Gain insight into regulations for the physical environment of long-term care settings with the goal of protecting the health, safety, and welfare of building occupants.

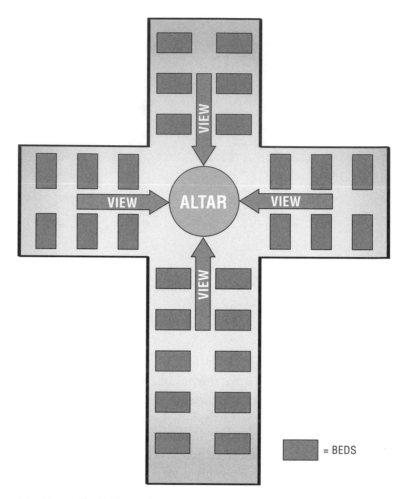

Figure 4.1   Monastic Hospital Concept Floor Plan
Source: Adapted from Eppstein Uhen Architects, Milwaukee, WI, 2014.

knowledge was very basic, and treatment consisted of food, shelter, and faith in God. The treatment was performed by ensuring that all patients were given shelter and food, and had a view of the altar from their bed. This resulted in a crucifix floor plan with the altar placed at the center of the intersecting halls (see Figure 4.1).

Military hospitals have existed for centuries. The Romans first established military hospitals to contend with the great number of wounded soldiers from their conquests. The Romans were also the first to adopt a ward-style arrangement for efficiency, which was similar to military barracks: large open rooms with rows of cots facing one another to provide ease of access and supervision for those providing care (see Figure 4.2).

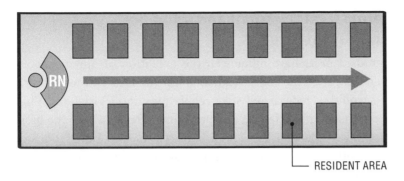

RESIDENT AREA

Figure 4.2   Roman Hospital Concept Floor Plan
Source: Adapted from Eppstein Uhen Architects, Milwaukee, WI, 2014.

In the late 1800s in the United States, the aftermath of the Civil War introduced a need for organized hospitals and long-term care settings. The influx of veterans who were wounded or disabled and who needed ongoing long-term benefits led to societal pressure on the government to provide for those who served their country. The government began providing benefits for wounded veterans, but fraud involved in distribution of these benefits led to the need for more restrictive governmental oversight; in addition the federal government began constructing hospitals and long-term care communities for use by veterans. During this time there remained an unclear delineation of hospital care and long-term care with many aged and infirm individuals in hospital settings; see Figure 4.3 for a concept floor plan from a traditional hospital-type setting.

POST–CIVIL WAR ERA WARDS

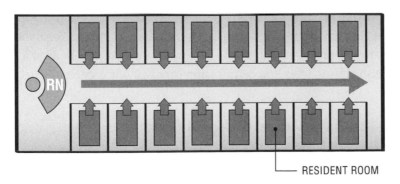

RESIDENT ROOM

Figure 4.3   Post–Civil War Hospital Concept Floor Plan: Beginning of a Traditional Institutional Double Loaded Corridor With Shared Rooms and Shared Bathrooms
Source: Adapted from Eppstein Uhen Architects, Milwaukee, WI, 2014.

Governmental Oversight and Influence on Long-Term Care

Numerous aspects have influenced the evolution of nursing home environments through the years. Arguably, not the least of these contributing aspects would be federal and state regulations and legislation. While each piece of legislation had lasting and profound effects on both the design and operational aspects of nursing homes, they also contributed to institutionalization with the influence of hospitals (see Chapter 1). They were enacted on the foundational thinking that those who required long-term care could be stereotyped and compartmentalized, and would be best served by a medical model of care in which staff efficiency outweighed individualized care.

As legislation in the middle of the 20th century provided funding for new hospital settings, many of the old hospital buildings remained in place and were converted to nursing home use. In addition, legislation specifically passed for the construction of nursing homes in the early 1950s also promoted design guidelines based on hospital settings.

Medicare and Medicaid: Following a series of tragically fatal nursing home fires between 1952 and 1963, coupled by an alarming increase in government payments for aged care through the Social Security Act, Congress passed Title XVIII and Title XIX in 1965, creating **Medicare** and **Medicaid** to provide health coverage to older adults and low-income individuals. As a result of this bill the **Centers for Medicare and Medicaid Services (CMS)** were created to oversee funding and regulate the quality of care and the physical environment. In 1967 the Moss Amendments were passed, which put into place complete regulations requiring nursing homes receiving payments from Medicare and Medicaid to comply with conditions of participation, including the physical environment, life safety codes, and quality of care standards.

Omnibus Reconciliation Act (OBRA): OBRA established the Resident's Bill of Rights and provided a massive overhaul of federal regulations for both the operation and physical environment of nursing homes. This law established the survey and certification process that is currently in place.

The Medical Model of Aged Care

The continued development of the acute care hospital eventually established a standardized floor plan also adopted by long-term care settings and utilized extensively during the latter half of the 20th century. The typical floor plan is characterized by numerous corridors with rooms on both sides, often referred to as a **double loaded corridor**. Most of the resident rooms are shared rooms, with little space on the unit dedicated to activities and socialization. The center of the floor plan is always reserved for the nursing station to promote visual access to the resident rooms and supervisory control over the unit. The organization of care settings around staff efficiency and the ability to control the environment is the medical model of care and the fundamental organizing factor in the design of both the acute care hospital and traditional long-term care settings (Johnson & Grant, 1985).

The acute care hospital is designed to assess patients, provide treatment, and then release them back into the community. However, the traits of an acute care environment do not meet the needs of individuals with chronic illnesses because of the length of stay: The average length of stay in a hospital is approximately 5 days, while the average in long-term care is 2.29 years (CDC, 2010, 2013).

Traditional Nursing Home Components

The unit: The basic building block of a traditional nursing home is the "unit." A unit is the living space for 40-plus residents and is typically composed of identical doors along a double loaded corridor.

Control points: The medical model promotes the adoption of **control points** in the physical setting as typical of "total institutions," such as prisons, in which hierarchical authority is mandated (Johnson & Grant, 1985). Control points are used for monitoring, and in a traditional model long-term care environment this is typically the nursing station. The ever-present nursing station is a constant reminder that the resident is in an institutional medical environment, not a home, constantly watched, and most importantly under the control of others.

Unit activity: The units usually have a small multipurpose lounge. The unit is not designed for the accommodation of residents in numerous social spaces over a long period of time. A minimum amount of resident activity is generally present, with residents spending a large amount of time getting ready or having staff assist them to move to the next meal or activity. Most dining and activity events take place in a large centralized space that residents need to access by leaving the unit.

The typical layout of a medical model environment does not offer many spaces for residents to gather or for activities to occur on the unit; they are usually designed for limited activities, such as crafts, not those associated with living in a place. Most activity on a unit occurs at the central nursing station, where residents and staff tend to congregate and which is often the only source of stimulation for residents. To support staff efficiency, the bathing room and other service areas are usually centrally located near the nursing station. This may reduce travel distances and be advantageous for staff, but it diminishes the residents' right to privacy and dignity.

Unit finishes and furnishings: Interior spaces on the units are generally very institutional in appearance, with fluorescent lighting creating a harsh glare off of highly polished floors. The floors and walls are constructed of non-porous tile and concrete masonry units (Hiatt, 1991). These environments reflect the intention of the medical unit to quickly treat a patient and release him; therefore the finishes support cleanliness, efficiency, and control of infection.

Storage: Storage space is always a problem on the units, which often results in the blocking of hallways with ambulatory-assistance devices, such as wheelchairs and lifts. In addition, the presence of various service carts in the hallway is associated with lingering unpleasant smells from soiled garments and linens.

Interior environmental quality: Noise is often a problem due to the reverberation of the hard surfaces and the presence of numerous televisions, radios, and intercom systems (Hiatt, 1991). Because resident bedrooms line the exterior walls, natural light is absent from the interior corridors. Typically natural light is present only in the centralized multipurpose area and at the end of a dead-end corridor.

Resident bedroom: Residents lack a sense of privacy or control over their environment, and typically share sleeping space and a bathroom with one or up to three individuals. The resident bedrooms were designed for temporary occupation since they were based on the acute care model. In addition, the bedrooms were never meant for living; residents were supposed to use the room for sleeping only, and were expected to be outside the room in the multipurpose area during the day, where nurses would have an easier time monitoring them.

Many long-term care units are located in a physical structure based on a decades-old acute care hospital model; therefore the implementation of contemporary operational methods results in a misfit between the "bricks and mortar" and the functions it houses. In a medical model, the patient is identified by her ailment, even though that is a minor part of whom she is. In order to eliminate this kind of thinking, a new model of care was introduced, called resident-centered care.

Resident-Centered Care Model

As the model of care moved away from organization and staff-centeredness, operational changes began to support resident-centered care. The goal of resident-centered care is to support the preferences of the resident, with the organization of daily routines around the resident's desires. This model also introduced a social component, with the goal to enhance **quality of life** and build relationships. Quality of life includes other aspects in addition to physical wellness, such as dignity, usefulness, independence, and control (Johnson & Grant, 1985). The quality of care an individual receives is still part of the resident-centered model of care, but the primary focus changes to supporting the resident as a unique individual.

A large focus of resident-centered care is supporting the individual's autonomy, giving residents the opportunity to have control over decisions about their daily routines, such as when they wake, when and what they eat, and what activities they partake in. Staff members are expected to organize their patterns around the preferences of the individual. The resident-centered care model is drastically different from the medical model's focus on staff efficiency and a hierarchical structure, making this contemporary operational structure incompatible with many existing long-term care buildings.

Development of Contemporary Long-Term Care Environments

The medical care model changed due to the evolving view of long-term care in American society, spurred by increased awareness of Alzheimer's disease and other related dementias (Weisman, 1997). The progression away from environments for the aged based on the medical model toward environments based on the resident-centered care model is evident in an examination of buildings that have been constructed over the past 25 years.

The earliest innovative long-term care buildings began as an attempt to directly counter the negative aspects of traditional nursing homes by changing one or two major characteristics, such as a lack of social and living spaces on the units and the use of institutional-style finishes and furniture. The later innovative projects concentrated on changing multiple environmental and operational features reminiscent of an institutional environment.

Exploded Corridor Floor Plans

One of the first steps to contemporary long-term care settings occurred with the implementation of *exploded corridor floor plans* in the early 1970s. The exploded corridor arranges residents' rooms around a large central activity space designed to serve as both a way-finding landmark and encourage resident involvement in activities (see Figure 4.4). Some aspects of traditional institutional environments were also present, including a large nursing station, a large unprogrammed floor area, shared bedrooms, and institutional furnishings and fixtures. It was, however, a significant

EXPLODED CORRIDOR

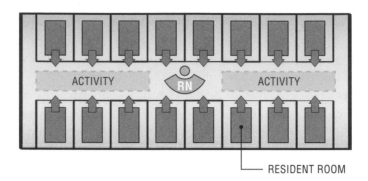

RESIDENT ROOM

Figure 4.4   Exploded Corridor Concept Floor Plan
Source: Adapted from Eppstein Uhen Architects, Milwaukee, WI, 2014.

step toward moving away from traditional institutional long-term care environments.

Household Model Development

The next step toward a contemporary long-term care setting occurred over several years, with dozens of projects slowly building upon one another. The basic change was that residents were given private rooms and the environment (finishes, lighting, and furniture) was modified to a more familiar residential scale and character (see Figure 4.5). Most importantly

DIVIDED HOUSEHOLD

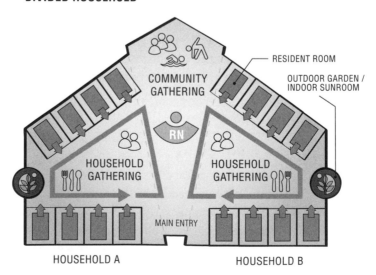

Figure 4.5   Divided Household Concept Floor Plan
Source: Adapted from Eppstein Uhen Architects, Milwaukee, WI, 2014.

the number of residents living together was reduced and the traditional nursing station was reduced in size or eliminated. It is important to note that the new environments were all developed and implemented in conjunction with intensive staff training aimed to break down the hierarchical model of staff care. The altered environment is less effective without organizational/procedural changes.

As opposed to a medical model, the foregoing models were designed to promote comfort, quality of life, and a more meaningful connection between residents and staff.

Contemporary Nursing Home Components

The household: The basic building block of contemporary long-term care environments is the **household** or a smaller-sized grouping of residents, typically 10 to 16 people who live together and share a kitchen, dining room, living room, and other service spaces.

Household activity: The household model emphasizes socialization and supports the development of personal relationships. Activities occur in the household and often involve everyday events, such as preparing a meal in the household kitchen. In addition, households promote a connection to nature; there is ample natural light indoors, and residents have complete access to a secure outdoor garden and walking path.

Household finishes and furnishings: Furniture and finishes have a more familiar residential appearance and often include materials associated with a private home, such as carpet and natural woods.

Household bedrooms: The majority of residents have private rooms with private three-piece bathrooms. If a shared resident room is used, it has a clearly defined personal space for each occupant and they share a three-piece bathroom. Residents are encouraged to personalize their space with their own furniture and display personal memorabilia.

Contemporary household layouts: A variety of contemporary household configurations exist based on individual organizational, contextual, or care population needs. However, the vast majority of the layouts can be classified according to the presence or absence of a clear **public to private gradient**. A public to private gradient mimics the location of spaces in a typical private residence, with the public spaces, such as the living room and kitchen, easily accessible from the front door. The private spaces, such as the bedrooms, are usually located the farthest away from the front door. The two typical household layouts are referred to as a "short corridor household" and a "living room household."

Short corridor household: The short corridor floor plan maintains a traditional residential-style public to private gradient. Most public spaces (kitchen and dining) are located at the entrance to the households, while

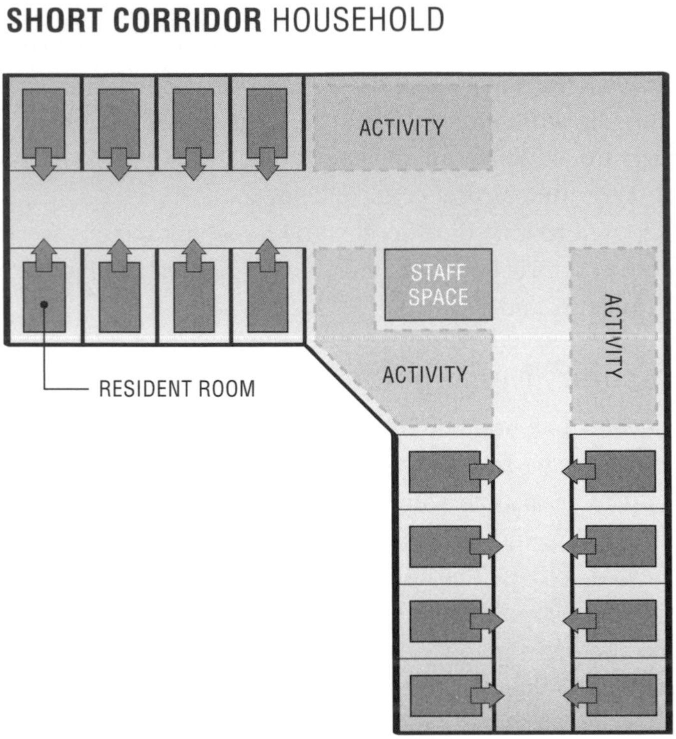

SHORT CORRIDOR HOUSEHOLD

Figure 4.6   Short Corridor Household Concept Floor Plan
Source: Adapted from Eppstein Uhen Architects, Milwaukee, WI, 2014.

the private bedrooms are located as far from the entry as possible. Staff and service spaces are decentralized throughout the household (see Figure 4.6).

Living room household: The living room household does not have a clear public to private gradient because the resident bedrooms are gathered around a central space containing the kitchen, dining, and living room. A majority of the bedrooms have direct visual access to activities on the household. Staff and services spaces are decentralized (see Figure 4.7).

The model/philosophy of care in these environments is based upon flexibility and meeting the individual needs of the residents. The flexibility allows residents to exercise personal choice and retain familiar routine schedules (waking, sleeping, eating, bathing, etc.). The flexible schedule of routines and activities is in contrast to the strict adherence to schedules in the traditional nursing home (Silverman et al., 1995).

Households may be designed as stand-alone buildings or for larger communities; households are grouped to make up a neighborhood. The facility as a whole may be composed of multiple neighborhoods, administrative spaces, back-of-house functions, and possibly an activity-based town center. The resident has access to a variety of social spaces, providing

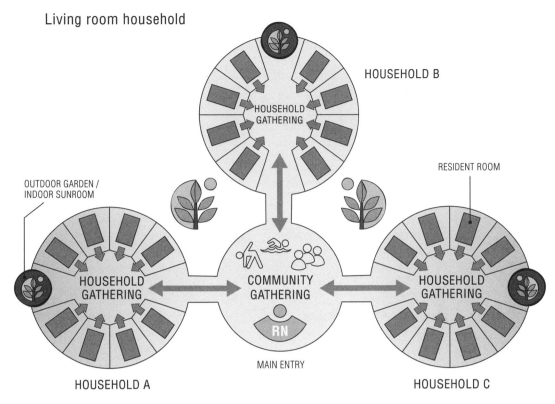

Figure 4.7   Living Room Household Concept Floor Plan
Source: Adapted from Eppstein Uhen Architects, Milwaukee, WI, 2014.

varying degrees of socialization to support many desires and comfort levels. In addition to the number of social options, each space offers a varying level of privacy (spaces for one person, spaces for eight people). The town center usually has a variety of options to choose from, including library, bank, gift shop, chapel, bistro, beauty/barber, and PT/OT, which provide residents the opportunity to enjoy an outing, leaving their households for larger community activities.

The Long-Term Care Culture Change Movement (Resident-Centered Care)

The culture change movement is based on the resident-centered model of care, where the choices of residents are respected to enhance quality of life and importance is placed on the relationships between residents and caregivers. Culture change supports the efforts of early innovation to eliminate the institutional atmosphere of a nursing home, with a more comprehensive effort that includes both the physical environment (see Table 4.1) and operations (see Table 4.2).

Table 4.1   Physical Environment Comparison: Models of Care

Traditional long-term care model	Contemporary resident-centered care model
Large centralized activity space	Small decentralized activity spaces
Large centralized dining space	Small decentralized dining spaces
Large centralized staff space (nursing station)	Small decentralized staffing spaces
Centralized resident care and service spaces	Decentralized care and service spaces
Institutional style finishes and furnishings	Residential interior finishes and furnishings
Lack of natural light and exterior views	Natural light and options for exterior views
Majority of multiple occupants (two, three, or four people) resident rooms with shared two-piece bathrooms and limited number of private rooms	Majority of private rooms with private three-piece bathrooms, limited number of companion rooms, "smart doubles"
Monochromatic interior colors and no textures	Variety of interior colors and mixture of textures
Limited outdoor access and gardens	Outdoor access with a variety of spaces

Table 4.2   Operational Comparison: Models of Care

Traditional long-term care model	Contemporary resident-centered care model
Ailment/disability focus	Resident as individual focus
Staff control of daily routines	Resident choice and control of daily routines
Maximization of staff efficiency	Optimize resident quality of life and independence
Rotated staff assignments	Permanent staff assignments
Specialized job tasks (hierarchical)	Wide range of tasks (team oriented)
Quality of care emphasis	Quality of care and quality of life emphasis
Majority of food preparation and plating of food behind closed doors	Majority of food preparation and serving of food at decentralized dining spaces in view of residents

Technology of Long-Term Care

Recent technological advancements have worked to support culture change efforts by supporting staff efficiency, quality of care, and quality of life. There are several kinds of technology used by staff and residents in long-term care environments.

Behavioral Monitoring

Behavioral monitoring refers to technology utilized to monitor and analyze routine daily activity or **activities of daily living** (ADLs); these devices can identify when residents may need help without the resident needing to press an emergency call button. An example of a behavioral monitoring device is one that is placed in a resident room to continuously and automatically sense and track movement. If a change in behavior is sensed, such as an extended period of time spent in the bathroom, which could mean that a fall has occurred, the device will automatically report the potential hazard to staff. This device is not a camera, which helps the resident to retain a sense of privacy and independence while still feeling safe and secure.

Ambulatory-Assistance Devices

In addition to canes, walkers, and wheelchairs, technology is improving to aid in **mobility assistance** and **transferring** of residents. Staff are often needed for transferring, such as in and out of bed or on and off the toilet, or moving from a sitting to a standing position. This can affect a resident's dignity and create a sense of dependence, and can cause numerous health problems for staff, such as musculoskeletal disorders, as a result of manually lifting and repositioning residents. According to the Bureau of Labor Statistics, in 2010 nursing aides, orderlies, and attendants had the highest rates of musculoskeletal disorders of all occupations, at 249 per 10,000 employees compared to the national average of 34 (OSHA, 2015). In an effort to decrease the negative effects of transferring, floor and ceiling mount **lift equipment** is used.

Lifts are a type of equipment used to help move, lift, or reposition a person who cannot do so on his own. A ceiling-mounted lift has a track fastened to the ceiling with a trolley-like device that moves along it. Floor lifts are portable devices that are moved easily on wheels. Many facilities require the use of lifts as opposed to manual lifting to protect staff; this is known as a **no-lift policy**.

Communication Technology

Wireless communication devices: In long-term care and nursing home environments, staff must be in frequent communication with each other. This used to be accomplished through overhead paging systems; however, the constant noise these systems produce can be very disruptive and can contribute to an environment's institutional image, leading to decreased quality of life for residents. Centralized corded telephones are not much better because of the noise from ringing, and the extra staffing required to answer the phone and relay information. Wireless communication devices, such as portable phones, can mitigate these negative factors.

Electronic charting: Traditional paper charting can take up a significant portion of a staff member's day and can require a large amount of secure storage space to maintain confidentiality and archiving of records. New electronic charting technology supports a streamlined reporting process by allowing point-of-care reporting and increasing accessibility to resident history. Electronic charting systems increase flexibility and support a switch to decentralized staffing and the elimination of institutional nursing stations.

Communication devices for residents: Not only can communication technology support staff efficiency and effectiveness, but also it can enhance safety and security for residents. Medical alert devices, called a nurse call system, can be placed by a resident's bed so he can push a button to call for help if needed, and can be linked to mobile staff devices for faster responses.

Building Code Requirements

History and Importance

Building codes are developed as a method to regulate the design, construction, alteration, and maintenance of structures in an effort to protect the health, safety, and welfare of building occupants. Codes are a set of minimum standards for acceptable levels of safety in a building that are established by the **International Building Code (IBC)** and enforced by state and local governments (International Code Council [ICC], 2012). Typically building codes are implemented as a response to a deficiency that resulted in negative consequences for the user. For example, the Great Chicago Fire of 1871 demonstrated the need for stricter regulations for building construction in terms of **fire resistance** and **emergency egress**.

Building code requirements are determined based on the **building occupancy classification**, the category of structure being based on its usage. Nursing homes have the building occupancy rating *Institutional-2* or *I-2*, making them one of the most regulated and restricted environments.

Americans With Disabilities Act

The **Americans With Disabilities Act (ADA)** is a civil rights law established in 1990 to ensure fair treatment and to prevent discrimination against individuals with disabilities. The act ensures the protection of the rights of the disabled, including the ability to access public spaces and buildings (ADA, 2010).

In 1991 The U.S. Architectural Transportation Barriers Compliance Board (the Access Board) published the Americans With Disabilities Act Accessibility Guidelines (ADAAG) to explain how to design and construct **accessible** spaces that comply with the act. Spaces that comply fully with accessibility guidelines still may not accommodate the needs of older adults.

Going Beyond ADA

The Americans With Disabilities Act (ADA) was initiated in the late 1970s largely to ensure that returning injured Vietnam War veterans would not face discrimination while self-navigating the built environment. Its implementation has significantly changed the way designers approach the creation of environments. However, the physical guidelines, initiated primarily for individuals who maintain good upper body strength, do not necessarily provide assistance for older adults, many of whom also have disabilities of a significantly differing nature. Additionally, many older adults, particularly in a care situation, may require assistance by caregivers in their activities of daily living, such as toileting transfers.

Designing spaces with older adults in mind requires designs that comply with ADA and go beyond those requirements to address, specifically, the unique abilities and care needs of an older adult. As an example, the established ADA maximum slope for a wheelchair ramp is 1:12; however, this may be too steep for an older adult with limited upper body strength, necessitating a shallower ramp.

Fire-Resistance Rated Construction

Codes and regulations for the design and construction of a building in case of a fire are numerous, and can help prevent potentially fatal consequences of fire and smoke through prevention, control, and containment. Codes are dependent on the type of construction material and assembly used, as well as the building occupancy classification. The International Code Council sets standards that individual states can adopt for fire-resistance rated construction. State codes can be modified only to be more restrictive than the International Building Code (IBC), and facilities must comply with the more restrictive standards. As stated in IBC 2012 for nursing homes and other medical facilities, code dictates that any floor must be separated into at least two **smoke compartments**, each with an area equal to or less than 22,500 square feet. A smoke compartment is a space within the building that is protected on all sides by construction to prevent the spread of fire and smoke, including floor and ceiling. In a fire emergency, a facility can employ a **defend-in-place** strategy, which consists of moving residents into a different smoke compartment, but not leaving the building.

There are several categories of building separation assemblies to restrict the passage of smoke and fire, which are determined by the amount of fire and smoke protection needed and the hourly **fire-resistance rating** required for occupant safety.

Fire wall: A firewall has the highest level of protection from fire and smoke. A fire wall extends continuously from the foundation to the roof and is separate from the structure of the building on either side of the wall, so if the structure on one side is compromised or collapses, the fire wall will remain structurally stable.

Fire barrier: A fire barrier is typically a 2-hour rating, and is used to separate occupancies within a building, such as assisted living from skilled nursing.

Fire partition: A fire partition is used to separate sleeping units and corridors within an area of the building.

Smoke barrier: A smoke barrier is a fire-resistance rated assembly that provides less protection from fire but resists the passage of smoke.

Smoke partition: A vertical assembly will restrict the passage of smoke but does not have a fire-resistance rating.

State and Local Regulatory Agencies

International Building Code (IBC)

In 1994, the International Code Council (ICC) was formed to develop code requirements, presented as the International Building Code (IBC). Many states adopt the International Building Code, and are responsible for updating and enforcing compliance.

A large portion of the IBC consists of minimum standards for the safety of building occupants, such as fire prevention, emergency egress, accessibility, and structural stability; it categorizes standards based on building occupancy type, such as residential, assembly, and business. The IBC discusses in detail requirements for facilities with vulnerable populations, such as nursing homes, where the intended occupancy may have special needs, especially in times of emergency. For example, egress requirements are often stricter in facilities with higher-acuity residents who require mobility assistance and may not be able to evacuate a building on their own in the event of an emergency. The ability to exit a building independently is referred to as *capable of self-preservation.*

The ADA discusses standards for the design and construction of accessible spaces; in 2004 these and other federal standards were coordinated with the International Building Code to make compliance more consistent and easier to understand. The IBC enforces these codes and contains the scoping provisions (what, where, and how many) for accessibility. IBC references another ICC document, American National Standards Institute (ANSI A117.1) Accessible and Usable Buildings and Facilities, which provides the technical requirements for making buildings accessible.

ANSI developed the A117.1 standards through a public hearing process to include input from federal agencies and disability advocacy groups. ANSI A117.1 establishes the minimum percentage of units that must be accessible; however, just like other ICC established building codes, they vary by state. Other accessibility requirements include: handicapped parking spaces (how many and where located); how a person with a disability will get to, enter, and independently use a facility; and minimum standards for bathrooms and kitchens, including clear floor space, and access to countertops and storage.

Compliance with the International Building Code is enforced through inspections by a local government code official. Construction documents are analyzed for compliance, and inspections are conducted during the construction phase to ensure that no deficiencies exist. If an unsafe or illegal condition is discovered, the code official will report the issue and the deficiency must be corrected and approved before the building may be occupied.

National Fire Protection Association and the Life Safety Code (LSC)

The **National Fire Protection Association (NFPA)** established **NFPA 101: Life Safety Code** in 1913 to provide standards for the safety of building occupants (National Fire Protection Association, 2015). The Life Safety Code enforces requirements for construction and operations to minimize danger from fire, smoke, toxic fumes, and panic. In contrast to the International Building Code, the majority of the Life Safety Code addresses standards for after the building has been occupied, and applies to both new and existing structures. Building inspectors and fire marshals will evaluate facilities to ensure that they are in compliance with all LSC requirements, and violations can be used against the facility in legal proceedings.

Nursing homes and other healthcare facilities must protect residents who may not be able to evacuate quickly or at all during an emergency. Staff are essential in these circumstances to ensure that residents are protected not only from fire but also from the harmful smoke that travels quickly through a building and can have devastating health impacts. Because of the limited mobility of residents, and the possible inability for self-preservation, codes for nursing homes and other healthcare facilities are based upon the concept of defend in place. This concept incorporates many strategies for fire safety, such as sprinkler systems, alarm systems, and **compartmentalization**, to allow occupants enough protection and time to relocate to a safe part of the building.

Authorities Having Jurisdiction (AHJ)

On a local level, building code and safety requirements are mandated and enforced by the authority having jurisdiction (AHJ). For new construction and renovation, the municipality in which the project is located will have a designated AHJ to regulate and monitor the construction process and to ensure code compliance. After construction is completed, a final inspection must be passed by the local AHJ before an occupancy permit will be issued. In the case of an existing facility, if the building does not meet current codes to the letter, the authority having jurisdiction can judge whether the facility meets the equivalence of the safety requirement necessary for the protection of building occupants.

Occupational Safety and Health Administration (OSHA)

History and Importance

In the early 1900s, there were numerous work-related injuries and illnesses partly because of the hazards of working in the industrial age. In 1970, the U.S. Department of Labor decided that there needed to be federal administration and enforcement of workplace safety and health standards to support state efforts, which resulted in the implementation of the Occupational Safety and Health Act.

OSHA Components

There are currently three main parts of the act: the **Occupational Safety and Health Administration (OSHA)**, which administers the act; the National Institute of Occupational Safety and Health (NIOSH), which conducts research and makes recommendations for new standards; and the Review Commission, which was established to respond to contested penalties.

Standards and Compliance Requirements for Administrators

All facilities must comply with the General Duty Clause to maintain a work environment free from known hazards that cause death or serious injury. General guidelines include requirements for means of egress, emergency preparedness, and safety from chemical/electrical hazards.

Lockout/Tagout

Lockout/tagout is the OSHA standard for The Control of Hazardous Energy, Title 29 in the Code of Federal Regulations. It addresses practices and procedures to ensure that dangerous machinery and equipment are properly shut off and remain off while employees conduct servicing and maintenance work. A lock is placed on the device to ensure that hazardous power sources are isolated and rendered inoperative prior to the start of any repairs; then a tag is affixed to the lock, indicating that it should not be turned on. In some situations the lock has holes for up to six workers to apply their own padlocks, ensuring that the device cannot be turned on until all six locks are removed.

Recordkeeping Rules

Nursing home administrators with more than 10 employees must keep meticulous and up-to-date records of all work-related illnesses and injuries. If a work-related incident results in anyone's death or the hospitalization of three or more employees, the employer has 8 hours to report the incident by telephone to the OSHA regional director. In all other circumstances, the employer must fill out the forms provided by OSHA. These records do not mean that the employer was at fault or a standard was violated; it is merely a record of work-related incidents.

There are three forms to fill out:

1. *Form 301, the Injury and Illness Incident Report:* This report must be filled out within 7 days of the incident, to record the individual circumstances and why the incident occurred.

2. *Form 300, the Log of Work-Related Injuries and Illnesses:* This report is used to classify all work-related incidents, including how and why each happened, as well as the extent and severity of each case.

3. *Form 300A, the Summary of Work-Related Injuries and Illnesses:* This document is filled out at the end of every calendar year, showing the total incidents in each category.

The facility must post the "Summary of Work-Related Injuries and Illnesses" in the workplace for at least 3 months from February to April each year; current and former employees have the right to access these records at any time.

Citations and Penalties

OSHA inspections are conducted at a time determined by the inspector without advance notice, or at the request of an employer or employee. Employees who request an inspection can remain anonymous and are protected by OSHA from retaliation. Nursing homes that are found to be noncompliant with OSHA standards are subject to penalties, including fines and imprisonment (for very serious violations and negligence). Inspectors will go through the building, looking for violations, as well as all records of workplace injuries and illnesses, making it vital for nursing home administrators to maintain detailed records.

There are four types of workplace safety and health violations with the following penalty limits effective as of October 1, 2010:

1. *Serious violations:* A fine of up to $7,000 per violation is imposed for any incident causing serious physical harm or death.

2. *Non-serious violations:* If a violation does not cause death or serious harm but is related to workplace safety and health, a fine may be imposed up to $7,000.

3. *Willful violations:* If an employer knowingly commits a violation, there is a fine of up to $70,000, with a minimum $5,000. If said violation resulted in a death, OSHA may bring criminal action against the employer.

4. *Repeated violations:* Repeated violations found on subsequent inspections will result in a fine up to $70,000.

Each citation given will state a date before which the violation must be corrected. If an employer does not correct a violation within the allotted time period, a fine will be imposed of up to $7,000 per violation per day. If employers choose to contest a penalty, a notice must be submitted within 15 days of the citation.

Preventative Maintenance Programs

History and Importance

The Safe Medical Devices Act (SMDA) of 1990 was designed to ensure that all medical devices are implemented and used safely, and gives the U.S. Food and Drug Administration (FDA) the authority to track and recall medical products that are suspected to have caused a serious illness, injury, or death, either by mechanical or user error. This act promoted the necessity for facilities to implement regular inspection schedules called **preventative maintenance (PM) programs**.

Useful Life

An important factor in developing a preventative maintenance program is to determine the useful life of capital, such as a building and its equipment. The useful life of a product determines at what point it is best to replace a product rather than continue investing in its repair. The Internal Revenue Service establishes guidelines to determine a product's useful life; however, the actual life of a product can vary greatly from these guidelines.

Maintenance Items

Common items included in a preventative maintenance program are: heating, ventilation and air conditioning (HVAC) systems; equipment that regulates water; electrical outlets and emergency backup power systems; elevators; fire sprinklers, extinguishers and alarms; balcony and stairwell railings; grab bars; and lighting. It is also important for nursing home administrators to keep up-to-date Materials Safety Data Sheets (MSDS), which provide information about possible hazardous chemicals that employees may be using.

Preventative Maintenance Software

Preventative maintenance software, also known as a work order system, is used to keep track of building and equipment maintenance schedules and automatically generate a work order when preventative maintenance is needed. Preventative maintenance services can also be contracted to an outside company that will manage the work order system and provide regular inspections and maintenance when needed.

Although the administrator may not be fully versed in a building's equipment and engineering services, he must be able to recognize possible problems and establish guidelines for maintenance workers to prevent safety hazards.

Infection Control Programs

Healthcare facilities often struggle with the issue of infection control. **Nosocomial infections** are infections that an individual caught while occupying a care environment. Nursing homes are at particular risk for the spread of infection because of the vulnerable population's diminished immune response and increased susceptibility. In addition, functional impairments, such as incontinence, increased risk of exposure to infection, and cognitive impairments, may limit an individual's ability to protect himself from infection through thorough sanitary habits. Finally, the emphasis on social integration in nursing homes increases the potential for the spread of infection (Smith et al., 2008).

Federal and state codes require that all facilities implement infection control programs aimed to prevent the spread of infections to residents, staff, and visitors. The facility should have written documentation of the standards and training for all members involved in implementing the program.

There are three main parts of a comprehensive infection control program: prevention, surveillance, and control.

Prevention: The most important part of an infection control program is the implementation of multiple techniques to prevent an infection in the first place. Incoming residents and new staff should have baseline health assessments; there should be clear guidelines for all staff detailing sterile medical procedures and the sterilization of equipment; dietary services should have guidelines for food preparation; sanitary and hygiene practices should be emphasized, such as hand washing; all staff should wear hand and eye protection; there should be a clear procedure for the isolation and sterilization of soiled linens as well as for waste disposal; and there should be comprehensive housekeeping practices and isolation procedures for infected individuals. There are also physical environment requirements for prevention, including the placement of sinks and the availability of single-use soap and paper towel dispensers.

Surveillance: This important because outbreaks must be anticipated for effective control. Each facility will nominate an infection control practitioner, who will be in charge of assessing and monitoring residents for infections.

Control: The final step is the effective control of infectious outbreaks, such as influenza and tuberculosis. Suspected outbreaks should be immediately reported to the Centers for Disease Control and Prevention (CDC), and steps should be taken internally to confine and contain the infection, such as isolating infected individuals and designating specific staff to care for them, as well as further surveillance to check for additional unrecognized cases (CDC, 1989).

Emergency Preparedness

History and Importance

As discussed in earlier sections, it is essential for long-term care facilities to establish programs and procedures that address safety in times of emergency, including fires and natural disasters.

Federal law requires that facilities receiving Medicare and Medicaid funding have written plans for all potential emergencies that outline the duties and responsibilities of staff members, as well as regular and comprehensive staff training. Although influenced by national regulations, emergency preparedness guidelines for nursing homes vary by geographic location; states that are considered more at risk will have additional requirements (e.g., Gulf states at risk of hurricanes). Each state is required to establish a long-term care ombudsman program to monitor emergency preparedness levels and to advocate for residents. On a local level, each jurisdiction will establish an emergency operations plan to specify evacuation procedures and determine cases of **mandatory evacuation** versus allowable defend-in-place. All facilities must comply with state and national regulations, and compliance will be assessed during random surveys.

Steps for Emergency Preparedness

Hazard identification: Identify all potential hazards and whether they are facility- or community-based.

Hazard mitigation: Take steps to prevent the disaster or to reduce the potential severity of the consequences.

Preparedness: Develop a written plan discussing how the administrator and staff will meet the needs of residents in times of crisis, including continuing to provide essential medical assistance during an extended emergency situation. Preparedness includes staff training to ensure efficient and effective responses, and revising the plan if needed.

Response: Address the immediate effects of the emergency and execute the plan.

Recovery: Implement necessary activities after the response to return the facility to its normal operating state (Levinson, 2006).

Emergencies and Preparations

There are many types of hazards, and there must be adequate policies and training in place for how to handle each. A comprehensive emergency preparedness plan should utilize an "all-hazards" approach.

Fire is one of the most prevalent disasters to which a long-term care facility must be prepared to respond. A vital way to prepare for a fire emergency is to ensure that the facility and operations comply with all regulations under NFPA 101: Life Safety Code. Make sure that the locations of all fire alarms and extinguishers are posted in plain sight, including directions for how to use emergency equipment.

As part of an administrator's regular building inspections, there are a few important fire safety features to check:

- To block passage of smoke and fire, fire doors must be inspected to ensure that they latch without any additional force.

- Clutter should be removed from all corridors so building occupants can move unimpeded during an evacuation.

- Fire alarms and fire extinguishers should be regularly inspected for proper function. Staff should be trained on how to properly use a fire extinguisher.

- All exit signs should be lit at all times.

Disaster planning is another form of emergency preparedness that requires specific preparation and staff training. Natural disasters, such as tornados, hurricanes, floods, and earthquakes, can be devastating emergencies, especially in facilities with a population that needs medical and mobility assistance. An important strategy when planning for a natural disaster is to ensure the facility is connected to state and local **authorities having jurisdiction (AHJ)** for quick communication and notification of an impending disaster.

In addition to natural disasters, facilities must be aware of threats from manmade disasters, such as *bombs, terrorism*, and *bioterrorism*. An important procedure to establish in case of a bomb threat is a designated communication structure, including who will be in charge of calling the local authorities and family members. Determine how residents will be informed of the danger and where they will go. In cases of terrorism and bioterrorism, the best way to prepare is to seek professional assistance and contact state agencies for guidelines and requirements.

Water outages can be an independent crisis or a result of another emergency. Determine what emergency water will be used until the normal supply is reconnected, how emergency water will be delivered to the facility, and how to tell the difference between potable (safe to consume) and non-potable (not safe to consume) water.

Power outage: Before a power outage occurs, have on hand a list of numbers to contact for maintenance. Test the capacity of the backup generator to make sure that necessary medical equipment can continue working. During the power outage, keep medication and food storage areas secure to avoid spoilage. The facility must also have a plan for extended power outages.

Resident elopement may not always be considered an emergency scenario, but the facility must have procedures for staff to follow in such a situation. Throughout an individual's stay in a nursing home, regular resident assessments must be performed to establish a care plan, including an evaluation of a resident's risk of wandering and **elopement**. Elopement occurs when a resident who could be a potential danger to himself due to cognitive decline or physical impairment leaves secured areas without staff supervision. If a community has residents who are at risk of elopement, a **wander detection system** that utilizes **delayed egress** (delays opening the door) while alerting staff can be installed.

To establish procedures for resident elopement, first decide how to confirm that an elopement has occurred. Create a code word that staff will use to communicate that a resident elopement has taken place, and establish protocol for looking for the resident, including who will be part of the response team. Determine if the facility is in a state that requires state agencies be notified in such a situation. The National Council of Certified Dementia Practitioners provides resources to prevent and respond to resident elopement (http://www.nccdp.org).

Checklists are provided by the Centers for Medicare and Medicaid services, listing important tasks to establish a comprehensive emergency preparedness plan (http://www.cms.gov).

Egress Procedures

In emergency situations, some facilities may be under orders to evacuate, while others may have the option to defend in place. There are many factors that influence a decision to evacuate or to defend in place. The most influential factor for determining the strategy used is the health and safety of residents, and whether evacuating would cause more negative consequences than the potential emergency situation. Frail older adults have impaired physical mobility and functional limitations, diminished sensory awareness, and mental health conditions that hinder their adaptability during an emergency, and may make it difficult to evacuate. The defend-in-place strategy may be preferred because moving frail older adults in an emergency may cause health impacts, such as stress and psychological distress that can lead to increased morbidity, mortality, and hospitalization in the years following the evacuation (Brown et al., 2012; Kuba, Dorian, Kuljian, & Shoaf, 2004). If the decision is made to defend in place, residents will be directed and assisted to a safe portion of the building until the emergency situation is no longer a threat.

If the decision is made to evacuate the building, a host facility and alternative shelter site must be established in advance. Written evacuation procedures should go into detail about specific resident needs. Plans should be made to protect and transfer confidential medical records, ideally with the resident. Finally, procedures must be discussed for returning to the facility after an evacuation. Evacuation procedures should be coordinated with family members as well as state and local emergency management agencies.

Assisted Evacuation

For facilities that have a vulnerable population, the design of the building integrates areas of refuge for assisted evacuation. An **area of refuge** is a space separated from other spaces, and must be protected from the hazards of smoke and have direct access to a building exit. For example, stairwells that are rated for fire protection and release to an outdoor public area must have an area where a person in a wheelchair can safely stay for a period of time while waiting for assistance from the fire department.

Testing

As part of a facility's preventative maintenance program and an administrator's daily inspections, a building's safety features should be regularly inspected for proper function.

Training and Drills

Long-term care facilities must regularly review emergency preparedness procedures with staff and conduct random, unannounced drills to test staff readiness. Train staff members in Rescue, alert, confine/contain and extinguish (RACE) protocol to prevent the spread of a small fire (Guideone Insurance, 2008):

- R: Rescue anyone in immediate danger of smoke inhalation
- A: Alert/Alarm
- C: Confine/Contain the fire within the room by closing windows and doors
- E: Extinguish the fire and evacuate if necessary

It is essential that staff know their individual responsibilities and duties during a disaster event. Provide written procedures, and go over with each staff member what he will be expected to do in each type of emergency. Also establish a code phrase that staff members can use to communicate that an emergency situation is taking place, which can be used in case the alarm system malfunctions. In all cases, it is important for staff to know that they must remain calm and avoid further distressing residents, especially residents with dementia.

Drills are important training tools to assess how staff respond to an emergency situation, and should also include awareness training for residents and family members. Fire drills are a good way to practice fire evacuation/relocation procedures with residents. There should be at least one fire drill per month, with each shift experiencing a fire drill at least once per quarter. In addition, a disaster simulation drill should be conducted once a year to rehearse and coordinate staff responsibilities.

Survey Process

Nursing Home Oversight

Nursing home oversight is an integral process to ensure proper code compliance and the safety of building occupants. The Code of Federal Regulations is the general and permanent rules that nursing homes must follow to participate in federal funding programs, such as Medicare and Medicaid. In order to obtain federal funding and state certification, compliance with these codes is inspected by local code officials during the survey process. Surveys are unannounced mandatory building inspections that occur annually or due to a complaint about the facility. They may be conducted at any time 24 hours a day, including weekends, meaning that the facility must be prepared for an inspection at all times.

There are four main types of surveys: standard, abbreviated standard, extended, and post-survey revisit. During a standard survey, the inspection team follows the eight survey tasks, including interviews with residents, family members, and staff, to determine the quality of care processes, staff and resident interaction, fire safety, and the quality of the environment. An extended survey is conducted after a standard survey if the facility is deemed to have a substandard quality of care. An abbreviated standard survey may be chosen to respond to specific complaints about the facility, or to evaluate the facility after a change of leadership, rather than complete a full standard survey. The post-survey revisit is conducted to reevaluate any citations of noncompliance to ensure they have been corrected.

Summary

Contemporary long-term care environments are very different from traditional settings, which were based on the medical model of operations and mimic an institutional acute care hospital in shape and form. Long-term care has evolved to be resident-centered and assume a familiar residential scale in shape and form. The *household* and *neighborhood* are the new basic building blocks of long-term care communities, and in conjunction with an operational model often referred to as "resident-centered care" allow greater resident choice, privacy, dignity, and autonomy in daily life.

The operational methods and physical settings of long-term care environments will continue to evolve in the future as the resident demographics change and expectations of what an elder care setting should be also change.

People provide care for residents, but the physical environment is a valuable component in that endeavor by providing a space for those actions to occur, and hopefully thrive. The environment should support resident abilities for as long as possible, and when, or if, additional care is needed the environment should allow the care to be given and received with dignity.

Key Terms

Accessible is a general term used to describe the degree to which a product (e.g., device, service, and environment) is manageable for use by as many people as possible, including those with physical and cognitive disabilities.

Activities of daily living (ADLs) are routine activities people tend to do every day without needing assistance. There are six basic ADLs: eating, bathing, dressing, toileting, transferring, and continence.

Americans With Disabilities Act (ADA) is a wide-ranging civil rights law that prohibits discrimination based on disability and influences the design of public facilities.

Area of refuge is a space located in the path of travel leading to an exit that is protected from the effects of fire, to permit a delay in egress travel from any level.

Authorities having jurisdiction (AHJ) are organizations, offices, or individuals responsible for enforcing the requirements of a code or standard, or for approving equipment, materials, an installation, or a procedure.

Behavioral monitoring refers to using technology to monitor daily activities to identify when residents may need help without the resident needing to signal for assistance.

Building occupancy classification is a determination of the type of usage in a structure, used for the implementation and enforcement of building and fire codes.

Centers for Medicare and Medicaid Services (CMS) is an agency within the U.S. Department of Health & Human Services responsible for administration of several key federal healthcare programs.

Compartmentalization is the act of subdividing a large building area into separate spaces, by means of a structural assembly, such as a fire wall, fire barrier, or smoke barrier.

Control points are centralized locations used for monitoring by staff, and in institutional-style environments the control point is typically the nursing station.

Defend in place is a strategy used when residents are unable to evacuate the building in case of fire. Residents are transported to a safe location on the same floor, which is created by subdividing the floor into two or more fire/smoke compartments, using fire-resistance construction techniques.

Delayed egress is a means of delaying people as they try to exit a building, which is often used in environments that care for the cognitively impaired to help minimize elopement, while maintaining a margin of safety in times of evacuation.

Double loaded corridor is a building design term for a corridor with rooms located on both sides.

Elopement is a dangerous result of wandering, where an individual, typically with dementia, leaves a secure unit without permission by staff.

Emergency egress is used to describe the means to exit a building in the event of an emergency.

Fire-resistance rating is the time period that the element, component, or assembly will withstand fire exposure and continue to perform its structural function.

Household is a setting for typically 10 to 16 residents to live together and share a kitchen, dining room, living room, and other service spaces. Groupings of households are referred to as neighborhoods.

International Building Code (IBC) is a published set of standards that provides minimum guidelines for design and construction of structures to ensure public safety, health, and welfare.

Life Safety Code is a set of standards used to ensure the protection of lives in all types of occupancies.

Lift equipment is floor- or ceiling-based equipment that is used to help move, lift, or reposition a person who cannot do so on his own.

Lockout/tagout is the OSHA standard for the Control of Hazardous Energy. Procedures include the placement of locks and tags on potentially hazardous equipment to notify that the equipment has been shut off and must remain off while employees conduct servicing and maintenance work.

Long-term care is a wide range of health and personal care, from simple assisted living arrangements to intensive nursing home care, for older or disabled person(s).

Mandatory evacuation is a state or local order that a facility cannot employ defend-in-place strategies and must evacuate all residents and personnel in the event of an emergency or natural disaster.

Medicaid is the United States health coverage program for individuals and families with low incomes and resources.

Medicare is a social insurance program administered by the United States federal government, providing health insurance coverage to people who are aged 65 and over, or who meet other special criteria.

Mobility assistance is an aid to help with movement and can be provided by another individual or by a device, such as a wheelchair or walker.

National Fire Protection Association (NFPA) is a nonprofit organization that aims to reduce the worldwide burden of fire and other hazards on the quality of life by providing and advocating consensus codes and standards, research, training, and education.

NFPA 101: Life Safety Code provides minimum requirements, with due regard to function, for the design, operation, and maintenance of buildings for safety to life from fire.

No-lift policy is a rule implemented in a care facility that mandates staff utilize ceiling- or floor-based lift equipment instead of manually lifting when transferring or repositioning residents.

Nosocomial infections are infections that are the result of treatment in a care environment, but secondary to the patient's original condition. Infections are considered nosocomial if they first appear 48 hours or more after an admission or within 30 days after discharge.

Occupational Safety and Health Administration (OSHA) is a government agency in the Department of Labor created to maintain a safe and healthy work environment.

Physical environment is the external, tangible surroundings in which a person exists and which can influence behavior and development.

Preventative maintenance program is a comprehensive schedule to regularly inspect and maintain buildings, tools, and equipment, and to conduct repairs in order to prevent more serious problems and equipment failure before they occur.

Public to private gradient mimics the location of spaces in a typical private residence, with the public spaces, such as the living room and kitchen, easily accessible from the front door. The private spaces, such as the bedrooms, are usually located the farthest away from the front door.

Quality of care is the degree to which health services for individuals and populations increase the likelihood of desired health outcomes and are consistent with current professional knowledge.

Quality of life is a descriptive term that refers to people's emotional, social, and physical well-being, and their ability to function in the ordinary tasks of living.

Skilled nursing facilities (SNF) provide 24-hour nursing care for persons who have significant deficiencies with ADLs.

Smoke compartments are sections of a building that are separated by fire-resistive construction to prevent the spread of fire and smoke and can be closed off to create a safe area for people who cannot evacuate a building.

Transferring residents involves relocating or repositioning a resident to a different posture or a different location.

Wander detection system is technology that can be used to notify staff if a resident has the potential for wandering or elopement.

Review Questions

1. What are the origins of long-term care environments and how did the original adopted model of care impact the historical physical environments?

2. In reference to the design of the physical environment of long-term care, what is the basic building block of traditional settings and contemporary settings?

3. Discuss what aspects of the physical environment contribute to a contemporary resident-centered model of care.

4. Describe the spaces typically included in a contemporary long-term care household setting.

5. How do contemporary operational models differ in comparison to more traditional long-term care operational models?

6. What is the purpose of regulations and minimum standards for the physical environment, and how can the nursing home administrator ensure compliance with these standards?

Case Studies

Case Study #1

Mr. Nader has started his first day as the administrator of a 200-resident nursing home. The building was built 50 years ago and has had numerous renovations and additions over the years. Mr. Nader reviews the documentation on the building and discovers that several previous inspections reported issues with infection control procedures. He realizes that an inspection is due at any time, and he must prepare his staff and get the building ready for the next inspection.

*   What are the three main parts of a comprehensive infection control program that Mr. Nader should review with his staff?

*   Describe the physical environment features for preventing the spread of infections.

Case Study #2

Mrs. Relli, age 85, is a resident of an institutional model nursing home built in the late 1950s with 100 residents in units with shared rooms and shared bathrooms. The community has obtained funding to construct a new nursing home. The new building will be based on a contemporary 10-resident household/neighborhood model with all private rooms and private three-piece bathrooms. The staff members are receiving training in a resident-centered model of care.

*   How would you describe the components of a household/neighborhood setting to Mrs. Relli?

*   What will the experience of a household setting be like for Mrs. Relli? Specifically, how will the operations differ in comparison to a traditional nursing home?

References

Americans With Disabilities Act. (2010). Retrieved from http://www.access-board .gov/guidelines-and-standards/buildings-and-sites/about-the-ada-standards/ ada-standards

Brown, L. M., Dosa, D. M., Thomas, K., Hyer, K., Feng, Z., & Mor, V. (2012). The effects of evacuation on nursing home residents with dementia. *American Journal of Alzheimer's Disease and Other Dementias, 27*(6), 406–412.

Centers for Disease Control and Prevention. (1989). Surveillance for epidemics. *MMWR Recommendations and Reports, 38,* 694–696.

Centers for Disease Control and Prevention. (2010). *National Hospital Discharge Survey: 2010 Table, Number and rate of hospital discharges.* Retrieved from http://www.cdc.gov/nchs/fastats/hospital.htm

Centers for Disease Control and Prevention. (2013). *Long-term care services in the United States: 2013 Overview.* Retrieved from http://www.cdc.gov/nchs/fastats/nursing-home-care.htm

GuideOne Insurance. (2008, April). *Fire safety: The R.A.C.E protocol.* Retrieved from https://www.guideone.com/SafetyResources/SLC/Docs/firesafety08.pdf

Hiatt, L. (1991). *Nursing home renovation designed for reform.* Boston, MA: Butterworth Architecture.

International Code Council. (2012) *International Building Code (IBC).* Retrieved from http://publicecodes.cyberregs.com/icod/ibc/

Johnson, C., & Grant, L. (1985). *The nursing home in American society.* Baltimore, MD: Johns Hopkins Press.

Kuba, M., Dorian, A., Kuljian, S., & Shoaf, K. (2004). Elderly populations in disasters: Recounting evacuation processes from two skilled-care facilities in Central Florida. In *Quick Response Research Report* (p. 172). UCLA Center for Public Health and Disasters, Natural Hazards Center., Los Angeles, CA.

Levinson, D. R. (2006). *Nursing home emergency preparedness and response during recent hurricanes.* Retrieved from the website of Office of Inspector General: http://oig.hhs.gov/oei/reports/oei-06-06-00020.pdf

National Council of Certified Dementia Practitioners. (2001). *Wandering and elopement resources.* Retrieved from http://www.nccdp.org

National Fire Protection Association. (2015). *NFPA 101: Life safety code.* Retrieved from http://www.nfpa.org/

Occupational Safety & Health Administration. (n.d.). *Safety and health topics: nursing homes and personal care facilities 2015.* Retrieved from https://www.osha.gov/SLTC/nursinghome/index.html

Silverman, M., Musa, D., Martin, D. C., Lave, J. R., Adams, J., & Ricci, E. M. (1995). Evaluation of outpatient geriatric assessment: A randomized multi-site trail. *Journal of the American Geriatrics Society, 43*(7), 733–740.

Smith, P. W., Bennett, G., Bradley, S., Drinka, P., Lautenbach, E., Marx, J., . . . Stevenson, K. (2008). Guideline: Infection prevention and control in the long-term care facility. *American Journal of Infection Control, 36*(7), 504.

U.S. Department of Labor, Occupational Safety and Health Administration (OSHA). (2015). Retrieved from https://www.osha.gov/

Weisman, G. (1997). Environments for older persons with cognitive impairments. *Advances in Environment Behavior and Design, 4,* 315–346.

CHAPTER 5

HUMAN RESOURCES

Managing Employees in Long-Term Care

Sonja Talley
Carissa Podesta

The provision of quality care, the maintenance of a safe and caring environment, and positive clinical outcomes cannot be achieved without qualified, well-trained, and dedicated staff. This chapter will present an overview of human resources concepts and functions in long-term care with an emphasis on skilled nursing facilities. First, it explores the unique challenges of finding and retaining qualified caregivers and managing a diverse workforce that serves a fast-growing patient population with similarly diverse characteristics. Next, it looks at the employee selection and training processes necessary to identify and prepare new employees to provide safe and appropriate resident care. Several sections are devoted to the importance of positive and strong employee-management relations as a means to help long-term care operators retain good workers in a high-turnover and high-burnout environment. These sections address employee communications and engagement. Key legal rights and benefits afforded to the skilled nursing workforce are also presented to provide a firm understanding of employers' legal obligations.

Core Human Resources Functions in Long-Term Care

The human resources (HR) function may assume different levels of responsibility based on the organizational

LEARNING OBJECTIVES

- Identify factors to be considered in manpower forecasting/staffing.

- Define managing diversity and its importance in the long-term care setting.

- Identify preemployment screening requirements that apply to the long-term care workforce.

- Describe the requirements for and benefits of long-term care workforce orientation, training, and continuing education.

- Describe protected concerted activity and how it applies to employees in the long-term care setting (a) in a union environment, (b) in a non-union environment.

structure, management philosophy, and/or size of the facility but also based on the HR practitioner's area and/or level of expertise, experience, and education. The following core HR functions provide a basic overview of the different roles HR provides. The responsibilities within each core area are not rigid, and HR might function as a partner in any of these areas.

Administrative Partner

HR as administrative partner takes on an administrative, clerical role, and is responsible for maintaining legal compliance with all federal, state, and local laws, which include processes to recruit, screen, and onboard applicants, and monitoring, reviewing, and implementing regulatory changes. HR might also assist administrators and supervisors with the implementation of performance improvement plans, processing disciplinary actions, and administration of **employee benefit programs**.

Business Partner

HR as a business partner may act as the single point of contact for management by developing and maintaining relationships with managers and employees. The emphasis of this level of HR is support as internal consultant, aiding managers with employee relations, improving awareness of business goals, and mitigating litigation risks.

Strategic Partner

HR as a strategic partner helps to achieve organizational goals by identifying and implementing ways to enhance innovation, increase productivity and efficiency, and creating a highly competitive work environment. HR as a strategic partner helps to gain or maintain the company's competitive advantage through the management of **human capital**. Human capital reflects the knowledge, skills, and experience of individuals in terms of the cost or value to an organization.

Outsourcing Human Resources

Outsourcing the HR function is a way to gain HR expertise while controlling costs by converting fixed costs into variable costs. Reasons for outsourcing HR services are (a) to increase **productivity**, which is the measure of quality and quantity of produced work within the framework of cost; (b) to fill a need for which in-house expertise is absent when full-time or senior-level HR support is not financially feasible; (c) to fill a short-term need; or (d) as strategic measure (e.g., to save on cost). Some HR functions that are more frequently considered for outsourcing are payroll, benefits, training, and/or leave of absence management.

Human Resources Challenges in Long-Term Care

Managing the diversity of personnel (e.g., culture, age, gender, education) and residents (e.g., culture, gender, ethnicity) is only one of the challenges HR faces in long-term care. Recruiting and retaining an adequate **talent pool** to deliver quality care are also crucial.

Direct care staff are those employees who personally deliver patient care, such as licensed nurses and nursing assistants, and make up the majority of employees in long-term care. Direct care employees are most likely to be unmarried, non-White women with children (Scanlon, 2001). Most choose to work in a direct care setting because they love to help people and have a general interest in working in health care (Mickus, Luz, & Hogan, 2004). Although direct care work has a sense of intrinsic reward, direct care staff often face heavy workloads, lack of control over their jobs, limited training, and below-average pay as compared to other occupations (e.g., clerical or sales positions). The following highlights the unique challenges HR faces in recruiting, retaining, and managing the long-term care talent pool.

Workforce Availability

A general shortage of healthcare workers who possess the requisite skills and qualifications needed to perform direct care duties makes it difficult to follow federal and state staffing regulations, let alone ensure the quality of care strived for by administrators and nursing executives. The following statistics from the American Health Care Association (2012) are more than concerning. Full-time direct care staff vacancies in America's skilled nursing facilities in 2010 were at about 70,000, reflecting a 16.8% increase from 2010. The nursing staff vacancy nationwide is predicted to exceed 450,000 in 2015.

Contingent Workforce

Contingent workers are those individuals who are temporarily assigned to a job through a staffing agency and often referred to as **registry**. Registry staff is utilized as a way to fill openings until a regular employee can be hired or to fill additional staffing needs due to increased census, fluctuating acuity, or temporary planned or unplanned staff absences. Temporary staff allows the facility to maintain adequate staffing levels when regular staff is unavailable.

The use of registry staff also reduces the legal liability associated with selection, discipline, and termination. Temporary workers may also reduce certain fixed payroll and benefit costs since temporary workers are paid only when they work. The use of contingent workers, however, is not without problems.

Registry staff require additional time for training and have a higher rate of pay. Temporary workers also do not have the ready knowledge of established resident plans of care, making them less efficient and presenting a potential risk for medication or other care-related errors. Temporary workers may be a good source to consider for a current or future vacancy due to turnover.

Turnover

Turnover is defined as the departure of employees who will need to be replaced. Employee turnover can be attributed to two basic reasons, job satisfaction (or rather the lack thereof) and organizational commitment to its workforce (or rather the lack thereof). Turnover can be calculated as cost for each position, per building, or as corporate turnover and could have a significant impact on the facility's budget, especially when high turnover is present.

Not all turnover is bad. New employees bring fresh and innovative ideas to the workplace. The goal, when hiring new employees, is to select those applicants who possess the requisite job skills and whose values best fit the **organization's culture**. High turnover almost always indicates the existence of a problem. The reasons why employees leave often have common denominators in poor working conditions, heavy workloads, stress, burnout, and lack of appreciation. Employee turnover is always associated with significant costs to the facility (American Health Care Association, 2010).

Composition of Workforce

According to U.S. Bureau of Labor Statistics (BLS) (2013b) data, the skilled nursing facility workforce is made up largely of female workers (84%). The racial/ethnic breakdown of this predominately female workforce is White (66%), African American (29%), Asian (5%), and Hispanic (10%), and provides a glimpse into the changing demographics of the U.S. workforce. The U.S. Census predicts that by 2050 minorities will represent the majority of workers while White workers will represent the minority.

Diversity of long-term care workers extends beyond race and ethnicity; diversity embraces culture, education, family status, age, and gender—in short, the differences between the workers. Assessing the existing workforce is a critical first step for employers to identify skills gaps, facilitate the transfer of knowledge, and predict future staffing needs. Designing effective programs for retention, recruitment, and training must take the diversity of the workforce into account.

Managing Diversity

Today's U.S. workforce enjoys four generations, known as the Silent Generation, Baby Boomers, Generation X, and Generation Y, working side by side, intertwined in an unmatched web of cultural and ethnical diversity. Diversity in the work environment also embraces an increasing number of women and single parent workers. According to the BLS (2012), approximately 33% of today's workforce is considered a minority. Following current trends, it is predicted that by 2050 there will not be a racial/ethnic majority. U.S. immigration during 2000 and 2050 will represent 83% of the growth in our working population.

Diversity. **Diversity** is the recognition that differences among people exist. The challenge is to manage the diversity of the workforce with efforts that value employees equally regardless of their differences in order to build and maintain a collaborative workplace through team cohesion, but also to be compliant with the law. A diverse workforce will most likely increase organizational performance when diversity is embraced. Diversity efforts have been shown to help with recruiting and retention efforts of minority employees. Recognizing and managing diversity increase morale and may reduce potential discrimination complaints and the cost associated with such claims.

Generational differences. The four generations working side by side in today's workforce are Silent Generation (1925 to 1945), Baby Boomers (1946 to 1964), Generation X (1965 to 1979), and Generation Y or Millennials (1980 to 1999) (Alsop, 2008). Each generation brings distinct values, beliefs, attitudes, and expectations to the workplace. Organizations must be cognizant of the needs and expectations of the employees who deliver patient services in order to provide safe, high-quality, and cost-effective health care (Piper, 2011).

Cultural diversity. **Culture** affects the values, beliefs, and actions of specific groups of people. Cultural diversity in the workplace is even more evident when we consider that the U.S. welcomes about 1 million immigrants on average each year (Office of Immigrant Statistics, 2010). Approximately half of direct care workers are made up of ethnic or racial minorities. This cultural mix includes 33% of direct care workers of

African American descent and another 15% of Hispanic or other persons of color (Harahan & Stone, 2009). Human resources must be aware of the various cultures within the workplace in order to recognize what practices, trainings, and policies may need to be altered to be effective.

English-only policy. In order to promote resident dignity and the right to communicate and be communicated with in a language that is understood, skilled nursing facilities may choose to implement a policy that only English be spoken within the facility environment. The English-only requirement may be applied universally or only at certain times or in certain situations, such as in areas where residents are present, as long as the employer can justify a clear business necessity. In skilled nursing, the business necessity lies in the duty of the operation to protect resident rights, provide appropriate care, and protect against the risk to residents in a health or other emergency.

Employers may administer English comprehension and spoken English clarity tests as a preemployment screening. However, an English testing policy should be adopted that clearly establishes which positions are subject to the English-only policy and the minimum passing score for the preemployment English tests. All candidates for the designated positions must be tested equally.

Workforce Planning

Quality clinical outcomes in long-term care communities require appropriate numbers of staff. As discussed in the previous section, long-term care faces many obstacles when it comes to staff retention. Successful organizations engage in some level of regular workforce planning and provide an orientation experience that motivates and prepares staff. Workforce planning is a strategic component of managing the current and future workforce of the organization. It includes specific strategies for establishing current and long-term staffing needs and matches those needs with specific recruiting, retaining, training, competitive pay and benefits, and employee-management initiatives. Workforce planning links these strategies to desired clinical and business outcomes.

Direct Care Staffing

The most challenging component of staffing in skilled nursing facilities is establishing and maintaining the appropriate nursing staff-to-resident ratio. Management constantly struggles to find the proper balance between providing the right number of staff to meet resident care needs and the desire to be fiscally responsible. Management must also factor in the limitations of lesser experienced or stressed staff due to a workforce with extremely high turnover rates.

In addition, facilities must comply with federal and state regulatory staffing standards while managing the day-to-day realities of workforce unavailability due to illness, vacation, and leaves of absence. A study commissioned by the Centers for Medicare and Medicaid (CMS) in 2000, and numerous studies since, has established that better clinical outcomes are directly related to higher direct care staff-to-resident ratios (Kramer & Fish, 2001; Schnelle, Simmons, Codogan, Garcia, & Bates-Jensen, 2004).

It would seem, then, since sufficient staffing is such a critical component to skilled nursing care that the federal regulations would set clear standards in this area, but this has largely been addressed at the state level. The federal regulations provide only a generalized directive. Actual staffing levels are left to the discretion of management. In the absence of a federal staff-to-resident standard, some states have set direct care staffing standards (e.g., California, Florida, Massachusetts, Maine, Oregon, Wisconsin) by requiring minimum staff-to-resident hours per day. Skilled nursing staffing is measured by using the ratio of the number of direct care staff hours divided by the number of residents as measured by the facility's census during the same day. For example, if a facility's census is 100 on a given day and the total number of direct care staffing hours worked that day was 264, then the direct care hours on a per resident basis was 2.64 ppd (per patient day).

In addition to the regulatory staffing requirements, the acuity of residents is considered when determining staffing levels. As the healthcare system attempts to control costs, skilled nursing organizations care for residents who are more medically complex. For example, a resident who requires a feeding tube or intravenous medication needs more direct nursing care than residents without intravenous needs. Other considerations, such as continuity of care (staffing the same employees with the same residents to promote consistency) and prevention of staff burnout, also impact staffing decisions.

Recruiting

Recruiting efforts are time-consuming, especially when recruiting for hard-to-fill specialty or high-skill positions. A required minimum set of experience and/or skills to match the open position is critical, but perhaps equally critical is employee-organization and employee-job match, especially when working with patients and residents. Employee-organization fit refers to the match between an employee's behaviors, attitudes, and expectations and the organization's culture. Typically, HR handles the bulk of recruiting and ensures that recruiting practices do not violate equal employment opportunity (EEO) regulations.

Job Descriptions

Job descriptions are dynamic documents that need to be revised based on evolving job duties. It is good practice to review job descriptions on an annual basis or at a minimum at the time job duties change. Job descriptions spell out the job duties of a job and include information about the competencies, knowledge, and skills needed to perform the job, the physical demands, types of equipment that is used, working conditions, and the relationship with other jobs, as well as the chain of command. Many state regulations require that skilled nursing facilities maintain written job descriptions in the personnel file of every employee. Job descriptions also help attract qualified job candidates by describing the requirements of a position, serve as the basis for compensation decisions, and outline performance expectations. Writing job descriptions in a manner that imbeds accountability mechanisms and organizational behaviors and values will help promote the organization's culture.

Referral Programs

Internal recruiting can be one of the most effective methods to recruit qualified individuals due to low cost, quick vacancy-to-hire time, and higher retention rates of newly hired candidates. This is especially true when it comes to **tight labor markets** containing more jobs than workers to fill them. The actual cost per hire through employee referral depends on the employer's program design. A typical component of referral programs is a cash **bonus** to the existing employee who refers a new employee. Many employers opt to stagger the bonus payout by paying the referring employee an amount upon successful hire, a further amount at the completion of a conditional period of employment, and perhaps an additional bonus at the completion of the new hire's first annual anniversary.

Screening and Selection

Once qualified applicants are identified, interviews of those applicants are used to select candidates for employment. The purpose of conducting job interviews is to select the best qualified candidate for the job. Interview questions must comply with federal and state laws, meaning that any question pertaining to age, race, national origin, gender, religion, marital status, or sexual orientation should be eliminated as the answers could reveal discriminatory information. Interview questions should relate to specific occupational qualifications.

Once a candidate is selected for hire, certain initial preemployment screenings should be performed before an employment offer is made. Certification or licensure credentials should be verified with the state. Medicare- or Medicaid-certified entities must check the state nurse aide registry to confirm that negative findings against the candidate do not exist. Verification of the candidate's employment history listed on the employment application and professional reference checks may also be performed.

Assuming these screenings do not result in any negative findings, then an offer of employment is the next step. Only after making a **conditional offer of employment** are employers able to initiate more in-depth background screenings that may yield information about an applicant that identifies membership in a protected class as defined under federal and state EEO laws. For example, a preemployment physical may cause disclosure of a disability or medical condition or a criminal background check may require the applicant to provide a date of birth.

Physicals, drug screening, and criminal background checks must be postponed until after a conditional offer is made and accepted so that such information cannot influence the employment offer decision. This makes rescinding conditional offers of employment very risky. Facts supporting retractions of conditional employment offers should be supported by clear, non-discriminatory reasons.

Preemployment physicals. All positions in long-term care require minimum health standards (e.g., free from active tuberculosis or other communicable disease). Preemployment physicals are necessary to confirm a new employee's general health and to obtain a tuberculosis screening. In addition, resident care positions have physical demands. For example, a certified nursing assistant must be able to assist residents transferring from bed to wheelchair. Determining the physical requirements for these positions and requiring that prospective employees receive preemployment physical demands assessment tests whether the candidate can safely perform the job.

Many long-term care employers include drug screening as a precursor to or component of the preemployment physical. Individuals who use illegal drugs are more likely to have worked for multiple employers within the last year, more likely to be absent from work, and more likely to have a workplace accident or injury (Slavit, Reagin, & Finch, 2009).

Exclusion and sanctions database. Skilled nursing facilities, home health and hospice agencies certified to provide services to Medicare and Medicaid beneficiaries are prohibited from employing individuals listed on the Department of Health and Human Services (HHS) Office of the Inspector General's (OIG) List of Excluded Individuals and Entities. People and businesses barred from participation in the federal healthcare programs due to criminal convictions or administrative determinations are placed on this list. This employment prohibition extends to parties on any exclusion lists maintained by state Medicaid programs as well. The OIG and most states make their exclusion databases available online and update it monthly. Because the obligation not to employ excluded parties is ongoing, employee names should be checked against the updated database on a regular basis. There are many third-party providers that will perform these services for a fee. Penalties for a violation of this requirement can be very costly, depending on the length of employment of the excluded individual.

Criminal background checks. Federal regulations prohibit Medicare-certified skilled nursing facilities from employing individuals found guilty by a criminal court of abusing, neglecting, or mistreating residents or who have had a finding made against them by a state nurse aide registry, which all states are required to maintain. The federal regulations for Medicare-certified hospices specifically require a criminal background check for employees who have direct patient contact or access to medical records.

State licensing regulations vary greatly when it comes to criminal background checks of prospective long-term care employees. Some states require that a state-managed criminal history system be used, while others require a criminal background check but do not specify how the employer should perform it.

Training

Most long-term care providers are obligated by law to provide new hire orientation to all employees, providing education regarding operational policies and legal requirements. A multitude of other laws make it mandatory that additional types of training be delivered to all staff or to specific job classifications, depending on the law requiring training. In addition, many long-term care providers have an ongoing obligation to provide regular in-service education to its staff to keep them current on developments related to the patient population to which they provide care.

Orientation

New employees are introduced to their job responsibilities, coworkers, and the organization during **orientation**. Orientation provides an opportunity to make a favorable first impression about the job and the organization. These presentations allow the employee to gather information about organizational culture, expectations, and job duties. Orientation introduces coworkers and accelerates socialization and integration of new employees into their work environment. Integrating into the work environment early on has proven to enhance employee tenure, job satisfaction, and person-organization fit. The key to an effective orientation program is the relevance of the information provided to the employee. New hire orientation should deliver relevant information regarding the organization and the job in a clear and stimulating manner, utilizing a variety of adult learning principles.

Peer mentoring programs. As with other forms of mentoring, peer mentoring provides the opportunity for the new employee to have a consistent contact person who can assist them with the functional and emotional aspects of starting a new role, make introductions to residents, and accelerate integration into the workplace.

Mandated Training

Mandated training is training that is required by law for the purpose of informing employees of important concepts and laws designed to protect residents as well as the employees themselves. In addition to federally mandated training, state-specific training guidelines vary from state to state and by provider type (e.g., skilled nursing facility, assisted living facility). The following highlights the required training for skilled nursing facilities pursuant to federal law.

Abuse, neglect, exploitation prevention reporting requirements. The federal skilled nursing facility regulations at 42 C.F.R. §483.13(c) require skilled nursing facilities to develop and operationalize policies and procedures for screening and training employees, protection of residents, and the prevention, identification, investigation, and reporting of abuse, neglect, mistreatment, and misappropriation of property. In addition, 42 C.F.R. §483.74(e) requires skilled nursing facilities to have procedures to train employees via orientation and ongoing in-services on issues related to abuse prevention. Training of all staff and volunteers must occur at time of hire and annually thereafter.

Resident rights. Training on **resident rights** must be conducted upon hire and annually for all employees and volunteers. 42 C.F.R. §483.13(c) requires skilled nursing facilities to develop and operationalize policies and procedures for screening and training employees, protection of residents, and the prevention, identification, investigation, and reporting of abuse, neglect, mistreatment, and misappropriation of property.

Elder Justice Act. The Elder Justice Act was enacted in 2010 and requires individuals employed by or associated with a skilled nursing facility to report any reasonable suspicion of resident abuse within 2 hours of forming the suspicion. Employee training is required upon hire and annually. Part A of Title XI of the Social Security Act (SSA) § 1150B(a)(1).

Dementia management and patient abuse prevention training. Part A of Title XI of the Social Security Act (SSA) §§ 1819(f)(2)(A)(i)(I) and 1919(f)(2)(A)(i)(I) requires that nurse aides receive initial and annual dementia management and patient abuse prevention training.

In-service education. A skilled nursing facility must complete a performance review of every nurse aide at least once every 12 months and provide regular in-service education of no fewer than 12 hours per year based on the outcome of the review that is sufficient to ensure continuing competence of nurse aides (42 C.F.R. §483.75(e)(8)). The deadline by which a nurse aide must receive annual in-service education is calculated by using the employment date, not the calendar year.

The Health Insurance Portability and Accountability Act (HIPAA). Section 164.530 of the HIPAA privacy rule requires workforce training on the policies and procedures protecting health information within a reasonable period of time after the person is hired. When a material change in the policies or procedures protecting health information occurs, training must be provided within a reasonable period of time after the material change becomes effective.

Emergency Action and Disaster Plan. The federal Occupational Safety and Health Act (OSHA) requires employers with more than 10 employees to have an emergency action plan. An emergency action plan is a set of procedures for employees to follow in event of an emergency and covers topics such as emergency contact information, evacuations, how to account for employees in the event of an evacuation, and alarm systems. In addition, federal regulations require that skilled nursing facilities have "detailed written plans and procedures to meet all potential emergencies and disasters" (42 C.F.R. §483.75(m)(1)). Employee training on emergency and disaster preparation and procedure must occur upon hire and annually.

Bloodborne pathogens. Bloodborne pathogens are microorganisms present in the blood that may cause diseases. Examples are the hepatitis B virus and the human immunodeficiency virus (HIV). Employees whose jobs require exposure to blood must be trained on how to take protective measures to avoid infection. OSHA regulations require training of all direct care staff upon hire and annually (within one year of prior training). Retraining must occur when an employee fails to follow standards or when changes in the workplace (new equipment, new procedure) make retraining necessary.

Tuberculosis. OSHA requires employers in the medical care industry to train all employees on tuberculosis (TB). TB training must occur upon hire and annually. In addition, most states require long-term care employers to test new employees using a skin test for TB on hire, annually, or when exposure to TB is suspected. If the skin test is positive or if the employee has an allergy to the skin test, a chest x-ray must be performed.

Infection control. OSHA requires training for employees whose jobs require exposure to chemicals (maintenance or housekeeping employees) or blood (nursing or housekeeping employees) on how to use personal protective equipment (PPE). PPE includes eye, face, and respiratory protection. The employee must demonstrate understanding of the training (pass a quiz) and the ability to use PPE. Retraining must occur when an employee fails to properly use PPE or when changes in the workplace (new equipment, new procedure) make retraining necessary. Infection control training is mandated upon hire and includes proper hand washing, linen handling, and prevention of communicable diseases.

Ergonomics. **Ergonomics** training, conducted upon hire of direct care staff, includes safe patient handling and the reporting of workplace injuries. Due to the high incidence of work-related musculoskeletal disorders (MSD), such as injuries causing low back pain, rotator cuff injuries, and carpal tunnel syndrome, in skilled nursing facilities, employees who lift or reposition residents or perform work that may involve risk of injury should be trained on safe patient handling and lifting techniques before performing such work. Training should include the organization's policies and procedures to be followed to avoid injury, including proper work practices and use of equipment; how to recognize MSDs and their early indications; the advantages of addressing early indications of MSDs before serious injury develops; and the process for reporting work-related injuries and illnesses as required by OSHA's injury and illness recording and reporting regulation (29 C.F.R. §1904).

Hazard communication. OSHA requires employers of employees who work with hazardous chemicals and/or in areas where hazardous chemicals may be present to provide training on hazardous chemicals used in their work area at the time of their initial assignment and whenever a new chemical hazard is introduced into the workplace. Training shall cover categories listed in 29 C.F.R. 1910.1200(h)(3)(i) to (iv), which include how to detect chemical releases, the hazards/effects of the specific chemicals used in the work area, and how to protect against and respond to accidental exposure. Safety data sheets (SDSs) are provided by chemical manufacturers and convey information about the chemical's hazards and risks. Employers must train employees on how to properly interpret SDSs. In 2012, OSHA adopted new regulations to increase understanding of SDS information by coordinating the pictograms used in SDSs with global standards adopted by the United Nations (UN).

Lockout/tagout requirements. OSHA's standard for the "control of hazardous energy" (referred to as lockout/tagout) at 29 C.F.R. §1910.147 establishes an employer's responsibility to protect its employees from hazardous energy sources (electrocution). The regulations require employee training to ensure that they understand and follow the employer's hazardous energy control program and the energy control procedures relevant to the employee's job duties. Retraining must occur when an employee fails to properly use lockout/tagout procedures or when changes in the workplace (new equipment, new procedure) make retraining necessary.

Employee Relations

The foundation of an organization's culture is the relationship between management and staff. Those relationships can be developed and maintained only through two-way communication. When staff perceives communication as one-way (management is inaccessible, managers are not present on the floor, and management does not listen or fails to respond properly, or at all, to staff concerns), they eventually stop hearing management's message and vision. Strong relationships between management and staff also play a role in making sure that employee rights are being respected. If staff does not have trust and confidence in leadership, they will not report problems. If management is unaware of potential violations of employment laws, they lose the opportunity to intervene and correct problems before it is too late. Moreover, a failure by management to listen and address workplace issues may encourage employees to seek union representation.

Employee Communications

Accurate and consistent communication is imperative for success in long-term care communities. Achieving effective communication, however, requires collaboration. While it is natural for organizations to have **top-down communication** that reflects messages that start at the top of an organizational structure and are relayed down to the rest of organizational audience, in health care it is critical that the organization and administration promote **bottom-up communication** as well. Bottom-up communication reflects messages that start at the bottom of an organizational structure and are communicated up to individuals in positions of high authority in administration. By promoting **circular communication** (top-down and bottom-up), an organization is much more likely to create a culture that is responsive to employee and resident needs. Hence, circular communication stimulates an environment geared toward continuous quality improvement and delivery of quality care.

Circular communication should take place both formally and informally. Examples of formal communication include memorandums, daily **stand-up meetings**, and weekly and monthly meetings.

Informal communication includes verbal communication, e-mail, and **rounding** (or making rounds) throughout the facility. Rounding allows administrative leaders to get to know residents and employees and monitor daily operations. Many organizations promote the idea of "rounding with purpose" (Riordan, 2010), suggesting that rounds be focused on improving patient, resident, and employee satisfaction rates. A great question to ask on these rounds is, "What can I do today to help you?"

Employee Suggestion Program

Employee **suggestion programs** are formal methods to achieve upward (bottom-up) communication and obtain employee input toward changes or operational improvement. Employee suggestion programs may enhance employee morale and commitment to the organization as employees feel empowered to help improve the operation of the facility. A well-documented procedure for processing incoming suggestions and communicating the organization's response is key to the program's success. Such formality of communication may not be necessary if employee-leadership communication is well developed. An open-door policy is a more informal way to enhance communication between management and employees.

Open-Door Policy

Effective communication is one of the keys to successfully managing a long-term care facility. Managers who learn of evolving employee and/or procedural issues may be able to resolve them at an early stage. An **open-door policy** allows any employee to talk with any level of management about any issue at any time. This accessibility, along with action by management in response to workplace concerns, fosters trust and encourages employees to continue to share ideas.

Legal Rights and Benefits

Employees enjoy many legal rights and benefits conferred under federal and state laws. These laws aim to protect employees from employment practices that are unfair or contrary to public policy. Employees have the right to freely discuss the terms and conditions of their employment or complain about their supervisor without fear of reprisal, they are to be protected from workplace hazards, and they must not be the subject of workplace discrimination or harassment, or the target of retaliation.

At-Will Employment

The term "**at-will employment**" describes an employment relationship that exists at the will of both parties and may be ended at any time for any reason or no reason at all. All states, except Montana, have a presumption that all employment is "at-will" unless there is clear evidence to the contrary. At-will employers may change the terms and conditions (wages, hours, benefits) of the employment relationship at-will with or without notice.

But even where employment is at-will, **adverse employment actions** (e.g., termination or layoff, decrease in pay, less desirable job assignment, and any other negative change to a term or condition of employment shift) that are motivated for illegal reasons are the exception to the rule. Therefore, the concept of at-will employment must always be considered with these other principles in mind.

Union Organization

The National Labor Relations Act (NLRA) provides non-supervisory/ management employees with a federal right to engage in concerted activity. **Concerted activity** is when two or more employees take action for their mutual aid or protection regarding the terms and conditions of employment or in order to form or join a labor union. A single employee may also engage in concerted activity if he is acting on the authority of other employees, bringing group complaints to the employer's attention, trying to induce group action, or seeking to prepare for group action for the purpose of collectively bargaining, other mutual aid or protection, or forming or joining a labor union. Workers opposed to such conduct have the right to refrain from such activities.

It is not necessary that a union be involved when considering the protections of the NLRA. The terms of the NLRA apply to and protect employee conduct related to discussing, changing, or opposing the terms and conditions of employment regardless of union involvement. Employers may not take adverse employment action against employees for discussing or opposing workplace conditions (e.g., complaining about their supervisor) and terms of employment (comparing wage rates).

When employees exercise their right to unionize and hold an election to appoint a labor union as their representative, an employer is required to enter good-faith negotiations for a **collective bargaining agreement (CBA)**. A **bargaining unit** must be identified and comply with NLRA rules. A bargaining unit must have two or more employees with shared interests. A typical bargaining unit is a job classification, such as certified nurse assistant.

CBAs define certain terms and conditions of employment for the bargaining unit for the duration of the agreement. Typical CBA terms in skilled nursing facilities include wage scales, progressive discipline policies (including the right to have union representation during disciplinary meetings), healthcare coverage, and pension plans. Once a CBA is reached between the union and the employer, employees must vote again in order to ratify the contract and become bound to its terms.

Today, only 9% of healthcare support service employees are members of a union (BLS, 2013a). This figure has decreased over the past decade, presumably because employees feel less need to form a union to protect their interests. Unions charge employees dues in exchange for representation. Therefore, lower-wage workers may feel less compelled to pay for representation unnecessarily.

National Labor Relations Act (NLRA) Requirements

Employers may not engage in **unfair labor practices (ULPs),** which are defined by the NLRA, in relevant part, as interfering with, restraining, coercing, and discriminating against employees who exercise their rights under the NLRA. A ULP charge may be made to the National Labor Relations Board accusing the employer of a violation. ULPs are frequently filed during the period of the union campaign and before a CBA is ratified. Examples of ULPs are threats by the employer to make working conditions worse if employees participate in union activity, questioning employees regarding their beliefs toward the union, or performing surveillance of union meetings to see which employees attend. Employers are permitted to act within the bounds of the NLRA while a union campaign is occurring in its workplace. Management may honestly communicate with and inform employees of facts, such as the rights and benefits they already have without union representation. Managers may also provide personal opinions or relate experiences that support why they believe a union is unnecessary. Employers should take care not to use words that appear retaliatory or threatening in nature. Written communications are sometimes the safest method of conveying the employer's message.

Just as with any other non-work-related conduct, employees may not engage in union activity during working hours. Because employees congregate while at work, "on-the-clock" concerted activity may occur. Employers should consistently monitor and enforce policies prohibiting non-work-related activity by employees during working hours as well as policies restricting entry by non-employees on company property before concerted or union activity occurs so that management policy enforcement during a period of concerted or union activity is not perceived as an ULP. Meal or rest periods are not considered work time, and employees may engage in union discussion during their breaks.

Workers may engage in a work stoppage or **strike** as a concerted activity. Whether an employee who participates in a strike must be returned to work afterwards is dependent upon the strike's purpose. If the purpose is economic in nature (e.g., workers are seeking wage increases), workers may not be fired, but can be replaced and are entitled to be returned to work when openings occur. Workers opposing ULPs may be neither terminated nor permanently replaced and must be returned to work at the conclusion of the strike. Fortunately, the NLRA contains a provision requiring that a labor organization provide at least 10 days' written notice prior to striking when the employer is a healthcare facility so that alternative arrangements may be made for patient care duties. There are no other industries that are entitled to advance notice of a strike.

Occupational Safety and Health Act (OSHA) Requirements

The Occupational Safety and Health Act (OSHA) was passed in 1970 and regulates occupational working conditions. OSHA standards establish minimum safety requirements that must be followed by employers and vary by industry.

OSHA contains many regulations that directly relate to the healthcare environment. Workers exposed to bodily fluids, air that may contain airborne particles that cause disease or infection (e.g., tuberculosis or influenza), or hazardous chemicals must be provided with personal protective equipment (PPE), such as face shields, masks, and latex gloves or respiratory devices (29 C.F.R. §1910.132 to §1910.134). OSHA also addresses exposure to bloodborne pathogens and other potentially infectious materials that may cause disease or illness (29 C.F.R. §1030). The hazard communications standard applies to all workplaces where hazardous chemicals (e.g., sanitizing cleaning chemicals) are present and requires labeling and safety data sheets that convey the risks of exposure to chemicals through a classification system that relies on pictographs as well as the proper protective measures for that substance and instruction on what to do in the event of a spill or exposure (29 C.F.R. §1200). There are also regulations that require proper procedures (lockout/tagout) to prevent the release of potentially hazardous energy during equipment and environmental maintenance (29 C.F.R. §1910.147).

Employers are subject to unannounced onsite inspections by officials from the Occupational Safety and Health Administration for compliance with its health and safety standards. Employees may also file a complaint alleging OSHA noncompliance. If violations are discovered, the employer is subject to fines and penalties.

Worker Safety Programs

Many states require employers to adopt injury and illness prevention programs to encourage proactive employer efforts to avoid injuries and illnesses. But even in the absence of state requirements, long-term care employers should have a safety program in place, given the inherent risks in providing patient care.

In 2012, OSHA released its National Emphasis Program for Nursing and Residential Care Facilities in response to the high incidence of injuries in the industry (OSHA, 2012, p. 4). In comparison to all other private industries, in 2010, nursing and residential care facility employees suffered injuries resulting in lost time from work and/or job modification at a rate nearly 3 times the national average (p. 4). Injuries resulting from slips, trips, falls, and overexertion when transferring residents were most common (p. 4). Workers are also more likely to be exposed to infections, such as hepatitis B, or multi-drug resistant infections (p. 5). Another common occurrence in nursing facilities was injuries resulting from accidental exposure to hazardous chemicals used in cleaning, such as sanitizers and disinfectants (p. 6).

The National Emphasis Program (NEP) has increased the focus of both federal and state OSHA investigators on the skilled nursing facility work environment and resulted in increased safety inspections by these agencies. Most state agencies will perform an inspection at the request of the employer to measure compliance and provide the employer an opportunity to correct any safety violations before a citation is written. These voluntary inspections are an excellent means by which to evaluate the strength of a facility's safety program and practices.

Americans With Disabilities Act (ADA) Accommodation

Federal and state laws require employers to make employment decisions without regard to an individual's disability or perceived disability. An individual with a disability must be qualified for the position (have the requisite licensing, experience, and education) and be able to perform the essential functions of the position with or without a reasonable accommodation. **Essential job functions** are those basic responsibilities that the employee must be able to accomplish in order to perform his job. Essential functions of the job of a certified nurse assistant would be lifting at least 25 pounds and the ability to read, whereas a nonessential job function for a typical certified nurse assistant would be typing 35 words per minute. A **reasonable accommodation** is any adjustment made to an employee's position or work environment that allows him to perform the essential functions of his job (42 U.S.C. 126 §12111(10)).

When an employee needs a reasonable accommodation in order to perform his job the employer and employee must engage in an **interactive process** to determine whether a reasonable accommodation exists that would enable the employee to perform the essential functions of the job without causing undue hardship to the employer. The interactive process is a two-way communication where the employee helps the employer understand the challenges he is experiencing (or anticipates if the employee is newly hired) in performing the essential functions of his job as a result of the employee's disability. The employee may recommend or request a specific accommodation. The employer then has the opportunity to ask questions about the employee's challenges and potential accommodations in order to receive feedback and direction from the employee to assist in making a final decision on whether to accommodate.

Simply because an employee requests a reasonable accommodation does not necessarily mean that a reasonable accommodation is possible. An accommodation is not reasonable when it causes an **undue hardship** on the employer (ADA, 1990). An undue hardship is a significantly difficult action or expense that is determined by consideration of the cost of the action, the financial resources of the employer, the size of the employer, and the type of operation (42 U.S.C. 126 §12111(10)). Requests to displace other workers, create an unsafe condition, or reassign essential functions of the job are not considered reasonable accommodations. However, the provision of a special keyboard, chair, or workstation would likely be considered to be reasonable accommodations in most workplaces. A failure to engage in the interactive process to find a reasonable accommodation violates the ADA. In addition, if a reasonable accommodation is not made by the employer, the employer must be prepared to clearly establish facts that demonstrate that the reasonable accommodation posed an undue hardship in order to defend claims that the employer violated its obligation to reasonably accommodate under the ADA.

Discrimination and Harassment

Equal treatment of employees is regulated by **equal employment opportunity (EEO)** laws, which prohibit **employment discrimination**. Simply put, employers must assure that all individuals have the same employment opportunities and receive the same treatment. The law protects groups of individuals who share certain characteristics referred to as a **protected class**. The following is a listing of protected classes based on federal, state, and/or local law.

+   Age (employees over 40)
+   Individuals with disabilities (mental/physical)
+   Marital status (depending on state)
+   Military service (Vietnam-era veterans)
+   Race, ethnic origin, and color (African American, Asian American, Hispanic American, Native American)
+   Religious beliefs and practices
+   Sexual orientation (depending on state and/or city)

   Employment discrimination means to deny employment or subject an employee to an adverse employment action because he is a member of a protected class. Examples of employment discrimination are to deny a promotion to an employee because he is a Muslim or a failure to hire an otherwise qualified applicant because she is pregnant. **Harassment** is a form of discrimination and, as defined under federal and state equal employment opportunity laws, means to subject an employee to repeated, unwelcomed, and objectively offensive conduct because he is a member of a protected class. Examples of workplace harassment are young employees calling a 65-year-old employee derogatory names based on his age or a male employee telling a female employee he finds her sexually attractive and subjecting her to unwanted touching because she is female.

Training employees, especially managers, on discrimination and harassment and how to report, investigate, and respond to suspected violations of the organization's policies creates awareness of what is and is not appropriate workplace conduct. Awareness helps employees avoid misconduct or stop discriminatory behavior before it escalates.

Employees must be protected from harassment within the workplace without regard to the source. This can create very difficult situations when a resident is the alleged harasser. Inappropriate conduct by residents (e.g., a male resident who is subjecting female nurse assistants to unwanted touching) should not be dismissed as less severe than conduct by employees. In the case of substantiated coworker harassment, the harasser may be terminated for violation of the organization's policies. When a resident is found to have harassed an employee, the organization must take into consideration the resident's rights when deciding on corrective action. Removing the resident from the community may not be a viable or swift option. Arrangements to separate the victim from the resident must be made as soon as possible that do not violate the resident's rights or result in adverse employment action against the victim.

At the same time, courts are sensitive to the limitations faced by long-term care employers in these situations. Thorough documentation of the organization's response to resident harassment (even when the response does not solve the problem completely) in the appropriate records is critical to demonstrating that the organization acted to the best of its ability under the circumstances.

Retaliation

There are a myriad of federal and state laws that protect healthcare employees from retaliation for raising an objection, making a complaint about, or participating in governmental proceedings relating to quality of care, patient rights, suspected fraud, or other illegal behavior. An employee's refusal to engage in conduct that the employee reasonably believes to be a violation of law, even if not an actual violation, is also protected. In addition, many other laws applicable in the healthcare and non-healthcare setting, such as wage and hour or EEO laws, also contain retaliation provisions.

The act of objecting or of refusing to participate in what the employee believes is illegal or improper conduct by the employer is referred to as **protected activity**. **Retaliation** occurs when the employee is subjected to an adverse employment action because he engaged in protected activity.

Summary

While working in long-term care can be very rewarding, operators face many obstacles in retaining direct care staff. High turnover, the availability of a small population of qualified applicants to replace departing workers, and emotional and physical demands of the work environment itself make recruiting and retention of highly qualified workers very challenging. To overcome these obstacles, leaders must develop HR strategies to effectively manage a workforce with rapidly changing demographics that serves a resident population that is equally as diverse and growing.

Long-term care operators must also develop meaningful recruiting, screening, and selection processes that comply with the laws and regulations addressing long-term care staffing as well as equal employment opportunity. Investing in orientation and training programs that engage employees in the organization's culture while also preparing them to safely serve a vulnerable patient population will serve the long-term care organization well. Operators should be equally well-prepared to avoid violations of numerous federal and state laws on equal employment opportunity, labor relations, and health and safety.

In this environment, the value of an organizational culture built on genuine, two-way communication between management and staff, which embraces the diversity of the long-term care workforce, cannot be overstated. Open communications allow long-term care employers to continuously engage their staff and help them develop professionally. Employees who feel that their voice matters are more likely to report concerns early to management and are less likely to feel the need to file legal claims. Most importantly, satisfied and happy employees help reduce turnover. Having a strong (internal or external) HR manager or staff not only takes pressure off of already busy managers with less expertise but also can keep long-term care operators focused on the importance of their HR strategies and employee relations. HR managers and staff function as a partner to both employees and management. HR helps to ensure that employee needs are being met while also protecting the organization through the proper administration of the recruiting, screening, hiring, orientation, and performance management processes.

Key Terms

Adverse employment action: A substantial adverse change in working conditions that is significantly more disruptive than an inconvenience or alteration of job responsibilities.

At-will employment: Presumption that employment is for an indefinite period of time and may be terminated by either the employer or employee at any time.

Bargaining unit: A group of two or more employees with shared interests such that collective bargaining by a labor union on their behalf may occur.

Bonus: A one-time cash payment that does not increase the employee's base pay.

Bottom-up communication: Messages that start at the bottom of an organizational structure and are communicated up to personnel who hold positions of high authority in administration.

Circular communication: A mixture of top-down and bottom-up communication efforts to ensure constant communication within a facility.

Collective bargaining agreement: A negotiated agreement between workers and management regarding wages, hours, and other terms and conditions of employment.

Concerted activity: A term used in the National Labor Relations Act to describe the conduct taken by two or more employees who action for their mutual aid or protection regarding terms and conditions of employment or in order to form or join a labor union. A single employee may also engage in concerted activity if he is acting on the authority of other employees, bringing group complaints to the employer's attention, trying to induce group action, or seeking to prepare for group action for the purpose of collectively bargaining, other mutual aid or protection, or forming or joining a labor union.

Conditional offer of employment: An offer of employment that is contingent on the successful completion of certain conditions.

Culture: Societal forces affecting the values, beliefs, and actions of distinct groups of people.

Direct care staff: Employees who personally deliver patient care, such as licensed nurses and nursing assistants, and who also make up the majority of employees in long-term care.

Diversity: The differences among people.

Employee benefit programs: Indirect compensation, such as healthcare, dental, or vision insurance, provided to an employee as part of total compensation.

Employment discrimination: Unfair treatment of an employee by an employer motivated by the employee's membership in a protected classification.

Equal employment opportunity (EEO): Employees should receive equal treatment in all employment actions.

Ergonomics: Study and design of the work environment that identify the physiological and physical demands of the employees and attempt to eliminate negative consequences.

Essential job function: Fundamental duties of a job.

Harassment: As defined by federal and state equal employment opportunity laws, means to subject an employee to repeated, unwelcomed, and objectively offensive conduct because he is a member of a protected class.

Human capital: The knowledge, skills, and experience of individuals in terms of the cost or value to an organization.

Job description: A stated record of the essential functions involved in the performance of a task.

Interactive process: Collaborative effort between employer and employee to determine if the employee can return to work subsequent to an occupational or non-occupational injury, disease, or disorder.

Labor market: An area of economic exchange in which workers seek to fill jobs and employers seek workers.

Mandated training: Training required by a law or rule.

Open-door policy: Policy that allows any employee to talk with any level of management about any issue at any time in order to foster effective management-employee communication.

Organization's culture: The behavior of an organization's employees and the meaning that is attached to those behaviors.

Orientation: A period of time spent to welcome a new employee in order to help familiarize the employee with the facility's operations, expectations, benefits, people, and policies and procedures.

Outsourcing: Arrangement between companies where one company provides services for another company that could typically be provided internally.

Productivity: The measurement of the quality and quantity of produced work within the framework of cost.

Protected activity: Employee engagement in activities protected by Title VII; i.e., opposing discriminatory practices and/or participating in an investigation, proceeding, or hearing under Title VII.

Protected class: Individuals who share certain characteristics that have been identified for protection under equal employment laws.

Reasonable accommodations: The modification or adjustment of a job application process or work environment to enable a qualified individual with a disability to be considered for a job or to execute a job.

Recruiting: The process of generating a pool of qualified job applicants to fill vacant positions.

Registry: A staffing agency that provides nursing staff on a temporary basis to provide direct patient care.

Retaliation: Punitive actions taken by employers against employees who exercise their legal rights.

Rounding, or making rounds, is a term that is used to describe when administrative or clinical staff members walk throughout the facility and inspect or evaluate the facility as a means of assessing performance and governing facility operations.

Stand-up meetings: Meetings that are attended by facility senior administrative staff, or department managers, that take place at the beginning of the workday.

Strike: Work stoppage where union members refuse to work in order to put pressure on an employer to make changes.

Suggestion program: A formal program for obtaining employee input and upward communication.

Talent pool: The number of people with the appropriate skills who are available to do a particular type of job.

Tight labor market: The existence of more jobs than qualified workers to fill those jobs.

Top-down communication: Messages that start at the top of an organizational structure and are relayed down to the rest of organizational audience.

Turnover: Process in which employees leave the organization and create a vacancy, which needs to be filled.

Undue hardship: Significant difficulty or unreasonable expense imposed on an employer when making an accommodation for an employee.

Unfair labor practice (ULP): Conduct by an employer or union that violates Section 8 of the National Labor Relations Act.

Review Questions

1. What are some of the causes of long-term care staff turnover? What actions may be taken to control turnover?

2. Discuss how the aging of the workforce and a shortage of qualified direct care staff contribute to changing the meaning of "retirement."

3. What are some of the preemployment screenings that a skilled nursing facility should perform before making a conditional offer of employment? Which preemployment screenings may a skilled nursing facility perform only after making a conditional offer of employment?

4. Review the areas of mandatory training for all skilled nursing facility staff and discuss the purpose of these trainings.

5. What are some claims that a long-term care worker could bring against an employer?

Case Studies

Case Study #1

Ms. Duncan, a registered nurse, recently moved to California and is the director of nurses of a 100-bed skilled nursing facility with 75 residents. On her first day, she meets with the assistant director of nurses, a nurse, who prepares the nursing staff (includes licensed nurses and nursing assistants) schedule, and the director of staff development, also a nurse, who assists with the staffing schedules, to discuss nursing department staffing. They tell Ms. Duncan that they are running overtime every day and have been short on nurses because three are out on medical leave. Many of the facility's nursing assistants are calling off with the flu, so other nursing assistants are working a lot of double shifts. In the past 24 hours, nursing staff have worked 240 hours.

- What are some additional questions Ms. Duncan should ask to assess the staffing situation?

- What are some possible solutions to reduce overtime and improve direct care staffing levels?

- California law requires skilled nursing facilities to provide at least 3.2 nursing staff hours per patient day. What was the facility's nursing staff-to-patient ratio in the last 24 hours?

Case Study #2

Mr. Thomas is a new nursing home administrator. In his first few weeks on the job, he has noticed that the nursing assistants seem unhappy. Mr. Thomas has tried to visit with as many of the nursing assistants as possible to get to know them and to assess their satisfaction with the work environment. Most of them tell him "everything is fine." A few are more forthcoming and mention that the director of nurses and other nurse managers do not seem to care about the nursing assistants. They tell him that the only time nurse managers really communicate with the nursing assistants is when they deliver disciplinary action notices.

The facility's HR manager advises that the majority of the nursing assistants are overdue on their annual performance evaluations. She tells Mr. Thomas that she heard a rumor that some of the nursing assistants have been speaking to a union representative. A few fliers were found in the break room, announcing a union information meeting held at a nearby restaurant last week.

- If you were Mr. Thomas, what would be your next steps?

- A nursing assistant approaches Mr. Thomas in the hallway and tells him she has been asked to sign a petition to form a union, but is unsure what to do. She asks Mr. Thomas for his advice. How should he respond?

- Mr. Thomas receives a notice that the nursing assistants will be going out on strike next week. How should he prepare for the upcoming strike?

References

Alsop, R. (2008). *The trophy kids grow up*. San Francisco, CA: Jossey-Bass.

American Health Care Association. (2010). *2010 annual quality report*. Retrieved from www.ahcancal.org/quality_imporovement/Documents/2010Quality Report.pdf

American Health Care Association. (2012). *American Health Care Association 2012 staffing report*. Retrieved from www.ahcancal.org/research_data/staffing

Americans With Disabilities Act of 1990. Pub. L. No. 101-336, 104 Stat. 328 (1990).

Bureau of Labor Statistics. (2012). Labor Force Characteristics by Race and Ethnicity, 2012. Retrieved from http://www.bls.gov/cps/cprace2012.pdf

Bureau of Labor Statistics. (2013a). *Economic news release: Union affiliation of employed wage and salary workers by occupation and industry, 2012–2013 annual averages.* Retrieved from http://www.bls.gov/news.release/union2.t03.htm

Bureau of Labor Statistics. (2013b). *Occupational employment statistics: NAICS 623100—Nursing care facilities (skilled nursing facilities).* Retrieved from http://www.bls.gov/oes/current/naics4_623100.htm

Harahan, M. F., & Stone, R. I. (2009). Who will care: Building the geriatric long-term care workforce. In R. Hudson (Ed.), *Boomer bust? The economic and political issues of a graying society* (pp. 231–253). Westport, CT: Praeger.

Kramer, A. M., & Fish, R. (2001). The relationship between nurse staffing levels and the quality of nursing home care. *Report to Congress: Appropriateness of minimum nurse staffing ratios in nursing homes*: Phase II, volume II, Chapter 2. Department of Health and Human Services.

Mickus, M., Luz, C. C., & Hogan, A. (2004). *Voices from the front: Recruitment and retention of direct care workers in long-term care across Michigan.* East Lansing: Michigan State University.

Occupational Safety and Health Administration. (2012). *National Emphasis Program: Nursing and residential care facilities (NAICS 623110, 623210 and 623311).* Retrieved from https://www.osha.gov/OshDoc/Directive_pdf/CPL-03-00-016.pdf

Office of Immigrant Statistics. (2010). *Immigrant statistics.* Retrieved from Department of Homeland Security website: www.dhs.gov/fites/statistics/immigratin.shtm

Piper, L. E. (2011). The ethical leadership challenge: Creating a culture of patient- and family-centered care in the hospital setting. *Health Care Management, 30*(2), 128–138.

Riordan, M. (2010). *Rounding with and for a purpose* [Web log post]. Retrieved from http://blog.ghs.org/2010/09/rounding-with-and-for-a-purpose/

Scanlon, W. J. (2001). *Nursing workforce: Recruitment and retention of nurses and nurse aids is a growing concern* (GAO-01-750T). Washington, DC: Government Accounting Office.

Schnelle, J., Simmons, S. Codogan, M., Garcia, E., & Bates-Jensen, M. (2004). Relationship of nursing home staffing to quality of care. *Health Services Research, 39*(2), 225–250.

Slavit, W., Reagin, A., & Finch, R. (2009). *An employer's guide to workplace substance abuse: Strategies and treatment recommendations.* Washington, DC: National Business Group on Health, Center for Prevention and Health Services.

CHAPTER 6

REIMBURSEMENT IN THE LONG-TERM CARE ENVIRONMENT

Robert Miller

Health care in the United States is a very large business, accounting for roughly 20% of the nation's Gross Domestic Product (GDP). Understanding the healthcare business model is critical for administrative and clinical professionals, as the success of their organizations in delivering high-quality care is tied directly to their ability to generate revenue and thus support and expand their operations. The days when healthcare professionals could let the accountants worry about finance and reimbursement are gone. Gone too are the days when healthcare providers could take the approach that it was their responsibility to deliver all needed/desired services, regardless of the cost. Today, the interconnection between delivery of care and finance and reimbursement, and their impacts on the financial health of an organization, is the responsibility of the clinical staff, the business office, and the administration in equal measure.

This chapter addresses cost and reimbursement issues relevant to long-term care providers. This includes those providers who are eligible to receive reimbursement from government programs and private insurance plans and those who rely on private payers. While there are many reimbursement issues that overlap between long-term and acute care providers, we will focus solely on the former in this chapter. Financial issues in acute care will, inevitably, impact long-term care providers, and these impacts will be pointed out; however, a detailed explanation of the costs and reimbursement issues impacting acute care providers is beyond the scope of this text.

LEARNING OBJECTIVES

- Identify different payers/payer types.

- Become familiar with various reimbursement methodologies.

- Explain how different reimbursement methodologies classify residents.

- Differentiate between routine revenue and ancillary revenue.

- Identify resident-related items, how these can impact the financial health of a facility and how they can be managed.

- Become familiar with the roles and responsibilities of long-term care staff in handling resident funds and resident financial issues.

- Identify ways to assess revenue enhancement strategies and sources of funds to increase a facility's financial position.

Payer Sources

The government, encompassing both federal and state agencies, pays for approximately 67% of the healthcare services delivered to residents in long-term care facilities. The federal Medicaid program is the single largest payer for long-term care services (SCAN Foundation; www.thescanfoundation .org). Sometimes the government pays providers directly, as with the traditional fee-for-service Medicare program. In other cases the government pays an insurance company, like Blue Cross or Kaiser Permanente, which in turn contracts with providers to pay for services rendered. The more common government payer types are described ahead.

Government Programs

Government programs are a significant source of revenue for long-term care facilities. These include the various Medicare programs, Parts A, B, C, and D, which are explained in more detail ahead, and Medicaid, a joint federal and state program, which pays for healthcare services for low-income populations. The importance of these programs varies with the particular demographic characteristics of a facility's resident population, but most facilities except those that provide only custodial care will deal with Medicare, at least, at some point. Therefore, a solid understanding of these programs, how they work and what they cover, is important for long-term care administrators, nursing, social services, and rehabilitation program managers.

Medicare

The Medicare program pays for a variety of services for adults aged 65 years and older and adults with disabilities. Medicare is a federal program, and benefits are earned by individuals who have worked and paid into the program through payroll deductions. Medicare is divided into parts: Part A, Inpatient Care; Part B, Physician and Outpatient Services; Part C, Medicare Advantage Plans; and Part D, Prescription Drug coverage; each part pays for a different set of services.

Part A, "Inpatient" Coverage. Medicare Part A pays for the bundle or group of related services and supplies provided to a resident with inpatient Medicare eligibility who requires skilled nursing or rehabilitative care. Billing for bundled (grouped) services, eliminates the need for the facility to list each specific item and service, and the associated cost for each, on bills that are submitted to Medicare. The following describes what Medicare pays for in the long-term care facility.

Routine services are those services provided by the nursing staff and other departments, such as social services, dietary, or laundry. These may be paid by Medicare if the patient meets eligibility criteria. These services are called routine because they are provided to all residents in the facility, regardless of the payer source—government, private insurance, or **private pay**. Every resident is seen and cared for by the nursing staff, all residents are provided meals by the dietary department, and the laundry department washes the laundry and linens of all residents. The departments that provide routine services include (but are not limited to):

- Nursing
- Social Services
- Activities
- Dietary
- Laundry
- Housekeeping
- Plant Operations and Maintenance
- Medical Records
- Administration
- Nursing Administration
- Personal Supplies

Ancillary services are not provided to all residents. Ancillary services are provided to residents who need specific services related to a medical condition. Residents who need rehabilitation may receive physical, occupational, or speech therapy. Residents with an infection may be given an antibiotic drug. Residents who have respiratory problems or who cannot breathe on their own may require breathing treatments or need a ventilator. The major categories of ancillary services include (but are not limited to):

- Physical therapy
- Occupational therapy
- Speech therapy
- Respiratory therapy
- Medical supplies
- Drugs
- Laboratory services
- Radiology
- Complex equipment

Medicare Part A covers most of the services provided to residents of skilled nursing facilities (SNFs) while they meet the criteria for eligibility. Eligibility for Medicare coverage is based on the resident's need for skilled nursing services or rehabilitative care services. Once the resident no longer meets one of these criteria, he is no longer eligible for Medicare coverage during that period of service. In addition, Medicare will pay for a maximum of 100 days of long-term care services in a calendar year (U.S. Department of Health and Human Services, www.hhs.cms.gov). Facilities have the ability to access a centralized Medicare database to determine whether the resident is eligible for Medicare coverage prior to his admission to the facility. The database, formerly known as the Common Working File, contains information on all Medicare beneficiaries and includes case histories, claims information, benefits, and other personal health information. The Common Working File was deemed to be noncompliant with the regulations for protection of Personal Health Information (PHI) as contained in the Healthcare Information Portability and Accountability Act (HIPAA) and is being replaced by a new, more secure service. A resident in a SNF covered by Medicare Part A is said to be "on a Part A stay." Important rules for Part A coverage include:

- The maximum number of days per "spell of illness" or "benefit period" (the period of time, beginning with the day of admission to a hospital or skilled nursing facility and ending on the day of discharge from the facility, that an individual receives Medicare benefits) is 100 days. It is possible for a patient to have more than one benefit period, but that patient must meet certain conditions to regenerate his 100-day eligibility period. To generate a new benefit period, the patient must have been discharged from the facility for at least 60 days and must have another 3-day qualifying stay in an acute care hospital (Centers for Medicare and Medicaid Services [CMS], www.hhs.cms.gov).

- In order for a stay in a skilled nursing facility to be paid for by Medicare, the patient must first have been admitted as an inpatient to a hospital for a minimum of 3 days. To qualify under this rule, the patient must be an inpatient for at least 3 midnights, with the day of discharge not counting as a day in the minimum stay calculation (hospital days, for determining patient length of stay, begin and end at midnight).

- Coverage is *not* automatic. A patient must meet specific skilled criteria in order to be covered by Medicare Part A, such as requiring skilled nursing services or rehabilitation. There are volumes of coverage rules that govern this area. (Additional information regarding Medicare coverages, including links to current and proposed regulations and interpretive papers, can be found at the Medicare website, www .cms.gov.)

- The 100-day maximum is *not* automatic either. Most patients covered by Medicare Part A are not covered by Part A for the entire 100 days. The average Part A length of stay in a skilled nursing facility has remained relatively consistent, from 26.3 to 27.4 days for the last 7 years reported (2006 to 2012) (Medicare Payment Advisory Commission, 2014, p. 114).

- Once the patient no longer meets skilled criteria for coverage, Part A coverage is discontinued and replaced by a different payer, which can be either the patient, through another insurance plan or through private funds, or Medicaid. The latter will pay for services only if the patient meets specific financial requirements (explained later in this chapter).

- From the 20th day through the 100th day of Part A coverage, the patient becomes responsible for a daily co-pay amount, which may be covered by a secondary payer source if available. The co-pay amount is determined annually by the CMS and may change from year to year.

Part B, Ancillary Services Coverage. Medicare Part B pays only for certain ancillary services. Part B does not pay for routine services. If Medicare Part A is in effect (with limited exceptions), Medicare Part B will not come into play. However, if Medicare Part A coverage is terminated and replaced by a different primary payer, such as Medicaid, Medicare Part B may pay for the covered ancillary services if there is a change in condition or if the services are provided in an outpatient setting. Since Part B coverage is for ancillary services, it is not intended to replace or substitute for Part A coverage if Part A coverage is terminated.

The ancillary services typically covered by Part B include:

- Physical therapy
- Occupational therapy
- Speech therapy
- Medical supplies
- Laboratory services
- Radiology services
- Some medical equipment

Here again, the patient must meet the coverage criteria before Medicare Part B will pay for any of these services. Also, patients are required to pay a monthly premium and an annual deductible for Part B coverage. These costs are calculated based on the patient's annual tax return and are set on a sliding scale based on reported income. For certain services, such as physicians, outpatient therapy, and durable medical equipment, the patient will be responsible for a co-pay equal to 20% of the Medicare allowed charge for each service.

Part C, Medicare Advantage Plans. Medicare Part C, generally referred to as Medicare Advantage (MA) plans, is plans that are offered by private healthcare insurance companies as alternatives to Medicare Parts A and B. These MA plans are required to provide the same coverages as are offered by Medicare Parts A and B. However, MA plans may also offer extra coverages that are not included with Parts A and B. Individuals may choose to enroll in an MA plan, in which case they will not be covered by regular Medicare.

Many of the available MA plans operate like health maintenance organizations (HMOs), requiring their members to receive covered services from network (contracted) providers. In this way, these plans seek to control physician, inpatient, and outpatient services costs, which was one of the goals established when MA plans were first created. Individuals who enroll in MA plans do so on an annual basis during what is referred to as an "open or annual enrollment period." During this time, which is generally in the fall, members may also choose to join a different MA plan, or may also elect to return to traditional (Parts A and B) Medicare coverage. Individuals who choose to enroll in an MA plan will also receive prescription drug coverage through the MA plan, and thus do not need to enroll in a Part D prescription drug coverage plan. In fact, if a person already enrolled in an MA plan mistakenly enrolls in a Part D plan, the MA plan coverage will be terminated and he would be able to reapply for Part A and B coverage (www.medicare.gov).

While there may be advantages with MA plans in terms of expanded coverage, there are also potential downsides, especially if the plan requires its members to receive services from network providers only. It is important that social services and business office staff in long-term care facilities understand the differences between the various forms of Medicare coverage, as residents making decisions about their options for coverage under the Medicare program may often come to them for guidance in choosing between the various coverage options. In these instances it is important that staff asked to address the question provide explanations or direct residents or their representatives to appropriate sources when asked about the various coverage options. In order to avoid the appearance of favoritism or conflicts of interest and to avoid potential liability if the resident or his family feel they have incurred unnecessary costs in obtaining coverage, staff should avoid making recommendations or advocating for one plan or coverage type over another. In these instances, their role should be that of a provider of information, not an advocate. **Managed care plans** are discussed in greater detail ahead.

Part D, Drug Benefit. Medicare Part D is the prescription drug benefit component of traditional Medicare. In order to receive Part D coverage, the individual enrolls in a prescription drug plan, unless, as noted earlier, he is enrolled in a Medicare Advantage plan. Part D payments are made directly to the pharmacy that provides the drugs prescribed for the resident. There are a variety of Part D plans, each with different combinations of benefits, co-pays, deductibles, and **formularies** (list of drugs covered by the plan). Plans also have different tiers in their formularies, often distinguishing between generic and brand-name varieties of the same drug. The decision on whether to prescribe a generic or brand-name drug is generally made by the prescribing physician. Generic (nonbranded) versions of prescription drugs generally have a lower co-pay requirement than do name brand drugs; however, not all prescription medications have generic versions. Many physicians will write prescriptions to allow for use of a generic version of a drug when it is available, since the difference in the patient's co-pay between generic and branded drugs can be substantial. Also, in many instances patients and residents can request their physician prescribe generic alternatives due to their lower cost. The ultimate decision of whether to prescribe a branded or generic alternative drug rests with the prescribing physician.

Enrollment in a Part D plan is done annually during the open, or annual, enrollment period. Individuals who do not enroll in a Part D plan during this period may be assessed a late enrollment penalty fee if they enroll later. Because there is considerable variety within Part D plans, long-term care facility staff need to be informed about these plans, where to get information about them, and how to assist their residents in choosing and enrolling in a plan.

Medicaid

Medicaid is a combined federal and state program that provides medical insurance to residents with low income. Residents who are eligible for Medicaid benefits have limited income and **assets**. When Medicaid pays for services in a skilled nursing facility, the resident is required to contribute most of his personal income toward his care. This contribution is called his **share of cost**. The share of cost is calculated on the cost of the service in question, what the state (as Medicaid payer) pays for the service, and the recipient's income as a percentage of the federal poverty level (FPL). In addition, providers may not refuse to provide services based on the recipient's inability to pay even the nominal share of cost. Individuals may apply for Medicaid coverage once they have exhausted their ability to pay privately for long-term care services. Their coverage will be based on their level of income as a percentage of the federal poverty level.

Medicaid is considered the payer of last resort. In other words, if any other payer is available, Medicaid will not pay for the services. For example, if a resident is eligible for Medicare benefits, Medicaid will not pay until the Medicare benefits are terminated or exhausted. As a general rule, Medicaid reimbursement levels are lower than Medicare or private insurance rates for almost all services. As such, it is important that administrators in long-term care facilities pay attention to their mix of payers—that is, Medicare, Medicaid, private insurance, and private pay. Having a payer mix too heavily weighted to Medicaid beneficiaries can reduce the amount of reimbursement the facility receives and have a negative impact on its financial health.

As with all programs, there are coverage criteria, which can be found on state Medicaid websites and at the federal site, www.cms.gov, that must be met before Medicaid will pay for services rendered. Medicaid assesses the resident's needs to determine whether the patient's stay meets the criteria for skilled nursing care or if his needs could be met with a lower and less expensive **level of care**.

Veterans Affairs (VA)

The Department of Veterans Affairs is a federal agency that administers a variety of programs and services, including healthcare services for veterans. The VA operates a large number of hospitals but also pays non-VA hospitals and other providers for services provided to veterans. These include long-term care and rehabilitative services, home health care, and durable medical equipment, as well as physicians, outpatient therapy services, counseling services, and supportive care.

Bed certifications. This is virtually a nonissue, but in the past and for a few providers that offer only custodial care not covered by Medicare, the facility designates certain beds as Medicare-certified beds and others as noncertified beds (such a facility is then referred to as a **partially participating facility**, and may accept Medicare patients only if it has Medicare-certified beds available for them). A resident on a Medicare Part A stay must be placed in a bed certified for Medicare participation, or risk having reimbursement for Medicare-covered services denied since the services were not provided in a certified setting. If all the beds in the facility are Medicare-certified (a **fully participating facility**), a Medicare beneficiary may reside in any bed in the facility.

Since the inception of the **prospective payment system (PPS)**, used by Medicare to pay providers set rates for patient care and services based on their diagnoses and acuity, almost all hospitals and SNFs, except some small rural and critical access designated hospitals and long-term care providers and those providing only custodial care, are fully participating facilities. The administrator is responsible for knowing the status of the facility's bed certification, since providing Medicare-covered services in a noncertified setting risks denial of payment for those services.

Managed Care

Managed care has been a significant part of the healthcare delivery system in the United States since the 1980s, although the concept of managed care and its most commonly recognized vehicle, the health maintenance organization (HMO), had its beginnings much earlier. The original HMO was started in the 1930s, as a means of providing medical services for industrial workers at a reasonable cost, and became prominent during World War II when the Kaiser Shipyards in Richmond, California, organized the first truly large-scale prepaid (providers were paid a set rate to care for workers when their services were needed, regardless of what these services entailed) healthcare program (Kaiser Permanente; www .kp.org).

The basic concept behind all managed care plans is that individuals enrolled in the plan receive their care from physicians and other providers (referred to as network providers) who agree to accept negotiated (usually discounted) fees for providing services to these patients. In turn, plan members will be charged lower, or no, co-pays if they receive services from network providers. Managed care providers come in three major forms: the **health maintenance organization (HMO)**, the **preferred provider organization (PPO)**, and the **point-of-service plan (POS)**. HMOs assign each insured member to a specific primary care physician from whom they receive primary and preventive care services. HMO patients needing specialized care, hospitalization, or other services beyond primary care must obtain these services from providers either employed by or contracted with the HMO. In this way, the HMO seeks to contain costs. Patients covered by a PPO may choose physicians, specialty care, and hospital services from a network of providers contracted with the PPO. They will generally be charged lower co-pays if they receive care from these "in-network" providers. Should they elect to see a provider that is not contracted with the PPO, the patient will have a higher co-pay and a higher deductible to pay. POS plans allow patients a wider choice of providers but do so at a greater cost to the patient in terms of deductibles and co-pays.

Managed care plans are private insurance companies that pay for healthcare services. Some of these companies (like Kaiser Permanente) operate their own hospitals and employ their own physicians and other providers—therapists, psychologists, and laboratory personnel. Others are simply insurance companies that pay for services provided by contracted network providers.

Managed care plans contract with employers, the states, and the federal government to coordinate services and pay providers based on agreed-upon amounts. Payments to managed care plans are based on per-member, per-month (PMPM) calculations, and all services provided for plan members must be paid from the funds received by the plan. These are referred to as "capitated contracts," and the payment methodology is referred to as "**capitation**." In turn, the managed care plan contracts with providers to deliver the services and pays them a negotiated rate for those services. The plan assumes the financial risk for providing care for that individual, and if it spends more than the employer or the government has paid it, it loses money. Conversely, if it can reduce its costs for providing care, by finding lower-cost suppliers, reducing payments to staff and/or contract providers, or eliminating potentially redundant tests, the plan can make a profit. It is important to note that managed care plans that contract to provide Medicare and/or Medicaid coverage must provide all of the benefits that are traditionally provided by these programs under fee-for-service provider contracts.

A recent development for managed care plans is the use of **shared risk arrangements** with contracted providers. In these contracts, the providers agree to share the risk associated with capitated contracts and try to control both **utilization**, the amount and variety of services used, and costs of providing those services. These shared risk arrangements are becoming a prominent feature of many **accountable care organizations** (ACOs) that have emerged as a result of passage of the Patient Protection and Affordable Care Act (PPACA), otherwise known as "Obamacare." Under shared risk arrangements, providers and health plans assume the risk of providing appropriate and necessary care, while accepting a specified level of reimbursement. If the care provided exceeds the amount received, both the plan and the provider lose, since payments are capped. The plan will lose because it has contractual obligations to its participating providers to reimburse them a specified amount for the services they provide, regardless of whether the amount it (the plan) receives covers these costs. Similarly, providers can also lose in this scenario if their costs for providing the services exceed the amount they have agreed to accept for the particular service(s). However, if the net cost—that is, the total amount spent for care for all plan members—is less than the net total payments projected for the services provided, the plan and the participating providers share in the savings.

Both state and federal governments are shifting more activity from traditional fee-for-service programs to managed care plans. The government sees this as an opportunity to save money or limit its risk. If the government (state or federal) agrees to pay only a specified amount to the managed care plan and the plan is responsible for ensuring that all of the appropriate services are delivered, the plan rather than the government has the risk of higher costs of care. It is then the plan's responsibility to manage the care and control cost. The cost can be controlled in two ways: (1) pay providers less money for the services they deliver or (2) limit the volume of the services that are delivered. In the former case, providers may be reluctant to offer or refer patients for services for which they may not be reimbursed, while in the latter case healthcare plans may limit the services that they will cover for reimbursement or restrict patients to a few in-network or contracted providers. In the case of a limited number of providers, patients may self-limit their use of healthcare services due to difficulties with getting appointments or scheduling procedures. While these methods may help reduce healthcare expenditures, the trade-off in quality of, and access to, care needs to be appreciated and understood by patients, providers, and administrators.

Private Pay

In some cases the individual resident pays the provider directly for the services he receives using his own funds. This is usually the case when the resident does not qualify for other payer sources. For example, if the resident does not have a medical condition complex enough to qualify for Medicare benefits or otherwise is not eligible for Medicare coverage, Medicare (Part A) will not pay for any services provided to him. If the resident has more assets or a higher income level than allowed by Medicaid (is ineligible for Medicaid benefits), Medicaid will not pay for the services provided. Similarly, if the person does not have insurance or the insurance policy does not cover long-term care, services will not be paid for the resident. In each of these situations, the resident would be responsible for paying the facility directly with his own funds.

Long-Term Care Insurance Plans

Many people who are employed have some sort of insurance policy that covers at least some of their healthcare needs. These health insurance policies cover a variety of services related to care and treatment for acute illness and injury, including physician services, therapy services, and acute care hospital services, as well as **post-discharge** care, such as home health nursing and therapy services, outpatient care, and durable medical equipment, such as wheelchairs, walkers, or specialized hospital beds. Even if an individual has health insurance, it does not automatically mean the policy will cover skilled nursing care. In fact, very few insurance policies cover skilled nursing services. To address this issue, insurance companies have developed a variety of long-term care insurance products. These policies are designed to pay for long-term care services provided in different settings, including independent and assisted living centers, adult day care, and skilled nursing facilities. People purchase these policies primarily so that they will not need to exhaust their savings should they require long-term care. However, it is important for these purchasers to be aware of the conditions and exclusions that are often contained in these policies. Chief among these is usually a **waiting period**, usually the initial period of the individual's stay in a long-term care facility that is paid for by the individual before insurance coverage begins. Waiting periods vary in length, and during these periods the policyholder will be responsible for the charges incurred for his stay. Once the waiting period is completed, the policy will assume the cost of care. Facility staff must address coverage issues with residents and track waiting periods closely in order to begin billing the insurance plan for covered services as soon as the waiting period expires. This is generally the responsibility of either a nurse case manager or the director of social services, working with the billing office to monitor waiting periods and initiate billing the appropriate insurance company when coverage becomes effective. Also, since not all plans are identical in either the length of their waiting periods or in the services they cover, these provisions need to be clearly understood and explained to residents. Again, this would be the responsibility of a case manager or the director of social services. While the number of people who have purchased long-term care insurance is growing, along with the number and variety of such products, these policies still constitute a very minor part of the payment system for skilled nursing care. The costs associated with long-term care are still not well understood by the general population, and this, combined with the perception that Medicare and other government programs pay for these services, has contributed to the relatively small number of long-term care insurance policies sold to date.

Supplemental Insurance Plans

As previously noted, residents who have Medicare Parts A and B coverage are responsible for certain co-pay or share of cost obligations. There may also be services that are either not paid for by Medicare or are partially paid for by Medicare. In these instances, the resident is said to have an obligation to cover the partial or nonpayment. Supplemental insurance plans, also referred to as **Medi-gap plans**, are designed and marketed to provide additional coverage over and above what is paid for by Medicare and thus cover these obligations. This may include coverage for the co-pay amounts specified for Part A– and B–covered services or for services such as mental health care, which are not covered by Medicare. It is important to distinguish between these plans, which are merely adjuncts to traditional Medicare, and the Medicare Advantage plans, which are alternatives to traditional Medicare. There are many different supplemental plans to choose from and a variety of sources, including the American Association of Retired Persons (AARP) and various state and federal websites, and the insurers' as well, that can assist individuals in assessing their needs and the costs associated with these various coverage options.

Reimbursement Methods

There are several different methods that payers use to provide reimbursement (payment) for long term care services. Long-term care facilities will typically utilize a combination of these methodologies to maximize resident composition and revenue in the facility. These methods, including **prospective** and **retrospective payment systems**, cost-based, price-based, and flat-rate reimbursement models, acuity adjustments, and resource utilization groups, are described ahead.

Prospective

A provider of healthcare services, either an acute care or rehabilitation hospital, a skilled nursing facility, a home health agency, or a hospice can be paid **prospectively** (in advance) or **retrospectively** (after the fact) for services provided. For these providers, Medicare Part A payments are made prospectively, and are based on **diagnosis-related groups (DRGs)**, a system that links payment for services to the diagnosis of the patient's condition, for acute care hospitals, **resource utilization groups (RUGs)**, a determination of the amount of care and services needed by the patient in a skilled nursing facility based on the assessment of his condition at the time of admission to the facility, or some other measure of diagnosis and acuity. Many insurance companies are now also moving to prospective payment systems, as these are seen to be a better way to control the growth of healthcare spending. By implementing prospective payment systems, payers are able to shift the burden of managing care to the providers. In addition, when payment amounts are established in advance, providers are incentivized to keep costs within the amount provided for the particular patient.

Prospective payment systems as described here, while having the ability to reduce or control costs, also create certain "perverse incentives" for providers, including the potential for limiting services to ensure that the funds received cover the cost of the care provided. In other cases, providers try to overstate the severity of the patient's condition and his need for services in order to gain a higher acuity score, thus increasing the prospective payment. To combat these activities, both private insurance and government payers routinely audit patient care records and utilize case managers to make regular visits to monitor the progress of the patients whose care they are funding. Understanding these processes is important for long-term care administrators to maintain their facilities' financial strength and their quality of care ratings.

While adjustments to payments can be made after the fact, increases for payment require significant documentation and justification by the provider of services. For example, changes to RUG levels can affect payments, positively by increasing payments, or negatively by decreasing payments. RUG levels need to accurately reflect the patient's condition, and the services required for that condition at the time that the determination is made to avoid an adjustment. Changes to RUG levels need to reflect actual **changes in condition** supported by appropriate documentation. It is also important to note that retroactive adjustments can reduce the amount paid to a provider. These adjustments, referred to as **recoupments**, repayments to Medicare for charges that were determined to be inappropriate upon later review, can reduce the amount paid for a particular patient's diagnosis, term of stay, or episode of care. Medicare may recoup payments as much as 3 years after the initial evaluation was made. It has been suggested that this adjustment provision be phased out in the future, but this has not been finalized. While in the past the adjustment process was more common, its use is contrary to the concept of prospective payment as a cost-control mechanism and is anticipated to continue to decline.

Retrospective

Retrospective payment systems, otherwise known as fee-for-service, were at one time the most common form of payment in the healthcare industry. In a fee-for-service system a healthcare provider renders services to a patient and then bills the patient's insurance company, or other responsible payer (Medicare, Medicaid) for these services. The fee billed is determined by the provider, but the reimbursement may be less than the amount billed because the reimbursement rate is negotiated between the provider and the payer, or as in the case of Medicare and Medicaid, established by the payer. In a true fee-for-service system, providers are paid for the services they provide based upon their best medical judgment. In such a system, concerns about the cost of care are not taken into account.

Cost-based. **Cost-based reimbursement** systems came into use as a means of providing some degree of cost control for healthcare services. The concept is based on the theory that the amounts paid to providers should be based on the actual cost of providing the care, with a small percentage added for profit. The amount paid to the provider could be based on the actual cost incurred by an individual provider or it could be based on the average cost for all providers of the same type in a particular geographic region. Cost of care averages are based on Medicare cost reports submitted by facilities and published by the Centers for Medicare and Medicaid Studies (CMS). In a cost-based system, payment rates may be determined prospectively but the actual payments (reimbursement) are made only retrospectively in the form of a fee-for-service model. Under a cost-based system, the provider's costs for providing services are covered but limited to those deemed medically necessary. Medically necessary services can be specified in contracts with private insurance companies, and a provider's bills for services provided are reviewed for medical necessity by the payer before reimbursement is provided. In this type of system providers need to monitor the services they deliver to ensure they meet the test of medical necessity since submitting claims for review for medical necessity will delay, or possibly even result in denial of, payment for services provided. Even if payments are ultimately received, delays can be as long 60 to 90 days before payment is received. Time frames for both payment and review for payment are typically established as contract provisions in agreements between payers and providers. There is no specific standard for these time periods, although the minimum time for payment of clean (no errors) and undisputed (no questions of medical necessity) claims is typically 30 days.

Price-based. In most cases today the amounts paid to providers are **price-based**. The amount paid per day, per item, or per unit of service is set at a predetermined level, referred to as a price. Examples of prices include:

- $200 per day for room and board services paid by Medicaid
- $27.33 for a 15-minute unit of physical therapy paid by Medicare Part B
- An all-inclusive rate of $567.41 per day for a Medicare Part A patient

Price-based reimbursement is another form of retrospective payment, since providers are paid only for the services delivered to patients and residents. In addition, since the price that is paid to the provider is set by the payer, it may fail to cover the actual cost of providing the service. Price-based reimbursement systems require facilities and providers to closely monitor their **patient mix**, the number of patients they admit and treat from the various payer categories (Medicare, Medicaid, private pay, and commercial insurance plans) since the reimbursement rates they receive from these various sources will vary significantly. Doing so will help to ensure that revenues are maximized.

Flat-rate methodologies. Under a flat-rate reimbursement system, providers are paid a predetermined rate for each of a variety of services (e.g., daily nursing care, various forms of therapy), are paid one rate for a group of "bundled" services, as in "per diem" payments to SNFs, or are paid on a capitation basis prospectively and must provide all necessary services required by the patient or patients in question. **Flat-rate methodologies** are designed to enable payers, insurance plans, and Medicare to better predict their costs of service since the flat per-patient rate can be multiplied by the number of patients receiving care to determine the expected daily, weekly, or monthly cost to the payer. Flat-rate methodologies shift the responsibility for cost control to the provider, since they must deliver services within the parameters of the funds they receive. Flat-rate methodologies include both prospective and retrospective payment forms, but all are based on the concept of a predetermined payment for a service or group of services. As discussed earlier, flat-rate methodologies can incentivize providers to limit or restrict care and services to ensure that the amount received for the patient is not exceeded by the cost of his care.

Acuity adjustment. The basic premise for acuity-adjusted payment methodologies is that while flat-rate systems are effective as reimbursement for most patients, patients with higher acuity require more complex care and services than can be adequately covered by a basic flat rate. Under an **acuity adjustment** reimbursement system providers are paid a flat rate for specified services. In the case of long-term care this is often an all-inclusive per diem rate, with an additional amount added to the per diem rate for patients with higher acuity scores. The acuity adjustment accounts for the impact of adding higher-cost services, such as ventilators, feeding tubes, or daily therapy services, on the provider's overall cost structure.

Acuity adjustments can also be used as a means of structuring reimbursement under cost-based structures where the adjustment factor is used as a means of determining a final cost. Again, the basic concept is that a patient's acuity is a primary causative factor in driving the overall cost of care. It is not unusual in long-term care settings for a patient to have a change of condition—a change in his acuity over time. Thus, the cost of care will change as the need for care and services is adjusted to meet the changing needs of the patient. These determinations, which are reflected in altered resource utilization groups (RUG) scores, are made by nurse case managers in consultation with the patient's attending physician, therapists, and other clinical staff involved in his care.

It is financially reasonable to pay a provider more for more complex services. To accomplish this, the facility assesses the resident's condition on a regular basis and based on that assessment places the resident in a category. These assessments are done weekly by the nursing staff and on a monthly basis by the attending physician. If based on the assessment, the resident requires more care and resources, he is assigned to a category associated with a higher resource utilization groups (RUGs) rate, which is used in the Medicare Part A program for SNFs.

Resource utilization groups. The resource utilization groups (RUGs) system uses an assessment tool to determine what types and amount of care and services a resident requires. This assessment tool is called the minimum data set (MDS) and is completed by members of the interdisciplinary team, which results in a payment category. The MDS includes items that measure physical, psychological, and psychosocial functioning. The items in the MDS give a multidimensional view of the patient's functional capacities and helps staff to identify health problems and plan courses of treatment. Currently (2015) there are 66 categories used in the RUGs classification system. The Current RUG IV classification, which can be found on the CMS website (www.cms.gov), begins with eight major RUG groups, providing a broad patient categorization. From there hierarchical classifications, ADL scores, and case mix indices for rural and urban facilities further subdivide the patient population and assign each patient to a category. Based on government studies the estimated amount of resources that residents in each of these 66 categories used has been established. Such resources include:

•   Nursing time

•   Therapy treatments

•   Drugs

•   Medical supplies

•   Lab and x-ray services

The system does not establish exactly how many resources each individual resident has actually used; rather it determines the average amount expected to be used by all residents in any given category.

Based on the expected resource usage, a rate (or price) is assigned to each category. Higher rates or prices are assigned to categories that are anticipated to use more resources, typically for sicker or more complex patient care or rehabilitation and for patients in urban as opposed to rural facilities. The difference in urban and rural reimbursement rates is attributed to higher labor costs seen in urban areas. In addition, since higher-acuity patients tend to cluster in urban areas, or be moved to those areas for care that is generally not available in rural settings, the costs associated with delivering that care are greater, and this is reflected in higher reimbursement rates.

Levels of care. While not nearly as detailed or technically complex as the RUGs system, a "level of care" system attempts to determine how much care is required by a resident. This method is often, although not exclusively, used by managed care plans when contracting with SNFs. In these instances, the plans will pay different amounts for different levels of care. The simplified example cited ahead illustrates reimbursement in a level of care reimbursement system. It is used here only to demonstrate this concept and should not be taken as a definitive example of such a methodology.

Level 1: Room and board only

- $200 per day

Level 2: Room and board plus 1 hour of therapy per day

- $250 per day

Level 3: Room and board plus 1 hour of therapy per day plus IV antibiotics

- $350 per day

Level 4: Room and board plus 1 hour of therapy per day plus IV antibiotics plus ventilator services

- $550 per day

Negotiated rates. Reimbursement rates established by government payers, such as Medicare and Medicaid, are established without negotiation in the traditional sense of a bargaining process between payers and providers. Because of the statutory authority given to these programs, they can set reimbursement rates to meet the goals of the programs, which generally include cost containment or even cost reduction. Providers wishing to participate in these programs must agree to accept the established rates as payment in full. While in many cases there will be co-payments or shares of cost that are the responsibility of the patient, providers may not collect more than the established amount as set by the program. Reimbursement rates for government payers are generally adjusted for inflation and variations in costs of labor, equipment, and supplies on an annual basis. These adjustments take into account not only the costs of delivering services but also variations in costs from one region of the country to another and variations in labor costs seen between urban and rural areas. This process of regionalizing reimbursement rates for government-funded programs is unique to the United States, and is, at least in part, a reflection of the lack of a true systems approach to healthcare delivery in this country. Reimbursement rates are also responsive to a host of outside influences, including hospital, physician, and long-term care trade associations and patient advocacy groups, such as the American Association of Retired Persons (AARP). This is most often seen when agencies, such as Medicare, seek to limit or reduce amounts that it will pay for various services. In these instances, the various advocacy groups will lobby both the agency and members of Congress who have oversight of the agency, to curtail reductions or limitations that would have a negative impact on their members. In this regard AARP has been especially successful in its lobbying efforts, which have been aimed at minimizing any reductions in Medicare benefits and services for its membership. AARP's actions have significantly reduced a number of proposed reductions in Medicare benefits for seniors and have had the indirect effect of maximizing revenue for providers. Thus, while government payers' reimbursement rates are not negotiated in the traditional sense, there are many parties and organizations that have input into the final rates that are set in any given year.

Government rates differ from contractual arrangements for reimbursement between health insurance plans and long-term care providers because these latter rates are determined through a process of negotiation. There are many factors that influence these negotiations, including the amount of service a provider can deliver, the length of time covered, and competitors' rates for the same set of services.

Coding. All of the reimbursement methods discussed here ultimately tie back to the process of billing a payer for services provided to a patient—one covered by a government program (e.g., Medicare, Medicare Advantage, Medicaid), a private healthcare insurance plan, or private pay. The process of billing for services has become increasingly specialized and standardized, through the use of resource utilization groups (RUG codes), diagnosis-related groups (DRGs), or Healthcare Common Procedure Coding System (HCPCS) or International Statistical Classification of Diseases and Related Health Problems (ICD). These latter two coding sets (HCPCS and ICD) are used for medical procedures, services, and equipment, generally in hospitals and physician and ancillary service provider settings. Long-term care administrators need to understand that correct and appropriate coding, whatever methodology is required, is vital to the financial well-being of their organization. Conducting regular audits of bills and charges is a useful means of ensuring that the coding process is functioning effectively and capturing the complete spectrum of services provided by the organization.

Resident-Related Items

The topics discussed in this section directly involve residents and/or their responsible parties, the overall financial health of the facility, and regulatory compliance. The long-term care facility is in a unique position to assist residents with financial matters that relate to their use of the facility's services. This fiduciary duty is a resident right and at this level of care particularly important because many residents may not have family or friends available to assist with these needs. The facility's obligation is dictated in national regulations and enforced by federal and state regulatory agencies through licensing and compliance surveys. In addition, residents often have need of other financial advisement services, and for these they should consult a qualified financial advisor. Estate planning, age-appropriate investment strategies, wills and trusts, and the use of reverse mortgages to generate additional income are all issues that may require professional advice and consultation. While these are not facility responsibilities, having lists of qualified referrals can benefit residents when seeking these services.

Medicaid

To establish a payer source for custodial care or to ensure an uninterrupted payer source (e.g., private funds or Medicare are no longer available reimbursement options), it is in the facility's best interest to establish a screening protocol to determine if a potential resident will be eligible for Medicaid to subsidize his stay. The screening tool should investigate income, savings, property, assets, and other items that are integral components of the Medicaid eligibility determination. Medicaid eligibility is state-specific, and it is recommended that the facility work closely with the appropriate regulatory agencies in that state to ensure the success of an application. Often Medicaid is the only tool an individual can use to get the care he needs. Even though Medicaid reimbursement is significantly less than private pay or Medicare, it is important to understand that these individuals should and do receive the same degree of care as people with other payer sources.

Applications. It is a federally mandated obligation of each long-term care facility to help individuals with the Medicaid application process.

Individuals are often admitted to the facility with the expectation that they will eventually qualify for Medicaid benefits, even though this has not been determined at the time of admission. Some facilities use the term "Medicaid pending" to describe the period of time in which the application has been submitted but not yet approved.

Using the term "Medicaid pending" can be misleading as the resident is either eligible or not. If found to be eligible, the facility will bill Medicaid for services rendered according to the Medicaid rules for that state. If the resident is found not to be eligible, the resident will be on a private or self-pay status. All issues related to payer sources and the cost of care should be discussed thoroughly with the resident (and responsible party) and documented according to facility policy prior to admission.

Unfortunately, many residents move in before they become Medicaid-eligible and do not have the family support or other resources required to successfully navigate the Medicaid eligibility process. It will then be the facility's responsibility to assist the resident in completing the process. There may be long periods of time before eligibility is granted, and in some cases eligibility may be denied. If eligibility is denied, the resident will have no payer source and the facility will lose money on care provided.

By engaging in a screening process, the facility can help ensure adequate payer sources and identify potential problems, which will help both the resident and facility. Once eligibility is confirmed, the facility can bill Medicaid.

Spend-down. Residents who are already in a nursing facility may be eligible to received Medicaid nursing facility benefits after they have exhausted their Medicare benefit by exceeding the annual length of stay limit (see earlier). However, in order to be eligible for Medicaid, the individual has to meet certain financial criteria. This is currently defined as having an annual family income less than or equal to 133% of the federal poverty level (FPL). This figure is adjusted yearly based on changes in the FPL. Calculation of a family's income includes funds that they receive (income), such as Social Security and pension distributions, and the amount of property and other assets, such as bank accounts, stocks, and bonds, the family may have.

If the individual seeking Medicaid eligibility has more property/assets than is allowed, he must "spend down" in order to reach a point where his assets are at the allowable level. It is important that residents in this position receive guidance, often from a trained attorney, so all Medicaid criteria are complied with.

Share of cost. Once the resident is approved for Medicaid, he will have to pay a **share of cost**. Just like paying a mortgage or rent in the community, the share of cost is a monthly responsibility based on the resident's income level that is paid to the facility by the resident or the resident's family, if they are financially responsible for the resident's debts. Because Medicaid is a joint federal and state program, states have the option of establishing share of cost requirements. These can include co-payments, deductibles, and other such charges. An individual is not required to contribute all of his income to this share of cost requirement. However, share of cost limits will vary from state to state and will also vary depending on the individual's level of income. It is important to keep in mind that although an individual may meet the financial requirements for Medicaid eligibility, this does not preclude him from having a regular income. The requirement simply sets a cap on the amount of income that can be received on an annual basis. Thus, with the exception of funds that the resident may keep for "personal spending money," the individual may be required to contribute a significant portion of his income toward his care. If the resident is married and the spouse resides in the community, the share of cost may be greatly reduced or even zero as there are federal regulations established to ensure that the community spouse has adequate funds available to pay bills and continue living at home.

Appeals. Residents or potential residents may be denied Medicaid coverage for long-term care services either based on a lack of medical necessity for such services, as determined by a physician, or by virtue of having income and financial assets in excess of federally established limits. States may set higher income thresholds for eligibility of either specific target groups or all Medicaid-eligible persons if they desire, but their limits cannot be less than the federally established limit. A denial of Medicaid benefits eligibility determination can be appealed; however, unlimited appeals are not allowed. To assist residents and potential residents, facilities should have a list of qualified attorneys who can offer assistance with such appeals. Medicaid plans also incorporate an appeals process for those instances when the plan denies payment or coverage for either lack of medical necessity or income in excess of established limits. Due to the importance of having a payer source established prior to the resident's admission or his exhaustion of eligibility for other payer sources (e.g., Medicare), it is important not only for the resident but also for the facility to assist with this process. Medicaid eligibility may be extended retroactively for up to 3 months from the date at which a determination is made, if the individual would have been eligible during that time had he applied for benefits. This retroactive provision is not a guarantee and should not be relied upon when transitioning a resident from an existing payer source to Medicaid. Addressing eligibility issues and appeals in a timely manner is the best course of action to help ensure uninterrupted payment and continuation of services.

Resident trust account. For residents in long-term care facilities, it may be logistically difficult to get to the bank and/or engage in financial transactions. The resident can choose to open a **resident trust account** in the facility, which will function as a bank account. However, federal regulations (CMS, 2012a) specifically prohibit a facility from requiring a resident to deposit his funds with the facility. This is consistent with the overall requirement, which states that residents have the right to manage their own financial affairs. If the resident chooses to deposit funds with the facility, the funds must be placed in a trust account for safeguarding. There are specific federal regulations (CFR 42 Part 483.10) that provide oversight of resident trust accounts. The facility must maintain separate interest-bearing accounts for each resident and send regular statements, on at least a quarterly basis, to the resident or responsible party. Residents must also be able to access these accounts upon request. The facility may set reasonable parameters for this access, but these must be published and made known to residents and/or their designated representatives. Reasonable parameters, as specified by CMS (F158, F159) (CMS, 2012a, 2012b), include how funds must be maintained in interest-bearing accounts, how residents may access their funds, how funds must be accounted for, and how and to whom they must be conveyed upon a resident's death. Social services and/or business office staff are usually assigned to assist residents with deposits and withdrawals of funds if family members or other individuals authorized to act on the resident's behalf are not available. Establishing a trust account is advised rather than keeping money in a resident's room due to potential theft and loss issues. The intent of these regulations and procedures is to ensure that residents are allowed to make their own decisions regarding financial matters whenever it is possible and they desire to do so.

Petty cash. When a resident requests money from their trust account, the facility can withdraw the money from the petty cash account. This account is used for withdrawals of small amounts, defined as $50.00 or less for Medicaid beneficiaries and $100.00 or less for those covered by Medicare and is managed by the administrator or business office. All transactions must be documented so each resident's individual trust account can be reconciled (Figure 6.1).

Representative payee. Residents in long-term care facilities may have income from various sources, but most will have Social Security or Supplemental Security Income benefits. Residents may need assistance managing their money, from the practical challenges of writing, mailing, and tracking checks to preventing the mismanagement of their money. Staff may need

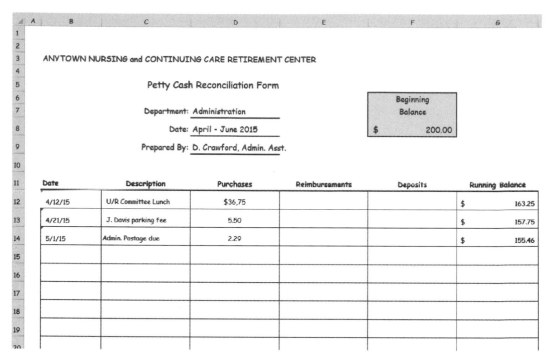

Figure 6.1   Petty Cash Form

to intervene to prevent fiduciary abuse and ensure that the monthly share of cost is being paid.

Early identification and intervention are important. One option the facility can exercise is to apply for approval as a **representative payee**, defined as "a person or organization appointed by the Social Security Administration to receive Social Security and/or Supplemental Security Income (SSI) benefits for someone who cannot manage or direct someone else to manage his or her money" (Social Security Administration). Once the representative payee is approved, Social Security will send the check directly to the facility to be deposited into the resident's trust account. The resident's share of costs can then be withdrawn from this account on a monthly basis.

Collections. The facility may encounter situations in which, despite everyone's best efforts, the amount owed to the facility goes unpaid. If the amounts are owed by third parties, such as Medicare or Medicaid, there are specific rules and procedures, published by CMS in the Federal Register and updated whenever changes are made, to follow to pursue payment. If the unpaid amounts are due from the resident, the facility must follow a collection procedure. The long-term care facility is required to establish a collection policy and procedure that will guide collection efforts. Common elements addressed in the policy and procedure include:

- Sending past due notices
- Making collection phone calls
- Writing more direct collection letters
- Turning the collection matter over to a collection agency
- Initiating a discharge process to evict the individual for nonpayment
- Reporting the individual and/or his responsible party to credit agencies
- Suing the individual or the responsible party

Collection efforts are a last resort, and a comprehensive understanding of the resident's financial and social situation prior to admission will help avoid this situation. Tracking progress and changes in payer source will also help avoid reimbursement issues throughout the resident's stay.

Notice of discharge for nonpayment. If the facility must initiate the discharge process due to nonpayment, it is imperative to follow the facility's policy and procedure as well as meet applicable federal and state regulations, such as F201§483.12(a) Transfer, and Discharge. Individual states may have different rules related to this process, but typically the following agencies and individuals must be notified:

- The resident's responsible party
- The ombudsman
- The Department of Public Health
- The facility's legal counsel

This process can be very difficult and disruptive, and all steps should be taken to avoid this situation. As a resident advocate (but not collection agent), the facility social worker plays an integral part of this process to ensure that all possible solutions have been explored and that the resident has a safe discharge plan.

Supplemental services. **Supplemental services** are those services opted for by the resident or responsible party that are not reimbursed by Medicare, Medicaid, or other third-party payer as part of the per diem. Private rooms are one of the most common examples of this type of situation, since private rooms are not covered unless a very specific medical reason exists, such as a communicable disease requiring isolation to prevent the spread of infection to other residents. If a private room is a personal choice, then the resident or responsible party can supplement the amount paid by the third party to pay for the difference in the private room rate.

Notice of noncoverage. When a resident is admitted with Medicare coverage for a skilled stay, that coverage will end when the skilled care is no longer needed. As the resident recovers and is approaching the end of his skilled care, the facility is required to inform the resident or responsible party that the payment for his care will cease soon by issuing a **notice of noncoverage** letter. Throughout the skilled stay, appropriate staff should be communicating with the resident and responsible party about the medical status and progress in therapy so by the time the noncoverage letter is issued, it is not a surprise.

Medicare has specific requirements for proper notification, published in the Federal Register and updated when changes are made, and the facility must use the correct form in order to avoid possible denial of payment. Additionally, the resident or responsible party has the right to appeal the decision to terminate coverage and must be informed of these appeal rights in writing. Typically, the facility social worker issues these letters and will assist with the appeals process if requested. Please see the CMS website (www.cms.gov) for examples of notices of noncoverage. It is also useful to note that in addition to the Federal Register, a number of other publications specific to long-term care facilities administration provide regular summaries and updates on both Medicare and Medicaid regulations pertaining to long-term care. These sources, which are often provided on a subscription basis, are available in both print and online versions.

Managed care plans often rely on plan case managers to issue similar letters, but in instances where the managed care plan communicates its decision of noncoverage directly to the facility, a staff member may be responsible for communicating this information to the resident. It is always good risk management for the facility to document that the notice was issued and to follow facility policy and procedure.

Summary

Long-term care facilities are facing increasing pressure to deliver solid financial performance even as they are required to provide high-quality care to an aging and medically more complex resident population. This means that administrators and managers in these facilities must be familiar with the various payer sources, what services each payer will and will not cover, and how to determine the optimal payer mix for their particular facility. As with health care in general, long-term care providers are being asked to maintain both their residents' health and the financial health of their organizations, in ways that were not known in the very recent past.

The goal of this chapter is to provide an introduction to the variety of financial and reimbursement concepts, issues, and methodologies that healthcare providers working in the long-term care arena need to be familiar with. It includes information on the various payer sources—government, private insurance, and private pay—that typically fund the provision of long-term care services.

To ensure this solid financial knowledge, the chapter also addressed the number of different payers that fund long-term care. These payer sources include government funding programs that cover a variety of services, as well as private healthcare insurance providers and private pay by the individuals receiving care, or their families. It is important to understand that, unlike other healthcare services, long-term care for any individual is often paid for by several different sources over the time that the services are provided. This multiplicity of payer sources makes it critical that administrators and managers learn to navigate the payment process.

Key Terms

Accountable care organizations (ACOs): ACOs are organizations that combine a wide variety of providers, physicians, hospitals, long-term care facilities, and associated ancillary service providers into integrated networks that assume responsibility for the care of a group of Medicare patients (www.medicare.gov).

Acuity adjustment: Adjustments in reimbursement rates made because of a change in the patient's condition. These adjustments may either increase or decrease the amount paid on a daily basis for the individual's care.

Ancillary services: These are services that are not routinely utilized by, or provided for, all residents. These include physical, occupational, and speech therapy services, as well as many others.

Assets: The assets of a facility are the things of value that a company owns or controls—that is, the asset can be sold, leased, or used in some way in its operations. Examples include equipment or buildings that the organization owns or cash in the bank.

Capitation: In the context of this chapter this refers to a payment arrangement between a health insurance plan and a physician or physician group to pay a set amount, on a monthly or annual basis, to that physician or group, for each individual patient covered by the health insurance plan who is assigned to that physician or physician group. These payments are made regardless of whether or not the patients actually receive services; however, the payments are intended to cover any and all necessary services that may be provided to those patients receiving services from the physician or physician group during the specified period. Capitation is a common feature of many managed care plans and is seen as a means of healthcare cost containment.

Changes in condition: This refers to the changes in a skilled nursing facility patient's condition that may be noted over a period of time and is typically associated with adjustments to the patient's RUGS score and reimbursement rate.

Cost-based reimbursement: Under cost-based reimbursement, providers are reimbursed (paid) for the cost of care provided, based upon documentation of the care provided. This methodology may include a markup percentage for profit. This method may also require providers to get prior authorization (approval ahead of time) in order to provide certain services to patients. Cost-based reimbursement is no longer the dominant model in the U.S. healthcare market.

Diagnosis-related groups: A prospective payment system used to pay hospitals for services provided to patients based upon the diagnosis of the patient's condition upon admission and including the various treatments, interventions, and resources that are typically utilized in caring for the particular diagnosis. The DRG system was originally used to pay for inpatient hospital services for Medicare beneficiaries but has now been expanded and is used by most private healthcare plans.

Flat-rate methodologies: Flat-rate reimbursement methodologies specify a single rate for a specified service or bundle (group of related) services. All providers receive the same rate for services deemed to be similar. Flat-rate systems often include a single rate for a daily stay in a hospital or SNF, to include all services related to that stay.

Formularies: Lists of drugs that are covered by will be paid for by a private health insurance plan, or government sponsored health plan when prescribed for a patient covered by that health plan.

Fully participating facility: This refers to a hospital or skilled nursing facility that has designated all of its licensed beds as "Medicare certified." Today most hospitals and skilled nursing facilities that accept Medicare covered patients are fully participating facilities, since they can accept non-Medicare covered patients in Medicare certified beds.

Health Maintenance Organization (HMO): A type of managed care health insurance plan that is based on a network of contracted primary care and specialty care physicians, as well as contracted hospitals and ancillary care providers (physical, occupational, and speech therapists, etc.). Patients enrolling in an HMO are assigned to a primary care physician (PCP) for primary care. Patients requiring specialty care must receive a referral from their PCP and must, except in an emergency, obtain specialty care from a physician or other provider who is part of the HMO's network.

Levels of care: This refers to a process used in conjunction with flat-rate methodologies to determine the amount of care required by a resident, and thus the appropriate amount of reimbursement. This method attempts to take the patient's condition upon admission into account when determining the cost, and thus the reimbursement, for caring for the patient. Many managed care plans contract with SNFs and pay different amounts for different levels of care.

Managed care: Managed care plans are a form of insurance plan in which individuals receive their care from physicians and other providers (referred to as network providers) who agree to accept negotiated fees, usually discounted from their usual and customary fees, for providing services to these patients. In turn, plan members will be charged lower, or no, co-pays if they receive services from network providers. Managed care providers come in three major forms: the health maintenance organization (HMO), the preferred provider organization (PPO), and the point-of-service plan (POS).

Medicaid: Medicaid is a joint federal and state program that pays for certain healthcare costs, including some that are not normally covered by Medicare such as nursing home and personal care services. Qualification to receive coverage through the Medicaid program is based on an individual's income and resources.

Medicare Part A, Routine Care: Reimbursement (payment) from Medicare for inpatient stays and services provided in acute care hospitals, subacute hospitals, rehabilitation hospitals, and skilled nursing facilities.

Medicare Part B, Ancillary Care: Reimbursement (payment) from Medicare for non-inpatient services, including physical, occupational, and speech therapies, and other services that may be required. These payments do not include room and care charges or other routine inpatient services. They may be provided for inpatients or on an outpatient basis.

Medicare Part C, Medicare Advantage Plans: Health insurance plans that are offered as an alternative to traditional Medicare Parts A & B for Medicare-eligible individuals. Medicare Advantage Plans (MA Plans) must include coverage for all the services covered under Parts A & B, as well as Part D Drug Coverage. They may include additional services. Individuals who choose these plans may pay an additional premium over the rate charged by Medicare.

Medicare Part D, Drug Benefit: Reimbursement for prescription drugs offered as an additional benefit that individuals who opt for Traditional (Parts A & B) Medicare coverage may elect. Part D coverage is not automatic, and individuals electing to have this coverage must select an insurance carrier who provides this coverage. There is an extra cost (premium) for Part D coverage.

Medi-gap plans: Private insurance plans offered to individuals covered by Medicare that are designed to pay the required co-pays and deductible costs that are the responsibility of the patient when Medicare covers the majority of the cost for a patient's care and treatment. These plans pay that portion of the cost of a patient's care that would otherwise be paid by the patient.

Notice of discharge for nonpayment: This is the process that a facility must follow if it has to discharge a patient/resident for failure to pay for services. There are various regulations that must be followed when a facility chooses to take this action. The notice must include the reason or reasons for discharge, when the discharge is to be effective, and the appeals process that is available to the resident.

Notice of noncoverage: This notice is issued to a patient/resident when it has been determined that Medicare or an insurance payer will not cover (pay for) his care and services. This notice informs the patient that he is now responsible for paying the costs of his care.

Partially participating facility: This refers to a hospital or skilled nursing facility that designates only a portion of its licensed beds as "Medicare certified." Partially participating facilities may only accept a Medicare-covered patient if they have a Medicare certified bed available for that patient.

Patient mix: This refers to the combination of patients covered by private healthcare insurance plans, Medicare, Medicaid, and other government plans, and private pay patients that are being served in a facility at a particular time. The patient mix is often represented as a percentage of private insurance, government payers, and private pay patients in a facility's census at or for a specified time.

Point-of-Service Plan (POS): A hybrid form of managed care plan combining elements of an HMO and those of a PPO. Patients coved by a POS plan are assigned to a primary care physician but do not need to have a referral from their PCP to see a specialist. Typically patients receiving care from an in-network provider will pay no deductible or co-pay. Patients may also go "out-of-network" for services, but these will require a co-payment or the payment of a deductible.

Post-discharge: Refers to events, services, interactions, or interventions provided to a patient after discharge from a hospital, skilled nursing facility, or other healthcare facility or provider's service and that result from the condition or diagnosis of the patient when they were discharged from that facility or provider.

Preferred Provider Organization (PPO): Refers to a group of physicians, hospitals and ancillary services providers that contract with a health insurance plan to provide care and services to that plan's insured members at a reduced rate. Insurance plan members may receive services from any provider within the PPO and do not require a referral from their PCP in order to do so. Providers in PPOs agree to accept discounted fees for service provided to insurance plan members in return for the opportunity to provide an increased volume of services. A PPO is a type of managed care plan.

Price-based reimbursement: Price-based reimbursement is a payment system that is based on the provider's cost of delivering care and services. In this model, prices are either negotiated or determined by the payer, based upon market basket indices in particular areas. In these systems the price of services may be agreed upon ahead of time in the form of a contract, and payment may be either prospective or retrospective.

Private pay: This refers to payment methodologies where the patient or resident who is receiving care and/or services pays for these services directly. This may be the result of a denial of coverage by an insurance plan or Medicare for lack of medical necessity, or the individual may elect services, such as in an assisted living facility, that are not covered by insurance plans or Medicare. In either case it is the patient/resident or his family that bears the responsibility for payment to the provider facility.

Prospective payment systems (PPS): Prospective payment systems provide reimbursement to hospitals, long-term care facilities, and individual providers in the form of up-front payments based upon the patient's diagnosis and expected length of stay. PPS places the burden of cost containment on the providers, who must manage the patient's care within a defined budget. PPS is now the dominant payment methodology in the U.S. healthcare market.

Prospectively: In the context of this chapter this refers to "prospective payment" of a payment made to a healthcare provider before services are provided to a patient. These payments are made on the basis of a physician or provider diagnosis and typically include a prenegotiated rate and discount for each service that will be provided. Prospective payment is a key feature in managed care plans.

Recoupments: This refers to reductions in reimbursement provided to a healthcare facility or healthcare provider for services ordered to a patient that have been reviewed and determined to be not medically necessary at the time they were provided. Recoupments are typically made by reducing the amount of reimbursement given to a provider for services that have been billed for a patient other than the patient deemed to have received the unnecessary services, since the latter services had previously been reimbursed to the provider.

Representative payee: The representative payee is a person or organization appointed by the Social Security Administration to receive Social Security and/or Supplemental Security Income (SSI) benefits for an individual who is unable to manage his funds or to direct someone to do this.

Resident trust account: The resident trust account holds funds deposited by the resident with the facility, which the facility holds for the resident. The facility is required to provide reasonable access to these funds for the resident. The facility is also required to maintain an accurate accounting of all resident trust accounts and can be cited for deficiencies if this accounting is deemed to be insufficient.

Resource utilization groups (RUGs): The resource utilization groups system uses an assessment tool, the minimum data set (MDS), to determine what types and amount of care and services a resident requires. The MDS is completed by members of the facility's interdisciplinary (nursing, social services, rehabilitation, dietary) team, which results in a payment category. The MDS includes items that measure physical, psychological, and psychosocial functioning. The items in the MDS give a multidimensional view of the patient's functional capacities and help staff to identify health problems and plan courses of treatment. Currently (2015) there are 66 categories used in the RUGs classification system.

Retrospective payment systems: Retrospective payment systems, which were once the dominant payment methodology, provide reimbursement to the provider after the patient has completed his course of treatment. Providers incur the initial cost of care and are then reimbursed by the payer.

Retrospectively: In the context of this chapter this refers to payments made to a healthcare provider after those services have been provided to a patient.

Share of cost: The share of cost is the percentage amount that a resident will pay for his care under Medicare. Medicare will pay for a certain percentage of costs, with the resident responsible for paying the remainder.

Shared risk arrangements: These are contract arrangements between managed care organizations and healthcare providers in which in which the providers agree to accept lower reimbursement rates for their services in exchange for the opportunity to split any payments that the managed care organization may receive for reducing the overall cost of services provided to all patients assigned to that organization. Shared risk arrangements are an integral part of accountable care organizations (ACOs).

Spend-down: A situation in which an individual seeking to become eligible for Medicaid coverage has more property/assets than is allowed, and thus must "spend down" or reduce his assets in order to reach the allowable level, currently defined as an annual family income less than or equal to 133% of the federal poverty level (FPL). This figure is adjusted yearly based on changes in the FPL. Calculation of a family's income includes funds that they receive (income), such as Social Security and pension distributions, and the amount of property and other assets, such as bank accounts, stocks, and bonds, the family may have. It is important that residents in this position receive guidance, often from a trained attorney, so all Medicaid criteria are complied with.

Supplemental services: Supplemental services are those services opted for by the resident or responsible party that are not reimbursed by Medicare, Medicaid, or other third-party payer as part of the per diem. Private rooms are one of the most common examples of this type of situation because private rooms are not covered unless a very specific medical reason exists, like the resident has a communicable disease and needs an isolation room to prevent the spread of infection to other residents.

Utilization: As used in this chapter this refers to a review or analysis of the healthcare services provided to a patient or a group of patients. Utilization reviews are done are performed after services have been provided.

Waiting period: Refers to the period of time between when a patient is admitted to a skilled nursing facility and the time that the services that the patient is receiving from that facility will be covered by either Medicare, Medicaid, or the patient's private insurance. Services provided during the waiting period are typically paid for by the patient.

Review Questions

1. A reimbursement system that pays providers a specific, fixed amount based upon the patient's diagnosis and projected length of stay is called

   _____.
   a. Cost-based reimbursement
   b. Acuity adjustment
   c. Prospective payment system
   d. Flat-rate reimbursement
   e. Capitation reimbursement system

2. The federal government's Medicare program pays for ancillary services under what part of the Medicare program?
   a. Part A
   b. Part B
   c. Medicaid
   d. Part C
   e. Part D

3. The resident's contribution to his cost of care under Medicare's payment system is referred to as the _____.
   a. Resident's deductible
   b. Resident's share of costs

   c. Resident's co-pay

   d. Resident's spend-down

   e. Responsible party contribution

4. Many accountable care organizations (ACO) established under the Patient Protection and Affordable Care Act include these as one means of cost containment: _____.

   a. Cost-based reimbursement

   b. Zero-based budgeting

   c. Acuity adjustments

   d. Shared risk arrangements

   e. Capitation payments

5. Resource utilization groups (RUGs) include the estimated resident usage of a variety of patient care resources, including _____.

   a. Therapy services

   b. Dietary services

   c. Medical supplies

   d. Physician services

   e. A and C

6. Facilities are required by federal regulation to maintain resident trust accounts into which residents must deposit their funds to meet share of cost obligations. True or False?

7. The term "Medicaid pending" is used to indicate that a resident has qualified for Medicaid coverage but the date that coverage will start has not yet been determined. True or False?

Case Study

Aurora Skilled Nursing Facility, with a capacity of 200 beds, is one of four SNFs located in Anytown, and has been operating profitably since it was opened. The facility admits an average of 1,000 patients per year with an average length of stay of 28 days, thus generating an average of 28,000 patient days with an average reimbursement of $185.00/patient/day. It has also maintained an 85% occupancy rate. During that time patients have been referred to all four of these facilities in roughly equal amounts by all three of the hospitals in the community. Anytown General Hospital and St. Mary's Hospital and Medical Center have each accounted for 30% of the referrals, while Comprehensive Healthcare System provided the other 40% of annual referrals. Now Comprehensive Healthcare System has decided to form an accountable care organization, and has asked Aurora Skilled

Nursing Facility to join it. The offer to join the ACO includes the following provisions:

1.   ACO members will receive priority referrals, with the expectation that patients needing SNF services will be referred to the ACO-affiliated SNF.

2.   All ACO members will be expected to discount their fees by 20% for all ACO patients.

3.   ACO members must provide priority admission to ACO patients over referrals from non-ACO-affiliated facilities, but may admit non-ACO patients when bed space is available.

Based upon these provisions, and assuming that the ACO will increase the number of referrals it sends to Aurora to at least 80% of the facility's patient population, should Aurora affiliate with the ACO? Your answer should address the following:

1.   Assuming that the facility's bed capacity cannot be increased, what will be the effect on the facility's census?

2.   Will the increased revenue from ACO patients, at discounted rates, offset the potential loss of revenue from non-ACO patients?

3.   Will the increase in ACO patient referrals increase the occupancy rate sufficiently to offset the loss of revenue due to required discounting?

References

Centers for Medicare and Medicaid Services. (2012a). *Ftag 158.* Retrieved from https://www.careplans.com/pages/master_ftag/ftag_show.aspx?id=9

Centers for Medicare and Medicaid Services. (2012b). *Ftag 159.* Retrieved from http://apps.ahca.myflorida.com/nhcguide/static/f_provisions.html.

Centers for Medicare and Medicaid Services. (2015). *Accountable care organizations.* Washington, DC: Government Printing Office.

Medicare Payment Advisory Commission. (2014, June). *A data book: Healthcare spending and the Medicare program.* Washington, DC: Government Printing Office.

Acknowledgments

With gratitude and deep appreciation I wish to acknowledge the assistance, thoughts and suggestions, and necessary criticism provided by Paige Hector, who brought me into this project. This work could not have been completed without her able assistance. I am also, and always grateful to my wife, Dr. Shereen Lerner, for her belief and support. Mazel Tov to you both!

CHAPTER 7

COMPLIANCE AND RISK MANAGEMENT

Rebecca Lowell

"Long-term care" is an often misunderstood phrase. For purposes of this chapter, long-term care (LTC) will be defined as any provider of resident care services, outside of the hospital acute care setting. This broad definition is intended to encompass both licensed and unlicensed healthcare service providers.

The term "licensed healthcare provider" is an equally broad definition and varies from state to state. Further, there is often significant overlap in the types of services provided in a long-term care organization. The licensed healthcare provider may be the corporation that provides long-term care services, yet the employees within the organization may or *may not* be individually licensed healthcare providers. For example, a nurse or therapist is a licensed healthcare provider but a certified nursing assistant or activities director may not be. These nonlicensed providers of healthcare services work for a licensed healthcare provider (e.g., a skilled nursing facility) and work under the authority of the licensed healthcare providers.

Individuals considering a career in the long-term care industry must be cognizant that it is one of the most heavily regulated in the nation. As more fully detailed ahead, failure to comply with the regulations may have disastrous results, including patient injury or death, significant financial burdens, and possible criminal prosecution. Complicating matters are the ever-changing interpretation of the regulations, advances in medicine and technology, and the promulgation of new legislation. This chapter will focus on how the LTC provider can incorporate these

LEARNING OBJECTIVES

- **To identify the risks associated with the provision of long-term care services.**

- **To understand the various laws governing the provisions of long-term care services.**

- **To provide guidance in creating and implementing systems to address the requirements of the law.**

- **To assist in creating systems to identify and investigate breakdowns in the systems.**

- **To provide an understanding of how long-term care providers can best protect themselves.**

changes into its organizational structure so that it may remain in substantial compliance. Further, it will address the systems that may be implemented to handle the daily challenges of providing LTC services.

Compliance Today

Overview of LTC Regulations

Understanding the structure under which LTC providers operate will assist in understanding the regulations governing providers and their obligations. The Department of Health and Human Services (DHHS) is the primary federal agency responsible for monitoring the provision of healthcare services. This department reports directly to the president of the United States. Within the DHHS, there are a number of related agencies that report to the director of the DHHS. One of these agencies is the Centers for Medicare and Medicaid Services (CMS). CMS is responsible for administering the federal monies that are used to pay for Medicare and Medicaid (www.usa.gov). LTC services are primarily provided to Medicare and Medicaid beneficiaries (elderly and disabled), and as such, CMS is directly involved in the oversight of LTC providers.

State governments have a similar structure. For example, in California, the Department of Health and Human Services (HHS) reports directly to the governor, and the primary agencies responsible for the provision of health-related services are within the purview of the secretary of the state. Such departments include the Department of Aging, the Department of Health Services, the Department of Rehabilitation, the Department of Community Services and Development, Emergency Medical Services, and the Department of Social Services.

Federal LTC Statutes

LTC providers must maintain "substantial compliance" with all of the federal regulations, including those that specifically govern healthcare services. Some of the most pertinent regulations include: **Health Insurance Portability and Accountability Act (HIPAA)**, **False Claims Act (FCA)**, **Anti-Kickback Statute (AKS)**, **Stark I and II**, the **Affordable Care Act (ACA)**, the **Elder Justice Act (EJA)**, and, for skilled nursing facilities, the **Omnibus Budget and Reconciliation Act (OBRA)**. Within these statutes, there are interpretive guidelines. These guidelines arise through published opinions from the judiciary (Department Appeals Board, Circuit Court decisions, or Supreme Court decisions), guidelines published by the Department of Health and Human Services, or opinions set forth by the

Office of Inspector General (OIG), as well as numerous publications put forth by the Centers for Medicare and Medicaid Services (CMS), the Federal Register, and other government-affiliated agencies.

State LTC Statutes

Most states have also adopted statutes that mimic and oftentimes expand the federal regulations. However, the interpretation of state statutes is often left to the state oversight body, such as the Department of Health Services or Department of Social Services, without standardized guidelines.

State statutes impose a separate set of criminal or monetary penalties for violations. The state statutes and regulations allow the state administrative agency to prosecute the LTC provider for violations and allow the LTC recipient (or his representative) to file a civil lawsuit for a perceived wrong and obtain monetary awards. In the civil arena, the statutes usually exempt or expand the limits on liability (thereby greatly increasing any monetary award), expand the time period for an injured person to bring a lawsuit, and often allow for the recovery of attorney's fees and punitive damages. Many of these statutes are fairly recent by legal standards (enacted in the late 1980s or early 1990s), and as such, the case law providing guidance on the interpretation is slowly emerging.

Despite the uncertainty in interpretation, all of these regulations exist to protect privacy in medical records; protect the elderly and disabled adults; and ensure that federal/state monies are being spent wisely and that fraud, abuse, and waste are eliminated.

Who Does the Long-Term Care Provider Serve?

LTC providers primarily exist to serve the resident. However, the LTC provider must also serve its employees, the regulatory agencies, visitors, family members, and contractors to the facility, all the while providing an invaluable resource to its communities.

Pursuant to OBRA regulations, skilled nursing facilities are required to assist each resident in attaining or maintaining his highest practicable physical, mental, and psychosocial well-being. An inability to achieve this goal, absent sufficient explanation, may have significant detrimental effects upon the resident and the provider's business operations.

The obligation to employees is equally important. LTC is a service industry, and with quality employees, the organization is better able to meet its regulatory goals. Further, disgruntled employees may lead to worker's compensation actions, civil litigation, or whistle-blower actions.

Surveying agencies are ultimately responsible for ensuring the provision of quality services to the residents and compliance with state and federal regulations. Failing to comply with the requirements of these agencies may result in deficiencies, civil monetary penalties, and denials of payments for new admission, withdrawal from the Medicare and/or Medicaid program, or referrals to the Office of Inspector General and prosecution by the Department of Justice.

Visitors to the organization also have rights that must be protected. Primarily these rights arise from ensuring that the premises are adequately maintained and that the visitor does not come to unavoidable harm. (This is of significant concern if the organization provides services to residents with a history of violence or sexual deviance; reviewing the potential resident's history to determine appropriate placement is critical.) In short, the organization is obligated to operate in a manner that allows for the environment to be as safe as reasonably possible.

Lastly, there is a duty owed to vendors, contractors, and other agents. These duties go beyond a safe environment and include fair dealings in business relationships and a measure of oversight and accountability.

Compliance and Accountability

The most obvious questions are: Why is health care so regulated? Why are there so many agencies and laws surrounding this profession? Why are LTC providers subject to perceived enhanced scrutiny? Why do people suing LTC providers often obtain significant monetary awards or penalties?

The questions are valid and the answers uncomplicated: (a) The government understands the value of health, and most individuals value their health above any other possession; (b) the government establishes/pays for programs that allow people access to health care and to maintain their health; (c) in establishing these programs, the government expects the delivery of quality care and compliance with reimbursement; (d) oftentimes, the recipients of long-term care services are some of the most vulnerable individuals in our society, deserving of protection; and (e) the U.S. Census Bureau has identified the elderly (age 65 and older) as the fastest-growing population group. As of November 17, 2012, the nation's 90-and-older population had nearly tripled in the last 30 years, and was approaching 2 million people. This number was projected to quadruple over the next four decades (U.S. Census Bureau, 2011). Therefore, in order to ensure the continued economic viability of government-sponsored healthcare programs, the laws are necessary to stop fraud, abuse, and waste.

Government Tools

So, how does the government ensure compliance with the laws? The existing statutes create tools for government entities to: audit the care, establish incentives to improve the care, require deficient practices be corrected, implement individual compliance programs, and provide monetary rewards to those who report abuses.

Surveys

One of tools utilized to ensure compliance is the survey process. Entities that are licensed by the state and/or receive state/federal monies through Medicare, Medicaid, SSI, SSD, and so forth are subject to the survey process. For SNFs, the survey is intended to review compliance with the OBRA regulations and any state governing regulations. For assisted living facilities, senior day care centers, and other providers of LTC services, the state certification agency conducts surveys to ensure compliance with the state regulations. The survey process is comprehensive, and deficiencies usually require the facility to submit a corrective action plan. The survey result is a public document, and the most current survey must be maintained by the organization and made available to the public. Further, a plan of correction (POC) is required for almost every deficiency identified during the survey process. The POC must address: (a) an action plan to correct the problem identified (corrective action); (b) a system to ensure that other residents will not be affected by the deficient practice (systemic changes); (c) a method for monitoring that the deficient practice does not reoccur (monitoring process); and (f) dates of completion for the POC.

Five-Star Incentives

For SNF LTC providers who receive federal monies, survey results are transmitted to CMS. CMS publishes the results on the U.S. government website. A "five-star rating" system exists so consumers may make choices for SNF providers depending upon how many stars a particular facility receives. The SNF is required to post the five-star rating in three different locations throughout the facility so that it is prominently displayed to members of the public. It should be noted that the five-star rating has received significant criticism from the LTC provider community. This is because the rating system is inherently subjective (i.e., it relies upon the interpretation of the regulations by the survey team), as well as factors that are outside of the provider's control—that is, the overall medical condition and needs of its resident population.

Corporate Integrity Agreement

A corporate integrity agreement (CIA) is part of a settlement agreement between the LTC provider and federal healthcare program following investigations that typically involve violations of the false claims statutes. With the CIA, the LTC provider agrees to certain obligations, and in exchange, OIG agrees not to seek its exclusion from participation in Medicare, Medicaid, or other federal healthcare programs.

CIAs have many common elements, including hiring a compliance officer/appoint a compliance committee; developing written standards and policies; implementing a comprehensive employee training program; retaining an independent review organization to conduct annual reviews; establishing a confidential disclosure program; restricting employment of ineligible persons; reporting overpayments, reportable events, and ongoing investigations/legal proceedings; and providing regular reports to the OIG on the status of compliance activities (Office of Inspector General, U.S. Department of Health and Human Services, n.d.).

Corporate Compliance Program (CCP)

The ACA, more fully outlined in Chapter 8, requires that every skilled nursing facility receiving federal monies must maintain a functioning corporate compliance program (CCP). The CCP is the facility's promise to comply with all of the laws that govern the delivery of healthcare services. The CCP expands the standard survey process (which may focus on OBRA and the specific state regulations) and encompasses quality of care, the submission of accurate claims, the Anti-Kickback Statute, HIPAA and privacy concerns, submission of false claims, physician relationships, and pharmacy services. The facility's CCP program is required to have a reporting mechanism for employees and members of the public, an internal auditing/reporting system, a method for initial education and ongoing education of employees, a reporting mechanism, disciplinary action plan for violators, and person(s) responsible for ensuring the efficacy of the CCP.

Whistle-Blower Litigation

Generally speaking, a whistle-blower lawsuit (also known as a qui-tam lawsuit): (a) is brought by a private citizen against a person or organization whom that citizen believes violated the law; (b) alleges that the person or organization failed to perform work for the government that it was contracted to do, *and* (c) *alleges violations for which the statute provides penalties.* In these lawsuits, the whistle-blower is authorized by the provisions in the statutes to prosecute a claim on behalf of the government and receive part of any recovery (DeLancey, Nash, Smith, & Allen, 2014). In some instances, the federal or state government will intervene and become a party to the suit in order to guarantee success and be part of any negotiations and conduct of the case ("Qui Tam action," 2015). Throughout this process, the identity of the whistle-blower is intended to remain confidential.

In the context of providing health care, whistle-blower actions are typically brought for alleged violations of the FCA—that is, a long-term care provider will submit billing under the Medicare or Medicaid program for services that were not provided or were far in excess of what the patient actually needed. Whistle-blowers are often current or former employees or contractors who have knowledge of the billing practices and protocols of the facility.

Primary LTC Risk Areas

Given the number of regulations, it is not surprising that LTC providers face significant exposure from a variety of sources. As such, healthcare providers who become the subject of scrutiny often will have challenges on many different fronts: criminally, civilly, and through some regulatory action.

Criminal Prosecution

In many cases, criminal prosecution and conviction of individuals or organizations who violate the law result in incarceration and the strong likelihood of being placed on national databases, such as the Office of Inspector General's Excluded Providers list. (Being placed on this list would preclude any further participation as a provider of services that would be reimbursed by the federal or state healthcare programs.) In addition, if the criminal conduct involved misappropriation of funds, restitution of the monies, including a multiplier, is often part of the penalty. For organizations that bill the Medicare or Medicaid programs, most criminal prosecution is brought for violations of the FCA or the Anti-Kickback Statute.

Regulatory Risks

During the survey process, deficiencies may be discovered. Depending upon the scope and severity of the deficiency (or deficiencies), additional surveys are conducted. If the problems identified are severe enough, monetary penalties (daily and/or cumulatively) are imposed by the state agency, and often CMS. CMS may also initiate the denial of payments for new admissions, implementation of interim management, or revocation of the Medicare provider number. In any of these situations, the provider is encouraged to seek legal counsel and involvement *before* the penalties go into effect.

Civil Litigation

State statutes may provide for a longer statute of limitations, the imposition of punitive damages, the recovery of attorney's fees (by the plaintiff only), and little to no cap on general damages. In addition to the damages recoverable, civil litigation distracts employees and organizational administration from their purpose of resident care by pulling facility staff members into the discovery process and subjecting them to depositions, written interrogatories, requests to produce documents, and trial as necessary. For many residents or their family members, civil litigation is a viable alternative for perceived wrongs, especially given the potential for significant monetary recovery.

Compliance Program Necessities

Many healthcare providers have been required to implement compliance programs, either by operation of a statute or submission to a corporate integrity agreement (CIA).

Under the Patient Protection Affordable Care Act (ACA), each skilled nursing organization receiving federal or state monies (Medicare or Medicaid) shall "have in operation a compliance and ethics program that is effective in preventing and detecting criminal, civil and administrative violations under this Act and in promoting quality of care consistent with regulations" (42 USC §1301 et seq.). Further, the burden of demonstrating the operational effectiveness of the compliance program rests upon the facility (Office of Inspector General, Department of Health and Human Services, 2000).

ACA Guidelines

Per the ACA, the compliance program must contain:

1. Established standards and procedures that are to be followed by employees and agents, that are reasonably capable of reducing the prospect of criminal, civil, or administrative violations;

2. Specific individual(s) who are high enough placed in the organization to have overall responsibility to oversee the compliance and

ethics program and have enough resources and authority to assure compliance;

3.   Standards and protocols *not* to delegate authority to individuals, whom the organization knows or should know have a propensity to engage in prohibited criminal, civil, or administrative conduct. This tenet requires that the organization have some sort of screening process to ensure that those with authority within the facility have not previously engaged in prohibited criminal, civil, or regulatory conduct;

4.   An effective means to communicate the compliance and ethics program to the employees and agents—either through training programs or distributing written materials in such a way that these individuals understand the basic tenets of the program;

5.   Reasonable monitoring/auditing systems to detect any criminal, civil, or administrative violations. This system of monitoring must include a system that allows employees and agents to report violations without the fear of reprisal;

6.   An enforcement process with disciplinary mechanisms for individuals who are violating the program and for those who know or should have known of the violations and did not report them;

7.   A means for the organization to respond appropriately to violations and take reasonable steps to report the event as necessary and take action to reduce the risk for reoccurrence;

8.   A system to reassess the program and make changes as necessary to reflect current regulation changes within the organization.

The OIG has also issued numerous guidelines relative to the implementation of compliance programs within the healthcare industry. As these guidelines pertain to skilled nursing facilities, the OIG has issued two notices as follows: publication of the OIG Compliance Program Guidance for Nursing facilities in 2000 (Office of Inspector General, Department of Health and Human Services, 2000) and OIG Supplemental Compliance Program Guidance for Nursing facilities in 2008 (Office of Inspector General, Department of Health and Human Services, 2008). These resources, in conjunction with other guidance from the OIG and review of CIA programs that have been developed, are the primary ones a facility utilizes to build a CCP in accordance with the ACA.

2000 Office of Inspector General (OIG) Guidelines

The overarching goal of the CCP requirement is "reducing fraud and abuse, enhancing operational functions, improving the quality of health care services, and decreasing the cost of health care" (Office of Inspector General, Department of Health and Human Services, 2000). To accomplish this, the government has enacted legislation that incentivizes the public sector to report misuse/abuse of government monies.

In the 2000 guidelines, the requirements for an effective CCP are very broadly drafted, and in many ways, the ACA mimics these guidelines. Specifically, the OIG calls for the following:

1. The development and distribution of written standards of conduct (a code of conduct) *and* written policies, procedures, and protocols that promote compliance. These policies must address specific areas of potential fraud, abuse, claims, quality, physician relationships, and relationships with outside contractors. It is expected that the code of conduct summarize the basic legal principles under which the organization operates, that it be written in a manner that is easily understood by staff members, and that it be distributed to all affected employees.

2. The designation of a compliance officer and other appropriate committees charged with the responsibility of developing, operating, and monitoring the CCP. This compliance officer must report directly to the owner, governing body, and/or the CEO of the facility.

3. Effective education and training programs for all affected employees concerning the CCP must be implemented.

4. Communication lines between the corporate compliance officer and employees must be in place. The OIG encourages a "hotline number" or similar mechanism to allow employees or members of the public to make reports anonymously and protect from retaliation. It is further recommended that any reporting mechanism be available 24 hours a day, 7 days a week.

5. An audit mechanism to allow for evaluation of the compliance techniques that have been implemented. The audit program should help identify problem areas and reduce the risk for further issues. Risk areas identified by the OIG include quality of care, resident rights, billing/cost reporting, employee screening, kickbacks, inducements, and self-referrals.

6. Policies and procedures to screen and preclude individuals/entities from providing services to residents if they have been excluded from the program. There must also be disciplinary protocols for individuals/entities that have violated the compliance program.

7.   A system, including policies and procedures, to investigate identified problems, create corrective action plans to reduce reoccurrence, and report/repay as required by law.

2008 Supplemental Office of Inspector General Guidelines

The supplemental guidelines were issued to provide further clarification/recommendations to skilled nursing facilities and expanded the discussion regarding particular focus areas, including: quality of care, submission of accurate claims, Anti-Kickback Statute, and other risk areas, including physician relationships, HIPAA, Medicare Part D, and anti-supplementation. Per the OIG, there had been sufficient changes in the delivery of health care in the skilled nursing setting, the manner in which relationships with vendors had developed, and the reimbursement process to warrant the supplemental guidelines. The supplemental guidelines are to be read and implemented in conjunction with the 2000 guidelines.

Quality of Care

Every provider of LTC services understands that "quality of care" encompasses more than clinical nursing care. It is a compilation of the skills and experience in every department: operations/administration, dietary, activities, social services, maintenance, medical records, and a host of consultants and other professionals. The CCP quality of care component must focus on the following areas.

Sufficient staffing

Most state and federal regulations concerning staffing have left much to be desired. Some states have attempted to define staffing requirements by using a formula to calculate minimum nursing hours per patient day (PPD). However, these formulas fail to consider the needs of each specific resident or the skills and abilities of each care provider.

Federal regulations relating to resident assessment protocols provide additional information regarding staffing. Specifically, 42 CFR section 483.20(k)(3) states, "(3) The services provided or arranged by the facility must—(i) Meet professional standards of quality and (ii) Be provided by qualified persons in accordance with each resident's written plan of care."

Interpretive guidelines from this section further advise that the services being provided are done so by appropriately qualified personnel.

Federal regulations provide that "The facility must have sufficient staff to provide nursing and related services to attain or maintain the highest practicable physical, mental and psychosocial well-being of each resident, as determined by resident assessments and individualized plans of care" (42 CFR section 483.30). Section 483.30(a) goes on to state that "the facility must provide services by sufficient numbers to each of the following types of personnel on a 24-hour basis to provide nursing care to all residents in accordance with the resident care plans."

The OIG's 2008 CCP guideline recognizes that skilled nursing facilities are required to provide sufficient staffing to assist each resident in attaining or maintaining his highest physical, mental, and psychosocial well-being and that the relationship between actual nursing personnel on the floor and the staff's competency and the quality of care being delivered cannot be reduced to a single mathematical equation. Therefore, the OIG requires that the skilled nursing facility's CCP have systems and procedures in place to: (a) monitor the resident population and their care needs; (b) continuously evaluate whether there is sufficient competently trained staff to perform the functions of providing resident care; and (c) revise the staffing models and approaches regularly in order to meet the objects set forth in the federal regulations. Only through the constant reassessment process can the organization account for resident acuity, staff turnover, and other challenges the facility encounters on a regular basis.

Comprehensive Resident Care Plans

The dissonance as to what qualifies as an adequate, comprehensive care plan has been debated for many years. In the past, the care plan was often treated as a formality—just another document that had to be created and placed in the medical record. Recently, there has been a substantial push by care providers and surveyors alike that the care plan: (a) identify the individual needs of each resident; (b) contain realistic interventions/treatment modalities created for each resident to address the identified needs; and (c) have goals and objectives consistent with the resident's overall condition. As such, the CCP's care plan policies must be consistent and bring together all of the disciplines involved in providing resident care: the physicians(s), nursing, dietary, social services, activities, rehabilitation, and so forth. The manner and method of accomplishing this task are left to the individual facility. However, it is recommended that the CCP policies and procedures reflect the need for regular care plan meetings (sometimes referred to as interdisciplinary team meetings) involving all necessary departments, as well as documentation of who attended and the nature of the discussion and intended interventions.

One of the most important themes addressed by the OIG, and often overlooked in the long-term care setting, is that the resident's physician is charged with overall supervision of the resident's care plan. Too often, the physicians defer to the nurses and care providers on staff at the facility in identifying the resident's needs, creating achievable goals for the resident, and then implementing procedures to carry out those goals. The OIG specifically states,

> Facilities must also include the attending [physician] in the development of the resident's care plans.... Nursing facilities should evaluate, in conjunction with the attending physicians, how best to ensure physician participation—whether via consultation and post meeting debriefing, or telephone or personal attendance at meetings with a focus on serving the best interest of the resident and complying with applicable regulations. (OIG, Federal Register, September 2008)

This is not to say that the physician is solely responsible for the care plan. Rather, the physician must be involved and aware of the needs that have been identified by the various disciplines involved in the resident care. The physician must also agree with the goals that have been articulated and the means of achieving these goals. Finally, the physician must confirm that the goals are reasonable in light of the resident's overall condition and disease processes.

From a litigation and regulatory enforcement perspective, failure in any of these areas creates the impression that facility did not address the individual needs of the resident. For example, a resident with severe dementia who has just suffered a massive stroke resulting in significant paralysis will unlikely achieve his level of physical functioning before the stroke. Rather a more realistic outcome is that the resident may learn to perform some ADLs with limited assistance. So, too, a resident who has some self-care deficits but is completely ambulatory may not need a turning and repositioning program. It is incumbent upon the facility to recognize the needs of each individual resident and create both short- and long-term care plans addressing those needs.

Medication Management

The phrase "medication management" is an effort to encompass all of the various entities involved in establishing the medication protocol for each individual resident, including the physician(s) and their designees, pharmacy, and the nurses providing the daily care. The multidisciplinary approach is necessary due to the significant concerns related to polypharmacy and the costs (both physical and monetary) associated with multiple medication use.

Polypharmacy (the use of multiple medications and/or the administration of more medications than are clinically indicated, representing unnecessary drug use) is common among elderly residents. Studies suggest that polypharmacy continues to increase and is a known risk factor in morbidity and mortality of elderly residents. For further explanation, see Chapter 12.

Medication therapy is often necessary in the maintenance and prevention of medical conditions that are common with the aging process. However, the use of multiple medications leads to complex drug regimens, which may further increase complications as well as the possibility of adverse drug and disease interactions. This is in large part is due to the existing frail/fragile nature of the elderly.

According to studies, "Individuals 65 years and older make up >13% of the population, but they consume approximately 30% of all prescription medications. Older individuals account for > $3 billion in annual prescription drug sales. Also, 61% of this specific patient population is taking one prescription drug, and most take an average of 3 to 5 medications. Nearly 46% of all elderly individuals admitted to hospitals in the United States may be taking 7 medications (Terrie, 2004). A study of 33,301 nursing facility residents found that an average of 6.7 medications was ordered per resident, with 27% of residents taking nine or more medications" (Tobias & Sey, 2001).

Research findings suggest that between 35% and 53% of assisted living residents receive one or more psychotropic medications. Further, more than half of community-dwelling older adults who are admitted to nursing homes receive psychotropic medications within 2 weeks of their admission. In a study of older adults with dementia in nursing homes and acute care geriatric units, 87% of patients were taking one psychotropic medication, 66% were taking two, 36% were taking three, and 11% were taking four or more.

Federal OBRA regulations address "unnecessary drugs," noting that "Each resident's drug regimen must be free from unnecessary drugs." An unnecessary drug is any drug when used:

1. In excessive dose (including duplicate therapy); or

2. For excessive duration

3. Without adequate monitoring or without adequate indications for use; or

4. In the presence of adverse consequences that indicate the dose should be reduced or discontinued;

5. or any combination of the reason above (42 Code of Federal Regulations § 483.25(l)).

OBRA interpretive guidelines on the subject emphasize the organization's requirement to regularly reassess the medication protocol on a monthly basis or more often if necessary for each resident in conjunction with the resident's physician and pharmacist. Utilization of nonpharmacologic interventions, such as ice or hot packs, range of motion exercises, or pillows for comfort, to either reduce or eliminate medication is preferred.

The OIG guidelines emphasize the use of licensed pharmacists within the LTC setting. Pharmacists should specialize in the needs of older adults and work with the organization to review the medication regimen of each resident, note any irregularities, establish a system of records to account for controlled drugs and the disposition of same, and be involved in assisting the facility in reducing the medications taken by each resident so that unnecessary drugs are not given.

> Relationships established with pharmacists or any outside consultant must be compliant with other statutes addressed in this chapter.

To achieve the objectives set out in the OBRA regulations and the OIG guidelines, the organization's CCP must have policies and procedures that address the pharmacists' duties and obligations within the organization, an interdisciplinary approach to medication management, including physician involvement, and a system for staff to identify negative medication interactions and communicate with the physician.

Appropriate Use of Psychotropic Medications

A psychotropic medication is defined as a medication that affects mental activity, behavior, or perception, as a mood-altering drug and is often used as a tranquilizer, sedative, or antidepressant. These medications are commonly administered to individuals who exhibit behavior and/or psychiatric symptoms (MedicineNet, 2012).

In the skilled nursing setting, OBRA regulations and the OIG guidelines emphasize appropriate use of psychotropic medications. Both address the concerns of utilizing psychotropic medication as a chemical restraint or to treat a medical condition that is not specifically documented in the resident's clinical record. Analysis of antipsychotic use by 693,000 Medicare nursing home residents revealed that 28.5% of the doses received were excessive and 32.2% lacked appropriate indications for use (Tobias & Sey, 2001).

Because of this problem and the consequences for overuse/misuse, it is incumbent upon the skilled nursing organization, in conjunction with the resident's attending physician, to ensure appropriate use of these medications.

> Staff may not use psychotropic medication as a discipline or for their own convenience in order to address a resident behavior problem.

The CCP program and the policies and procedures implemented must use an *interdisciplinary approach* to psychotropic medication use. This means that the mental health therapist (psychiatrist or psychologist) must work in conjunction with the primary medical doctor, the pharmacists, nursing staff, and the other professionals on the interdisciplinary team. To the extent that psychotropic medications assist each resident in achieving or maintaining their highest practicable physical, mental, and psychosocial well-being, the use of these medications may be appropriate. However, if modalities may be implemented that forgo the use of such medication, it is incumbent upon the facility to attempt these approaches.

Resident Safety

Resident safety within the confines of the OIG CCP guidelines is quite limited. Resident safety as addressed in the OBRA guidelines speaks to a much larger obligation upon the skilled nursing facility staff.

> Pursuant to the OBRA regulations, resident safety encompasses a host of adverse events: falls, medication errors, and injuries of known and unknown origin. The facility must maintain policies and procedures in compliance with OBRA regulations to ensure resident safety.

The 2008 OIG guidelines require that the facility have policies and procedures in place to address any mistreatment (abuse or neglect) within the organization. This requirement addresses mistreatment or neglect by staff *and other residents* and the policies and procedures that must be implemented to reduce the risk to the residents and promote their safety. These policies and procedures must include a mechanism whereby staff and contractors are advised of the prohibition against abuse or neglect of residents and are screened prior to working with the elderly/disabled residents.

Secondarily, the organization must have established means of collecting information concerning abuse and/or neglect in a confidential manner (i.e., an effective reporting system that operates both internally through a chain of command and externally through a toll-free call-in "hotline"). Individuals who report problems must be assured that such reports are taken very seriously and that the organization maintains a no-retaliation policy. Finally, the facility must have procedures to investigate and report allegations or suspicions of abuse and neglect pursuant to both state and federal regulations. It is recommended that legal counsel be consulted as the organization designs the means and methods of investigating and reporting elder abuse and neglect.

In order to achieve these objectives, the organization must have a mechanism for recruiting and hiring appropriate individuals. Employees must be regularly trained on the policies and procedures, including what constitutes abuse and neglect, prevention, and the reporting obligations of any suspicions or allegations of abuse or neglect. Documenting the training and education should be maintained in a manner that is accessible should issues arise. Staff must also be screened through the OIG database, reference checks, nursing board reviews, and, for some organizations, background checks. The screening process for employees must be done on a fairly regular basis to ensure that new violations/problems are identified.

There should also be a screening process for residents so that the organization admits only those residents who are appropriate for placement and will not cause harm to other residents. Potential residents may be screened through review of medical records, interviews, and review of national databases, such as Megan's Law. For example, review of a potential resident reveals that he has a known history of violence and sexual deviance. If the resident is mobile, he may require a specialized care plan, including 1:1 monitoring.

Submission of Accurate Claims

The submission of false and/or fraudulent claims is prohibited. Submission of such a claim may result in the individual or entity being subject to criminal prosecution, civil liability, treble damages, penalties, and possible exclusion from the federal and/or state healthcare programs. Due to the interdisciplinary approach to resident care, the organization must be acutely aware of the risk associated with false/fraudulent billing and implement mechanisms to reduce their occurrence. For example, a therapy company providing services within an LTC setting must be attuned to patient needs and provide the services best suited for the individual patient, regardless of insurance benefits or billing rates. The organization, which has the contract with the therapy company, must also be aware of the therapy services being provided, ensuring that they are consistent with the patient's overall treatment plan. To ensure that all members of the interdisciplinary team are aware of the interplay between services and false/fraudulent billing, there must be appropriate training, a means of double- and triple-checking the billing, and an independent auditing system.

The OIG guidelines focus on ensuring that organizations properly report the resident case mix. There must also be appropriate accounting for therapy services (ensuring appropriate utilization and billing) and that individuals or entities that are excluded from the federal healthcare program are not employed by the organization and the organization. Finally, the organization is also prohibited from maintaining any contracts with excluded individuals or entities and those that provide restorative and personal care services.

- Resident case mix: The organization is reimbursed by the federal healthcare program in accordance with the resident's assessment of needs and services or RUG score. As such, the importance and accuracy of the resident assessment must be an integral part of the compliance program, which should include training of the interdisciplinary team members.

RUG stands for resource utilization group. Since July 1, 1998, RUGs are at the core of the SNF payment system under Medicare Part A. The MDS is used to capture resident clinical and functional characteristics, to generate/determine payment categories.

- Therapy services: These services may be billed under both Medicare and Medicaid and are at significant risk for abuse. Specifically, if the resident receives too much therapy—that is, beyond what is necessary for the resident's medical condition—the facility may have engaged in the submission of false claims. Further, if the resident does not receive sufficient therapy, the organization may found at fault for failing to assist the resident in attaining or maintaining his highest practicable quality of life. The compliance program must address appropriate utilization of therapy services and RUG classifications and ensure that therapy services are provided to residents who need the services and in a manner delineated by the provider orders and resident care plan.

> Therapy services are appropriate only when: (a) There is a physician order; (b) it is performed under the direction of a licensed therapist; (c) the resident's care plan identifies realistic goals; and (d) the resident is discharged from therapy when he has reached his goal *or* he has plateaued and no further improvement is expected.
>
> Bottom line: Therapy cannot drive patient care.

- Screening for excluded individuals and entities: Organizations may not hire, retain, or contract with individuals/entities that have been excluded from participation in the federal healthcare program. As such, the organization must implement policies and procedures to: (a) screen prospective employees and contractors and (b) create/implement systems for ongoing screening on at least an annual basis; however, more often is recommended. This is particularly true for any owners, officers, directors, and agents within the SNF or who provide services to the SNF.

- Restorative and personal care: The services that are provided within the skilled nursing organization and for which the facility gets paid are intended to assist each resident in maintaining/attaining his highest practicable physical, mental, and psychosocial well-being. To achieve this goal, the facility should implement systems to address the quality of care being provided. These systems may include employee interviews, resident/family member interviews, analysis of quality indicators, review and analysis of medical record keeping, and/or consultations with physicians and other contractors—in other words, a self-auditing system that is consistently reviewed.

Anti-Kickback Statute (AKS)

The AKS prohibits remuneration to or from any business entity, in order to induce or reward for a referral or generation of federal healthcare program business. This includes providing gifts, money, or anything of value, as a reward for business that will be billed to the Medicare or Medicaid programs. Many LTC providers fail to recognize the significance of this prohibition and how it pertains to organizational "practices." For example, during the holidays, many LTC providers give gifts to hospital discharge planners, or receive gifts from vendors as part of the "holiday spirit." Regardless of how "innocent" the intentions, the giving/receiving of gifts may be perceived as inducements for referrals and may be violative of the AKS. Such a violation often results in liability under the False Claims Act, civil monetary penalties, criminal prosecution, and exclusion from the Medicare and Medicaid programs.

There is a presumption that a violation of the AKS results in the submission of a false claim. Specifically, if referrals are being made to the federal healthcare program in exchange for a kickback, the necessity of the referral is automatically questioned.

Of particular concern are the following:

- The provision of free goods and services in exchange for referrals.

- Service contracts with nonphysicians (pharmacies, durable medical equipment, laboratories, diagnostic testing, rehabilitation services, home health services, etc.) at a reduced or discounted rate to generate referrals.

- Service contracts with physicians; physicians must be available to skilled nursing facilities to perform a variety of services, such as guiding specific resident care, providing medical director services, and assisting with quality assurance and infection control. However, physicians are directly able to generate referrals to the federal healthcare program or increase RUG scores. Therefore, these relationships must be closely monitored to ensure compliance with the AKS.

- Discounts/swapping; the government wants to encourage competition between providers of healthcare services. For example, if a radiology company is able to offer a quality service for a reduced price, the government encourages such behavior. The difficulty is that in some instances, discounts or swapping of services in exchange for referrals to the federal or state healthcare programs cannot be factored into the contract or negotiated price. Further, any such discounts must be reported through cost reports.

- Hospices; arrangements with hospices are subject to close scrutiny. Hospice by definition is designed for end-of-life care. According to guidelines enacted in 2013, "end of life" is considered 6 months or less to live. Hospice services are not intended to provide "additional nursing services" to residents who are not diagnosed with a terminal illness. Skilled nursing facilities must pay close attention to ensure residents receiving hospice services meet appropriate criteria and that the relationship with the hospice provider is not simply a conduit for future referrals.

* Reserved bed payments; contracts whereby a referring entity, such as a hospital, reserves beds within skilled nursing facilities may easily violate the AKS conditions—specifically, the contracts must be closely scrutinized to ensure that it is not contingent upon the volume of residents referred to the facility, or that the organization is failing to keep the beds open (i.e., receiving payments for reserved beds and also receiving additional payments because the beds are occupied; double dipping).

Because of the close monitoring of these relationships, facilities are encouraged to seek specific guidance from a qualified healthcare lawyer to determine if a business relationship violates the AKS or if an exception (often referred to as a safe harbor) exists (U.S. Department of Justice, n.d.).

Physician Relations

Physicians are in a position to easily generate referrals to the federal or state healthcare programs. As such, physicians are prohibited from engaging in certain behaviors (also referred to as the Stark laws; refer to Chapter 8 for further explanation). Because skilled nursing facilities must comply with physician orders unless contraindicated, organizations should monitor referral habits of the physicians providing care to residents. For example, physicians who refer directly to a laboratory company or a therapy company may be doing so because the physician maintains an inappropriate relationship with that laboratory or therapy company. For this reason, the organization may want to investigate further to determine if the physician is violating AKS, FCA, or the Stark laws. It is further encouraged that some form of screening program for physicians be created. Such a screening program may be modeled on those currently used by acute care hospitals and involve ensuring physicians are appropriately qualified to provide services to the organization's residents, that they have appropriate licensure and liability insurance, and that they agree in writing to comply with the federal and state laws governing the provision of services. With such a program, skilled nursing facilities retain the ability to "remove privileges" from physicians who fail to comply with these parameters.

Anti-Supplementation

In receiving a contract to provide services to Medicare or Medicaid beneficiaries, skilled nursing facilities also agree to accept as full and final payment the amounts paid under these programs, for the covered services. As such, the organization may not seek further payment from the resident, family, or referring entity (e.g., hospital), for items that are part of the covered service(s) and for which the organization has or will be paid. (The organization may seek reimbursement for services that are not part of the covered services, including the portion of the services that is the responsibility of the resident. This is also known as the "share of costs.")

Medicare Part D

Residents of skilled nursing facilities have the right to choose a Medicare Part D plan. The facility's obligation in this regard is to assist the resident in choosing the best plan that meets his medication profile. Under no circumstances may the facility accept any payments from any plan or pharmacy in exchange for influencing a resident to sign up for a particular plan or service.

HIPAA

The guidelines relative to securing protected health information (PHI) are extensive. Skilled nursing facilities and other healthcare providers have long been required to protect this information; however, with the advent of electronic medical record keeping, mobile devices, extensive use of social media, e-mails, and texting, it is incumbent upon the organization to develop protocols to guide employees, contractors, and agents on appropriate behavior. There must be methods of encryption and means of ensuring the safe storage, transmission, access to, and disposal of PHI. In the event of disaster the organization should have protocols that can be followed. The facility must have business associate (BA) agreements with noncovered entities relative to ensuring HIPAA guidelines are being met. Finally, there must be auditing systems to ensure compliance. More details concerning BA agreements and covered and noncovered entities may be found in Chapters 8 and 10.

The CCP envisioned by the ACA and the OIG must reflect an interdisciplinary approach, including all of the professionals providing care within and to the SNF. Fortunately, the OIG also recognizes the unique nature of the services provided to skilled nursing residents and understands that each facility may have particular circumstances that need to be addressed.

The OIG states, "A nursing facility should tailor its compliance measures to address identified risk areas and fit the unique environment of the facility (including its structure, operations, resources, the needs of its resident population and prior enforcement experience. In short, OIG recommends that each nursing facility establish policies and procedures reflecting the OIG guidelines and organization's commitment to a culture of ethical behavior" (OIG, Federal Register, September 2008).

Effective Risk Management

Quality Assurance and Risk Management

In the past, risk management was supported by the general/professional liability insurer. Efforts were made to reduce negative events because such events would impact insurance rates and reinsurance efforts. Given today's litigious environment, the organization must take control of risk management efforts, work internally with staff, externally with consultants, and incorporate advice from legal counsel to create a robust risk management structure.

Some well-known risk areas are:

- Weight/nutrition/hydration
- Wounds
- Fall/safety
- Infections
- HIPAA/privacy rights
- Medication management/ psychotropic drug use
- Billing
- Utilization review/rehabilitation services
- Staffing (hours/overtime/turnover)
- Business relationships/contracts
- Disaster prevention/ preparedness
- Marketing tactics

But what is risk management (RM)? In short, it is management's understanding of the scope of risks that exist in the LTC setting, and efforts made by management to reduce that risk. RM encompasses an immediate response to an incident or occurrence as well as review of the facility's system to prevent the incident/event from occurring. The QA component involves taking the lessons learned from the individual incident and analyzing the systems that led to the incident to determine if modifications/changes need to occur on an organization-wide basis (see Figures 7.1 and 7.2).

In establishing effective RM programs (that incorporate the CCP), the organization needs to create a structure that addresses: Who will be primarily responsible for the program(s)? What will the chain of command look like? Who will have responsibility relative to: (a) identifying incidents or breakdowns in the system; (b) conducting an investigation/analysis of the incident/breakdown; and (c) making a determination of whether the event is reportable to the state governing agency and/or the insurer? Once the structure is created, an analysis needs to be done to determine: (a) what

QUALITY ASSURANCE

An analysis of systems in order to improve the quality of care provided within the facility.

- A skilled nursing facility is required to maintain a quality assessment and assurance committee. (42 USC section 1396r (b)(1)(B).
- The purpose of the QA committee is to identify and develop plans to correct deficiencies in the quality of care provided to the residents. (42 USC section 1396r (b)(1)(B)
- Quality assurance committees are "key internal mechanisms that allow nursing homes to deal with quality concerns in a confidential manner and help them sustain a culture of quality improvement." (Quality Assurance in nursing homes, January 2003 at p 2.)
- Documents prepared by QA or gathered at the request of the QA department, are usually not discoverable.

QUALITY ASSURANCE DOCUMENTS SHOULD NOT BE DISCLOSED TO ANY PERSON OR COMMITTEE OUTSIDE OF QA. TO DO SO WOULD LIKELY WAIVE ANY PROTECTIONS.

INCIDENT REPORTS

An analysis of individual events in order to determine what occurred and reduce the risk of reoccurrence.

- In response to an adverse event/occurrence.

- Upcoming litigation is suspected.

- Investigations/interviews are done by or at the request of legal counsel.

- Information obtained is in anticipation of litigation and therefore may qualify as work product.

- Investigation may be privileged and not subject to disclosure to regulatory agencies or in civil litigation.

INCIDENT REPORTS SHOULD NOT BE DISCLOSED TO ANY PERSON/ENTITY THAT IS NOT IN PRIVITY WITH THE RM DEPARTMENT OR FACILITY ATTORNEY. TO DO SO WOULD LIKELY WAIVE ANY PROTECTIONS.

Figure 7.1   Quality Assurance Incident Reports

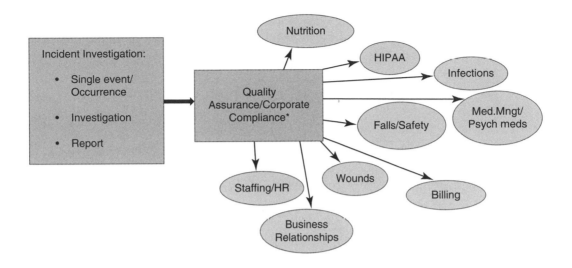

Figure 7.2   Incident Investigation

systems exist; and (b) what systems need improvement. Prioritizing those items needing immediate attention is recommended.

> It is recommended that each individual facility maintain a RM program, under the governance of the executive director/administrator. To the extent that the facility is part of a larger organizational structure, any RM issue may then be reported to counsel or a resource center for further guidance.

To facilitate this process, a root cause analysis (RCA) may need to be done by reviewing objective and subjective data. Sources of data include: events or incidents, survey results, audits, billing records, utilization review reports, quality indicators, staff turnover, interviews with staff and residents, resident council meetings, interdisciplinary meetings, pharmacy reports, laboratory reports, and contractors/vendors, as well as a host of other sources. Interviewing litigation counsel also provides insight into areas for concern.

Root Cause Analysis

1. Define the problem: What do you see happening? What specific symptoms are occurring?

    Example: Resident had a fall at 3 A.M.

2. Collect data specific to the issue.

    Example: Was the resident injured as a result of the fall? Is there a history of falls? A change in condition that contributed to the fall? What footwear was the resident wearing? What occurred immediately before and after the fall? Is the resident incontinent? Was there a change in medications? What was the staff doing before the fall, at the time of the fall, and immediately after?

    The situation must be fully analyzed. To maximize the effectiveness of the RCA, the staff directly caring for the resident must be interviewed, the resident (and possibly family members, guests, or roommates) need(s) to be interviewed, and documents must be reviewed, including the resident's medical chart, staffing records, call light logs, infection control records, maintenance records, and so forth.

Analyze the Data

Look for possible causal factors and patterns. Example: How many falls have occurred within the past few months? Are sleep cycle patterns being honored? What are the common themes between each of these falls? Has there been any increase in the number of falls? If so, are there any changes that might be contributing factors?

The focus of the questioning needs to revolve around what *possible* factors caused or contributed to the event. During this stage, identify as many causal factors as possible. Too often, people identify one or two factors and then stop, which is ineffective. Often, the root cause of the problem requires the investigator to drill down—breaking the problem into smaller, detailed parts to better understand the big picture.

Identify the Root Cause(s)

Example: Resident A fell attempting to get out of bed to go to the bathroom. Resident did not utilize the call light. Per resident interview, the call light was not within easy reach. The call light was found on the side of the bed, out of reach of the resident. Interviews with Nurse Assistant (NA) 1 reveal that the resident was assessed 15 minutes before the event. Per NA 1, resident did not need to use the restroom. Analysis of other falls in the preceding month reveals a 50% increase in resident falls during the night shift; 30% of these falls occurred with NA 1. Analysis further reveals that there was one "call-off" (one staff member failed to report for a scheduled shift).

In this scenario, what is the real reason the problem occurred? Is the issue staffing? Is the issue training? Is the issue resident noncompliance with instructions? Using the same tools to identify the causal factors, the roots of each factor need to be reviewed.

Recommend and Implement Solutions

Example: Disciplinary action of NA 1? Further training for NA 1? Further training for all staff regarding the issues presented? Implementation of a bowel and bladder program for Resident A? Identifying a means of ensuring the call light remains within easy reach? Providing Resident A with a bedside commode? Implementation of additional staff to account for call-offs?

Once the root cause is identified, measures must be implemented to reduce reoccurrence of the problem. Who will be responsible for implementing the solution(s)? Who will be responsible for training staff on the policies/procedures that have been designed to prevent reoccurrence? Training must be performed by qualified individuals, and the persons trained must be able to demonstrate an understanding of the new process.

Reassess to Determine Efficacy

Once a solution is determined, a monitoring/reassessment program must also occur. This audit of the program must ensure that the solution is working. In conducting the audit, many of the same tools are used: Analyze the cause-and-effect process, identifying changes needed for various systems. Analyze the effects of programs implemented. By doing so, potential failures may be identified *before* they occur (e.g., Has the rate of resident falls decreased? Are residents found with their call lights within reach? What is the status of staffing? Are staff arriving at their shifts prepared to provide professional resident care?).

An effective RM program in conjunction with the CCP is essential to any healthcare organization. By utilizing available data and staff with direct knowledge of residents and issues, the program is an effective tool as it leverages technology, existing resources, and information already being collected. Further, by identifying and responding to resident and family emotional needs through the RCA process, the organization demonstrates its resident-centered approach to healthcare delivery. In sum, a data-driven risk management program has demonstrated the ability to:

- Improve reimbursement accuracy
- Reduce survey deficiencies
- Obtain more accurate QI measures
- Reduce the occurrence of negative incidents
- Improve compliance with state and federal agencies
- Reduce professional liability premiums [and litigation]
- Improve public relations/marketing efforts (DeNatale, 2010)

Compliance Through Documentation

"The best defense is a good offense" is an old adage often used in sports and military endeavors. To weather the challenges of external investigations, litigation, or prosecution, it is best to keep the internal mechanisms as healthy as possible. This includes appropriate policies and procedures, mechanisms to train staff and perform regular audits, and implementing corrections as necessary. To create the offense, sufficient and accurate documentation is essential.

Medical Record

The resident medical record is a vital component in any organization that provides health-related services to the elderly. Too often, the medical record is simply overlooked when care providers are performing the more important task of actually giving the care. The recordation of what occurred may be done at the end of the shift and after the care provider has dealt with numerous other issues. As such, critical items that should have been recorded may not be.

Further, healthcare professionals typically "chart by exception"—that is, significant issues are noted, such as vital signs and the general condition of the resident, with some discussion about the specific issue being addressed. If there is no problem, nothing would be noted. This practice often gives the impression *to external reviewers* that nothing was done.

Another area of concern is improper medical charting. For example, a healthcare professional forgets to write a note or document a specific issue and then attempts to amend the medical record without noting the "late entry." Electronic medical record keeping is eliminating this problem.

To address the inadequate or inappropriate charting, many healthcare providers have implemented a chart review process. A comprehensive medical record review requires training and critical thinking skills with an ability to assimilate a large volume of information. A modified version involves a medical record clerk confirming that providers' orders were properly recorded and carried out, and that the nurses had charted accurately for their shift. Very rarely is the *content* of the notes reviewed to ensure accuracy. However, in the event of an incident or sudden change in condition, the medical record is the primary source of information. If the medical record is inaccurate, appears to contain "rote" information, or contains improper late entries, the organization will encounter deficiencies and litigation. The gravity of the errors is directly proportional to the significance of the penalty: the bigger the problems, the bigger the economic loss and loss to reputation.

Ensuring accurate medical record keeping begins with frontline staff who are charting.

- Staff *must* be trained that accurate medical record keeping is *as important a function* as dressing a wound or keeping a resident clean and dry. The training must be done upon hire (in order to acquaint the provider with the specific mechanisms within the organization), with continuous training throughout employment.

- An audit system must be implemented to check not only that there is documentation but also that the documentation is an accurate reflection of the resident's condition. Charting for each resident *at the end of the shift* is not a recommended practice because too much vital information may be lost from the time that the care is provided until the pen "hits the paper." Instead, charting should be completed after tasks are done.

- Identified errors must be immediately corrected *with the staff member who made the error, and a RCA should be done on what led to the error. Do not, under any circumstance, attempt to fraudulently alter the incorrect note.* Such an alteration will create an even larger problem. Specifically, the accuracy of the entire medical record may be called into question, issues of fraud will be raised, and reports to governing bodies, such as the nursing board or Department of Health Services, will be made. Such errors should be submitted to the quality assurance committee for evaluation, investigation, and further remedial action. To the extent that the medical record must be corrected to eliminate incorrect information, advice of counsel should be sought.

Employment Files

The best gauge for a how an LTC organization treats its residents is through a review of the staff working within the organization. This means that the staff must have the necessary qualifications to perform the specific task for which they are hired. The training they receive on an ongoing basis should be identified and recorded. Further, regulations require that staff be cleared through the necessary databases (OIG excluded provider system and some form of background check) to ensure that their background/history provides a reasonable basis that the staff member will not commit illegal activities within his employment. Finally, staff must have accurate documentation in their employment file to establish that they are legally able to work and perform the job duties for which they are hired. For further information concerning employee files training, please refer to Chapter 5.

Although many organizations already have mechanisms in place to conform to the foregoing guidelines, the system often breaks down in the documentation. Just like the resident medical record, the employees' personnel file may allow the facility to successfully defend civil or regulatory actions.

QA Studies and Audits (Often Referred to as Quality Assurance Performance Improvement or QAPI)

The QA process is one of the only mechanisms that a healthcare provider may use to identify and correct a problem and have that information protected from discovery. More importantly, the efforts to improve the quality of care must be documented in a confidential manner, available only to the members of the quality assurance team. (The quality assurance team is a regulatory mandate and is further discussed in Chapter 12.)

But what to document? First the problem must be identified. Thereafter, individuals and departments must become involved in investigating the problem. Documents/studies or audits created/used in the investigation process need to be identified as QAPI and, finally, the resolution to the problem. The resolution may be new or revised policies and procedures or training mechanisms.

By documenting the events, the organization can identify opportunities for improvement. Moreover, if the organization is subject to an investigation, state and federal agencies are more amenable to helping facilities work through problems that have already been identified internally if the organization can establish that it has been making efforts to correct the issues. Accurate and timely documentation supports those efforts.

Billing Records

As discussed earlier, LTC organizations face significant problems for failing to submit accurate claims. Such problems include potential prosecution for violations of the FCA or AKS, and litigation stemming from whistle-blower actions or other regulatory violations.

To better equip itself, the organization must have a comprehensive system of "checks and balances," whereby the organization can establish that the care provided was appropriate and billed correctly—both internally *and externally*. This means that systems must be in place to audit the delivery of services (e.g., therapy, hospice, diagnostics [lab and radiology], and durable medical equipment). In some instances, the organization may receive free or discounted goods or services. In the billing mechanism, the Medicare or Medicaid must be notified and they cannot be billed at a higher rate. (If the facility is receiving a benefit from a provider, it cannot be done so with the expectation of generating referrals to the federal/state healthcare program; see AKS.)

Finally, errors that are identified must be investigated and reported per state and federal regulations and, specifically, the FCA. (It is recommended that legal counsel be consulted in this regard.)

By creating the policies and procedures, training staff, and conducting internal and external audits, the facility is better able to identify problem employees' unintentional errors and everything in between.

Incident Investigation/Reporting

Incident investigation done by or through legal counsel, *in anticipation of litigation*, may also be protected from discovery (this is state-specific). More importantly, the incident investigation should involve an RCA whereby:

- Employees are identified and questioned concerning the events giving rise to the event.

- Documents are gathered and reviewed and critical memories/information is preserved.

Unanticipated external investigation or civil litigation often arises long after the specific event—months if not year(s) later. By preserving critical information (and possibly testimony) the organization is better able to defend itself. Further, if breakdowns in systems are identified, they can be corrected, reducing the risk of reoccurrence.

Contracts With External Resources

The business relationship between an LTC provider and the entities with whom it works is critical to the ongoing vitality of the provider. As noted earlier, numerous relationships are prohibited. However, the LTC provider must be aware that it may be liable for violations of the contracted providers. Some of the most common are HIPAA violations and unknowing violations of the FCA. For example, an external provider offers to run a diagnostic test at no charge. The test will assist the staff in providing better care. However, the LTC provider is unaware that the external provider is either billing a federal/state healthcare program or conducting the test for further business that will eventually be billed. In conducting the test, the external provider may review PHI and there may need to be a physician order and informed consent obtained (i.e., verification that the resident or legally responsible person has consented to the test). In this example, there are numerous potential concerns for an LTC organization.

To deal with the potential problems, the organization should have a comprehensive contract with the external provider. The contract would outline the duties and responsibilities of each, including indemnity clauses for breaches that would expose the organization. Such contacts should be negotiated through an "arm's-length" transaction, reviewed by counsel to ensure completeness, signed and dated, and reviewed annually to address any changes.

Summary

Regulations and their interpretations, as well as the manner in which health care is delivered and changes employment regulations, change constantly. LTC providers are required to remain abreast of these changes and incorporate them into their organization. By having an active and dynamic risk management/corporate compliance program, LTC providers can better improve the economic bottom line for the facility and provide better care to the recipients of the LTC services.

Key Terms

Affordable Care Act (ACA; also referred to as the Patient Protection Affordable Care Act or PPACA): The scope and breadth of the ACA are still being revealed. However, under the ACA, long-term care providers and specifically skilled nursing facilities must have in place an effective corporate compliance program that governs the employees of the facility and its external vendors, including other licensed and unlicensed healthcare providers.

Anti-Kickback Statute: The federal Anti-Kickback Statute (AKS) is a criminal statute that prohibits the exchange (or offer to exchange) of anything of value, in an effort to induce (or reward) the referral of federal healthcare program business. The Anti-Kickback Statute is broadly drafted and establishes penalties for individuals and entities on both sides of the prohibited transaction.

Elder Justice Act (EJA): The Elder Justice Act imposes further reporting requirements upon "covered individual" where there is a "reasonable suspicion of a crime" that is committed against any individual who is a resident of a long-term healthcare facility. The EJA does not supplant any reporting state requirements of abuse or neglect. Rather, the EJA places additional reporting requirements upon the provider.

False Claims Act (FCA): A series of statutes that creates liability for any person who (a) knowingly submits a false claim to the government, (b) causes another to submit a false claim to the government, or (c) knowingly makes a false record or statement to get a false claim paid by the government. Liability also exists where one acts improperly—not to get money from the government, but to avoid having to pay money to the government or who conspires to violate the FCA.

Health Insurance Portability and Accountability Act (HIPAA): This act addresses the access and disclosure of protected health information (PHI). HIPAA was promulgated under the Civil Rights Department of the DHHS. PHI is defined as "individually identifiable health information" held or transmitted by a "covered entity" or its "business associate," in any form or media, whether electronic, paper, or oral. HIPAA applies to health plans, healthcare clearinghouses, and any healthcare provider who transmits health information in electronic form (U.S. Department of Health and Human Services, n.d.).

Omnibus Budget Reconciliation Act (OBRA as it applies to SNF): A series of regulations that govern the provision of services and administration and employee duties and responsibilities within a skilled nursing facility that is licensed through the DHHS.

Stark I and II: The federal self-referral statute prohibits physicians from referring Medicare patients for designated health services to entities with which the physician (or an immediate family member) has a financial relationship, unless an exception applies. The Stark I and Stark II statutes are part of the Omnibus Budget Reconciliation Act of 1989 (OBRA 1989) codified at 42 U.S.C. § 1395nn.42 U.S.C. § 1395NN.

Review Questions

1. Why are LTC providers subject to enhanced scrutiny?

2. Why is "quality of care" one of the critical components of an effective CCP?

3. Explain the relationship between the AKS and the False Claims Act.

4. What is risk management?

5. What is quality assurance?

6. How do risk management and quality assurance interrelate?

7. Why is appropriate documentation so important?

Case Studies

Case Study #1

Facility LVN reports to the administrator that the medication room was unlocked and she found some resident medication bubble packs missing. The exact number of missing medication and residents affected was not reported by the LVN. Devise a plan for how the administrator will respond, keeping in mind the following: Is this abuse/neglect (theft of resident property)? Is there a violation of resident privacy (HIPAA)? Who needs to be informed (state/resident/pharmacy/physician/legal counsel)?

Devise a plan for the administrator to reduce the risk of reoccurrence.

Case Study #2

An organization's administrator receives an anonymous complaint that Resident A is sexually abusing Resident B. Both Resident A and Resident B are males and reside in the same room. Resident A has severe and advanced dementia but is ambulatory. Resident B uses a wheelchair for mobility and is developmentally disabled. Facility administrator immediately separates the residents, moving Resident A into another room and initiates an investigation. Outline and explain the administrator's requirements relative to:

1. Notifying family/legal representatives of both residents.

2. Notifying the state's oversight agency regarding the allegation and results of the investigation.

3. Notifying the facility's legal/risk management department.

4. Initiating a quality assurance review.

References

DeLancey, M. M., Nash, B., Smith, A. E., & Allen, C. J. (2014). *Alert: State false claims act enforcement explodes in 2014*. Retrieved from http://www.law360.com/health/articles/542555/state-false-claims-act-enforcement-explodes-in-2014

DiNatale, P. M., & Granger, B. (March 02, 2010). *Demystify risk management in nursing homes*. Retrieved from http://www.mcknights.com/guest-columns/demystify-risk-management-in-nursing-homes/article/164835/

MedicineNet. (n.d.). *Definition of psychotropic medication*. Retrieved from http://www.medicinenet.com/script/main/art.asp?articlekey=30808

Office of Inspector General, U.S. Department of Health and Human Services. (n.d.). *Corporate integrity agreements*. Retrieved from https://oig.hhs.gov/compliance/corporate-integrity-agreements

Office of Inspector General, Department of Health and Human Services (2000a). OIG Supplemental Compliance Program guidance for nursing facilities. *Federal Register*, *65*, No. 52.

Office of Inspector General, Department of Health and Human Services (2000b). Publication of the OIG Compliance Program guidance for nursing facilities. *Federal Register*, *65*, No. 52.

Office of Inspector General, Department of Health and Human Services (2008, Sep 30). OIG Supplemental Compliance Program guidance for nursing facilities. *Federal Register*, *73*, No. 190.

Qui Tam action. (2015). In *Legal dictionary*. Retrieved from http://dictionary.law.com/default.aspx?selected=1709

Terrie, Y. C. (2004). *Understanding and managing polypharmacy in the elderly*. Retrieved from www.pharmacytimes.com/publications/issue/2004/2004-12/2004-12-9094#sthash.crYD3gwZ.dpuf

Tobias, D. E., & Sey, M. (2001). General and Psychotherapeutic medication use in 328 nursing facilities: A year 2000 national survey. *The consultant pharmacist*, *15*, 34–42.

U.S. Census Bureau. (2011). *Census bureau releases comprehensive analysis of fast-growing 90-and-older population*. Retrieved from https://www.census.gov/newsroom/releases/archives/aging_population/cb11-194.html

U.S. Department of Justice. (n.d.). *The false claims act: A primer*. Retrieved from http://www.justice.gov/civil/docs_forms/C-FRAUDS_FCA_Primer.pdf

U.S. Department of Health and Human Services. (n.d.). *Health information privacy*. Retrieved from http://www.hhs.gov/ocr/privacy/index.html

CHAPTER 8

LEGAL AND ETHICAL ISSUES

Rebecca Lowell
Eduardo Gonzalez

This chapter will explore the state and federal laws governing the operation of long-term care (LTC) services and the numerous agencies involved in the oversight of LTC providers. This chapter will also discuss investigation, reporting, and prosecution (civilly and criminally) for violations of the laws, including violations of the **Health Insurance Portability and Accountability Act (HIPAA)**, the **Anti-Kickback Statute (AKS)**, the **False Claims Act (FCA)**, federal **Elder Justice Act (EJA)**, and the numerous state regulations. As the laws are discussed, ethical issues will be presented for consideration.

Health Care as a Business

Healthcare providers work with humans, and their impact on human lives often depends upon the providers' actions or inactions. This is especially true in LTC communities, where the providers address the complicated needs of aged, medically complex individuals. However, health care is also an industry made up of numerous businesses/business models, trying to make money. Just as in any other business, healthcare providers have expenses. They must hire and pay employees, procure insurances (workers compensation, professional liability, property), purchase supplies, pay rent (or mortgage), pay taxes and licensing fees, purchase/upgrade equipment, and generate revenue.

In generating revenue, LTC providers have an ethical duty to balance care and profit/surplus. Maximizing

LEARNING OBJECTIVES

- To gain knowledge of the scope of laws governing the provision of healthcare services to long-term care recipients.

- To understand the ramifications for failing to abide by the laws governing long-term care services.

- To understand the interplay of the legal and ethical decision making in the provision of long-term care services.

- To provide practical tools to help resolve potential legal and ethical conflicts.

- To consider the long-term care provider's obligations in balancing the laws that must be complied with, the ethical concerns, the provision of services to multiple patients, and the family involvement in care.

profit cannot be at the expense of providing marginal/substandard care. Rather, the LTC provider must eliminate waste, provide quality services, and use its ethical discernment in understanding the difference.

Payer Sources

As more fully explained in Chapter 6, there are numerous payer sources. However, most residents in LTC communities pay for their care with public funding (through their federal and/or state benefits). Private funding and long-term care insurances are less frequently used. Typically, the LTC community accepts residents with any payer source with whom they have a contract.

Medicare: Medicare is divided into four different benefits: A, B, C, and D.

- **Part A.** This benefit covers (Medicare.gov, n.d.a):
  - Hospital care
  - Skilled nursing facility care ("custodial care" not covered)
  - Hospice
  - Home health services

- **Part B.** This benefit covers (Medicare.gov, n.d.b):
  - Clinical research
  - Ambulance services
  - Durable medical equipment
  - Mental health
  - Second opinion before surgery
  - Limited outpatient prescription drugs

  These benefits are available regardless of whether the resident is living in an LTC community.

- **Part C. Health maintenance organizations (HMOs)** are a Part C benefit. HMOs have a contract with Medicare to provide "Part A" benefits to Medicare beneficiaries. The beneficiary has the choice of Part A or Part C coverage. Part C benefits may be greater than Part A (lower co-pays, x-ray, laboratory, non-emergency transportation, and eye and dental coverage).

  Medicare benefits Parts A, B, and C do not pay for the cost of an assisted living facility.

- **Part D.** This benefit, also known as Prescription/Drug Coverage, provides prescription medication benefits.

Medicaid benefits: As these benefits pertain to the provision of LTC services, they are reserved for individuals who have limited personal funds or no other benefit (e.g., private insurance) to pay for such services.

While Medicaid is considered to be a "state" program (because it is managed through and uses state public funds), the program is also funded by the federal government. For example, for the period of October 1, 2014, to September 20, 2015, California received from the federal government 50% of the total amount spent, by the state, in Medicaid (Office of the Assistant Secretary for Planning and Evaluation, 2015).

Medicaid benefits may change from state to state, but generally speaking, Medicaid will pay for long-term "**custodial care**." Other benefits may include nursing services, respiratory therapy, oxygen and other equipment, personal hygiene items, such as denture cleaners and dental floss, hair trims, wheelchairs, incontinence supplies, and non-legend drugs.

The Medicaid reimbursement rate is lower than any other payer source. As such, LTC community operators may be tempted to exclude/discharge Medicaid recipients to maximize profits. Such tactics are prohibited by federal regulations and are unethical. LTC operators are required to provide the same level of service (consistent with the individual resident care plan), regardless of the payer source. Further, the LTC operator is usually prohibited from transferring a resident to another room simply because of the payer source.

Finally, many state Medicaid programs do not cover assisted living services; however, some states have initiated a pilot program, experimenting with how the Medicaid funds may be used in this arena.

Long-term care insurance: Individuals may purchase insurance to pay for services in LTC communities. As with any other insurance, once the individual is admitted into the community, the resident, legal representative, and/or responsible party will make a claim to the insurance company. Payment is dependent upon the terms of the policy.

Private Pay

A private pay resident personally pays the LTC community's bill. Unfortunately, because LTC services are so costly, the majority of individuals run out of personal funds, eventually qualifying for Medicaid benefits.

Scope of Expectations

Regardless of who actually pays, the payer expects that the beneficiary will receive quality care. If the community is unable to provide this, the payer expects that the community will transfer the resident(s) to another provider(s) who is able to provide that care. (Federal and state regulations prohibit maintaining a resident in a setting that cannot provide care in accordance with the resident's needs and continuing to bill for these services.) More importantly, it is unethical for a community to keep a resident for whom they cannot provide appropriate care.

Legal Responsibilities

Initial State Licensure

All LTC facilities must be licensed by the state wherein they operate. Each state has its own agency responsible for licensing and conducting licensing reviews. As part of the initial licensing process, states obtain significant information from potential providers, often requiring them to submit an extensive application detailing the background of the applicant (or owners of the applicant); the financial resources of the applicant; and the legal right to possess the property of the facility. Assuming the applicant succeeds in this process, they are then subject to an onsite inspection to ensure compliance with the promulgated regulations governing the license.

Once an LTC organization is licensed (i.e., legally able) to provide the services, it then needs to obtain contracts with the various payer sources. The provider must then submit applications to the various payer sources for acceptance into their particular program (and often undergo additional screening/audits) to be paid by that program.

Contracts With Federal and State Governments

Many LTC communities provide services to Medicare and Medicaid beneficiaries, thereby receiving payment directly from the Medicare or Medicaid programs. Both of these programs cover only certain benefits.

Providers of skilled nursing services who participate in the Medicare or Medicaid programs must comply with a series of statutes as codified in the **Omnibus Budget Reconciliation Act** of 1987 (OBRA). Failure to adhere to OBRA, as determined by the state survey agency, may result in the organization not being granted initial certification. Assuming the organization initially meets the CMS standards, it enters into a Medicare provider agreement. Similarly, the provider must also enter into a Medicaid provider agreement with the appropriate state agency to participate in the Medicaid program.

OBRA requirements pertain to the following areas:

- Resident Rights (42 CFR 483.10 et seq.)

- Admission Transfer and Discharge (42 CFR 483.12 et seq.)

- Resident Behavior and Facility Practices (42 CFR 483.13 et seq.)

- Quality of Life (42 CFR 483.15 et seq.)

- Resident Assessment (42 CFR 483.20 et seq.)

- Quality of Care (42 CFR 483.25 et seq.)

- Nursing Services (42 CFR 483.30 et seq.)

- Dietary Services (42 CFR 483.35 et seq.)

- Physician Services (42 CFR 483.40 et seq.)

- Provisions of Services (42 CFR 483.45 et seq.)

- Dental Services (42 CFR 483.55 et seq.)

- Pharmacy Services (42 CFR 483.60 et seq.)

- Infection Control (42 CFR 483.65 et seq.)

- Physical environment (42 CFR 483.70 et seq.)

- Administration (42 CFR 483.75 et seq.)

Following initial certification, **skilled nursing facilities** undergo regular **surveys** to ensure continued compliance (42 CFR § 442.12).Failing any one of these surveys will result in administrative action against the skilled nursing facility, including deficiencies, appointment of a temporary manager, denial of payments for new admissions of Medicare residents (which is also typically followed by a denial of payment for new admissions of Medicaid residents), a directed plan of correction, closure of the facility, termination of Medicare and/or Medicaid participation, and civil money penalties (42 CFR § 488.330).

Other Federal Laws and Their Ethical Implications

Numerous other state and federal laws exist that govern the provision of LTC services. The enforceability of the laws arises from the organization's licensure, the organization's various contracts with payer sources, society's desire to protect the frail and vulnerable, and the need to eliminate criminal or unethical conduct. Some of these laws include the Anti-Kickback Statute,

False Claims Act, Stark law, the Patient Protection and Affordable Care Act, Health Insurance Portability and Accountability Act, Occupational Safety and Health Act, **resident rights** statutes, corporate compliance programs, and **qui tam** actions.

Agencies

Numerous agencies govern the LTC industry.

Department of Health and Human Services (DHHS or HHS)

As with most of the federal departments, this department has gone through several changes of duties and names. For LTC providers, the DHHS is responsible for creating the policies that reinforce all federal laws governing health care, as well as providing guidelines for all levels of healthcare providers. The department is also responsible for evaluating the care that residents are getting in the different LTC communities, through the survey process.

State Health Departments

In addition to the DHHS, every state has its own department of health that deals with and reinforces the state laws and regulations. In most cases the DHHS has contracted with these state agencies to enforce some of the federal laws (e.g., OBRA).

County health departments: On some occasions, local counties may have a department of health agency to enforce their local regulations. At times, the state healthcare department may subcontract with the county departments. A good example is Los Angeles County, California, where the Los Angeles County Department of Public Health is responsible for the survey process for skilled nursing facilities and home health and hospice services.

Department of Justice (DOJ) (Federal and State)

Federal and state DJs are primarily responsible for prosecuting organizations and individuals for violations of federal (or state) law. This is true in all areas of health care, including, but not limited to, healthcare negligence, fraud, and abuse. In many cases the department conducts its own independent investigations, bringing criminal charges separate from DHHS's findings.

In California, the Department of Justice has created the "Operation Guardian (Guardian) Program" with the intent to "improve the quality of care for California's elder and dependent adult residents residing in California's 1,340 skilled nursing facilities." Between 2002 and 2012, this program filed 890 criminal charges, convicted 617 individuals, and collected more than $4.7 million dollars (Elder Abuse Exposed.com, 2013).

The state DOJ functions in much the same manner as the federal DOJ, conducting state and local investigations and filing charges pursuant to state laws and regulations.

Office of Civil Rights (OCR)

The **Office of Civil Rights (OCR)** is part of the DHHS. The OCR helps to protect individuals from discrimination in certain healthcare and social service programs. Some of these programs may include:

- Hospitals, health clinics, nursing homes
- Medicaid and Medicare agencies
- Welfare programs
- Day care centers
- Doctors' offices and pharmacies
- Children's health programs
- Alcohol and drug treatment centers
- Adoption agencies

Mental health and developmental disabilities agencies (U.S. Department of Health & Human Services, n.d.) The OCR reinforces the privacy regulations under HIPAA.

Adult Protective Service (APS)

APS is a state-operated program but largely funded with federal monies under the EJA. Oftentimes, APS does not have any authority in the LTC community, but there are many opportunities in which APS can be relevant to the community. For example, if a resident is ready to leave the facility but there are questions of abuse (not necessarily physical) or neglect regarding the individual whom the resident is going to reside with or the individual responsible for the resident, APS should be called prior to the discharge.

The purpose of involving APS is to keep the resident safe after the discharge from the community.

Long-Term Care Ombudsman (Ombudsman)

This is a state agency, funded by public funds and tasked with protecting seniors in a skilled nursing environment. For example, in California the program goal "is to advocate for the rights of all residents of long-term care facilities. The Ombudsman's advocacy role takes on two forms: 1) to receive and resolve individual complaints and issues by, or on behalf of, these residents; and 2) to pursue resident advocacy in the long-term care system, its laws, policies, regulations, and administration through public education and consensus building." (California Department of Aging, 2012) Another service that the **ombudsman** provides may be to act as a witness for legal documents that the resident needs to sign.

The ombudsman program is staffed mostly by volunteers who visit the facility unannounced to evaluate residents' care. Under current regulations, the community must provide unregulated access to the ombudsman. This does *not* include access to protected health information.

For LTC operators, the ombudsman may be a good connection to the community. On many occasions, the ombudsman representative can defend the community when dealing with difficult or unreasonable residents, family members, and/or legal representatives.

Privately Funded Agencies

Privately funded agencies are also called "resident advocates" or "advocacy programs" and are intended to be a watchdog for the care provided in LTC communities. This appears to be a very noble idea; however, many of these agencies are hijacked by plaintiff attorneys and used to bring civil litigation or regulatory enforcement.

Employees

Although employees are not an agency, they are essential to delivering quality care. Most employees are very dedicated and compassionate in their duties and provide invaluable feedback concerning resident needs and services. For the operator, the value and power of staff input cannot be underestimated. Please refer to Chapter 5 for further information regarding employee/employer rights and obligations; qui tam actions are discussed ahead.

Court of Public Opinion/Media

It has been said that the best marketing is a happy customer, and the same applies to the worst marketing. An unhappy customer will be sure to tell everyone possible about the bad experience he has had in a community. Unfortunately, today's media (formal and informal) tends to focus on negative events, recalling the single event that went wrong, rather than the hundreds of events that were correct. As such, it is important for the LTC community to cultivate a positive public image, promptly addressing negative concerns, comments, or other action.

Principal Areas of Focus

Abuse and Neglect

One of the most important focus areas for LTC providers is the resident's right to be free from abuse, corporal punishment, involuntary seclusion, and restraints. Abuse takes many forms, including physical, mental, financial, and sexual, and has been defined as the "willful infliction of injury, unreasonable confinement, intimidation or punishment with resulting physical harm, pain or mental anguish." Community staff must also recognize and understand that the fact that the resident has sustained some form of physical injury does not necessarily mean the cause is abuse (e.g., a resident may be observed with a bruise and suspect abuse). In such instances, the facility must conduct an in-depth investigation where there is a suspicion or allegation of abuse. As part of the investigation, facility staff may learn that the injury was a consequence of medications, or the natural progression of aging (thin and frail skin).

Neglect is another area of increased focus by DHHS/CMS and consumers. CMS interpretive guidelines provide a broad interpretation of this regulation by expanding the regulatory language to include the "failure to provide goods and services necessary to avoid physical harm, mental anguish, or mental illness" (42 CFR 483.13). The definition of "neglect" is incredibly vague, and efforts to provide clarity have been offered by courts, plaintiff lawyers, families, and healthcare providers. What the healthcare provider must realize is that in a legal or regulatory forum, the standard of what constitutes neglect is dependent upon the subjective interpretation of the individual(s) examining the situation.

Specifically, some view neglect as instances when facility personnel fail to follow a nursing process. For example, the failure to prevent a resident-to-resident altercation has been cited by a survey team as neglect (*Haverhill*

Care Center v. HCFA, 1998). In other instances, neglect has been identified when clinical staff failed to give a resident his medications on a single occasion. And in yet other instances, neglect has been determined when there is a systematic failure—that is, the utter disregard for the resident's welfare and completely depriving the resident of the services necessary to sustain life, such as medication, food, water, or shelter.

Protecting the resident from abuse/neglect is such a focal point that facilities must have complete systems in place to identify, train, investigate, and report abuse.

Abuse/Neglect Investigation and Reporting

Federal and state regulations mandate that LTC communities and their employees abide by abuse reporting obligations. These individuals working in the community are called "**mandated reporters**."

Federal and State Requirements

The Elder Justice Act (EJA) was designed to "prevent, detect, treat, understand, intervene in and, where appropriate, prosecute elder abuse, neglect and exploitation" (Stiegel, 2010). The EJA has numerous requirements, including the oversight by the DHHS to develop and manage federal resources to protect seniors from elder abuse. This process was to include the establishment of various councils and advisory boards, grants for long-term care ombudsmen programs, and programs to provide training concerning elder abuse and exploitation.

Federal regulations require that when the community receives an allegation or forms a reasonable suspicion of abuse, an investigation must be immediately initiated, regardless of the operator's personal opinions. The EJA also requires a report to the authorities, regardless of whether the allegation or suspicion is unfounded.

Many communities have a policy that, if the alleged abuser is not another resident, once he is interviewed, the alleged abuser must be asked to leave the facility. If the alleged abuser is an employee, he must be suspended immediately until the investigation is concluded and a determination of abuse was proven to be true or not.

OBRA guidelines also require investigation by the LTC provider. The investigation should be comprehensive and include a statement of the alleged abuse by the individual making the report, interviews with the alleged victim, the alleged abuser, any witnesses, alleged victim roommate(s), alleged abuser roommate(s) (if the abuse is resident-to-resident), staff working during the alleged incident, and any visitors/family members in the community at the time of the alleged incident who may have witnessed the event. The investigation must be documented. Finally, the community must have policies and procedures to reduce the risk of the abuse occurring.

In addition to the federal requirements, most if not all states have implemented their own abuse reporting requirements. These state requirements are usually in addition to the federal requirements and are often more stringent. For example, in addition to the EJA, California requires that the community report the allegation to the LTC ombudsman for every single allegation; however, other states may only require an online report, with any additional evidence to be completed and submitted within the time frame given by the EJA.

Ethical Ramifications of Reporting

As important as it is to report abuse or neglect of a resident in an LTC environment, such a report carries great responsibility and ethical considerations. For example, consider that a consultant was called to assist a facility in investigating an allegation of abuse between a staff member and a resident. When the consultant arrived to the community and interviewed the administrator, the consultant learned that the incident occurred about one week prior. When asked if the report was submitted timely to the authorities, the administrator responded, "No, the employee is a good guy and a good employee and I don't believe he did anything." Further, when the consultant asked if the employee had been suspended after the investigation, the administrator stated, "No, he is a good guy, he didn't do anything, and my investigation was very simple because the resident has dementia and most of the time doesn't know what she is talking about."

Under the EJA regulations, the administrator is required to report any allegations of abuse regardless of his personal opinion. If the investigation reveals that the alleged abuse did occur, the administrator has placed himself in a position of being criminally and/or civilly charged with neglect.

In short, until a complete/thorough investigation is done, no conclusions as to the validity of the allegations should be made. Further, even after performing a the investigation, if the administrator is still not clear as to whether the alleged abuse occurred, the administrator must depend on independent investigations and results of the regulatory agencies before dismissing any allegations.

Residents' Rights

Residents living in healthcare communities, particularly in nursing homes, are endowed with rights, which the LTC community must protect. In addition to the prohibition on abuse and neglect, the resident rights that seem to regularly arise and result in regulatory action or civil litigation are: transfer and discharge rights, the right to adequate staff, the right to choose a physician and treatment and participate in decisions and care planning, the right to privacy and confidentiality, the right to form relationships and be visited by others, and the right to retain and use personal possessions.

As noted earlier, these rights pose challenges for the healthcare provider because what a resident chooses for himself may be contrary to physician recommendations or those of the resident's family member.

As it pertains to transfer and discharge rights, residents in LTC communities often have changes in their physical, mental, or social conditions that make their residency at a particular level of care inappropriate or dangerous for other residents or staff. For residents who do not want to leave the facility, discharge becomes very difficult despite notice, and regardless of the fact that a resident may pose a threat to others. In each of these instances (except where the facility ceases to operate), the resident's record must include appropriate documentation that reflects the reason and need for the transfer.

For example, assume a resident living in an skilled nursing facility begins to manifest psychiatric disorders, resulting in verbally and physically aggressive behavior. The facility cannot simply transfer the resident to a psychiatric facility regardless of whether such a setting is more appropriate. So, too, facility staff or his physician cannot simply medicate or restrain the resident. Rather, facility staff must abide by regulatory guidelines and provide sufficient notice to the resident (or his legally responsible party) stating the reason(s) for transfer or discharge, the effective date of the transfer or discharge, and the location to which the resident is to be transferred or discharged. (This requirement is often the most difficult, due to the fact that the facility may be unable to locate a facility willing to accept the resident.) The notice must also include a statement that the resident has the right to appeal the action, and the name, address, and telephone number of the state long-term care ombudsman (42 CFR 483.12).

The right to "adequate staff" has been the subject of extensive legislation and litigation. Many states have attempted to implement staffing guidelines and structures mandating the amount of training staff members are required to have as well as the number of staff members needed during a given shift or day. Whether these legislative measures have had significant impact on overall resident outcomes is the subject of extensive debate. However, as it pertains to the provision of LTC services, the provider must be very aware that failure to provide the adequate staff may result in regulatory and legal action.

As to a resident's right to participate in his own care and treatment and maintain his own personal possessions, providers may face numerous problems. For example, a resident may wish to maintain alcoholic beverages in his room. Such alcoholic beverages are part of the resident's custom, practice, and history (i.e., to have a glass of whisky every evening before dinner). The facility is obligated to allow the resident to participate and/or direct his own care, to provide a "homelike" environment, and to allow each resident to maintain his personal belongings. However, the alcoholic beverage contradicts physician orders and may prove fatal to the resident. Further, there is the risk of other residents getting access to the alcoholic beverage.

Other examples may involve residents' personal relationships. Such relationships may be objected to by the resident's immediate family and may create complications in providing privacy while pursuing such relationships. Or, a resident may exercise his right to refuse personal hygiene, thereby directly impacting the rights of other residents.

Compounding these challenges is that some residents have lost the capacity to make informed decisions and do not have advance directives in place or family members available to assist in the decision-making process. In each of these situations, the organization must address the legal and ethical conflicts that exist and resolve them in a manner that allows the resident to achieve and maintain the highest practicable physical, mental, and psychosocial well-being. In each of these situations, it is incumbent upon facility administration, together with the input of the resident's care team and physician, to address the issue directly, involving the resident, legally responsible party, family, and the local ombudsman (as available). Resolution may require some convincing skills and "out-of-the-box" ideas that protect each resident's rights. When there is some resolution, it must be documented in the resident's medical record, and time parameters created for follow-up to ensure that the problem/issue is in fact resolved. If it is not, the analysis begins afresh and a new resolution is crafted. In some circumstances, there is no resolution and a determination is made that the resident should be transferred or discharged, which, as noted earlier, creates its own set of challenges.

Civil and Regulatory Ramifications

There is significant regulatory oversight to ensure that the resident's rights are protected. State survey agencies regularly audit organizations, reviewing practices, policies, and procedures, and interviewing employees and residents to ensure that this is occurring. Further, agencies, such as APS and the ombudsman, receive and investigate LTC providers, providing information to the state regulatory agency if they believe that resident rights are being violated.

Moreover, many states allow residents or their family members to assert a private right of action, suing skilled nursing facilities over a resident rights violation. For example, in California, a current or former resident may file a lawsuit for a violation(s) of patient rights (Ca. Health and Safety Code section 1430(b)). This statute permits a civil action against a facility licensee "who violates any rights of the resident or patient as set forth in the Patients' Bill of Rights in Section 72527 of Title 22 of the California Code of Regulations, or any other right provided for by federal or state law or regulation." The statute states that the licensee "shall be liable for the acts of the licensee's employees. The licensee shall be liable for up to five hundred dollars ($500), and for costs and attorney fees, and may be enjoined from permitting the violation to continue."

This means that in California, the skilled nursing facility must protect every right of every resident as set forth in state or federal law, or face the very real prospect of litigation. Matters are further complicated by the simple fact that when one resident exercises his rights, it may very well impact and negate the rights of another resident.

Health Insurance Portability and Accountability Act (HIPAA)

In Chapter 10 HIPAA regulations are discussed in depth. However, many providers are often faced with the ethical responsibility for keeping or disseminating protected healthcare information (PHI) and/or electronic protected healthcare information (ePHI).

Covered Entities and Business Associates

Prior to 2013, the responsibility of protecting PHI belonged to covered entities (CE). With the expanded 2013 HIPAA regulations, both the CE and business associates (BA) are equally responsible and both must take the necessary steps to protect PHI.

Under these regulations, CEs and BAs must create clear policies and procedures to protect PHI and ePHI and have audits to identify vulnerabilities (where the PHI and/or ePHI might be compromised). If any PHI/ePHI is compromised, the CE/BA must determine how the **breach** occurred and implement measures to prevent reoccurrence.

Responsibilities and Requirements

The LTC community administrator is responsible for creating the HIPAA policies, training the staff on the procedures, and instructing them on how to prevent a breach as well as the need to report any breach.

Conducting audits and finding weaknesses are vital to protecting PHI and ensuring community viability. This is because a failure could subject the community to penalties, lawsuits, regulatory action, and damage to the reputation.

One of the common ethical dilemmas LTC providers face relates to providing PHI of a resident to his family member. The right to disclose PHI belongs to the resident or his legally responsible agent. As such, the operator cannot advise other close family members of the resident's condition, absent specific consent from the resident or his legal representative. By disclosing any such information, the operator may well have breached the resident's privacy and a report may need to be made in accordance with regulations.

It is critical that LTC operators understand the scope of their duty and authority relative to PHI and ePHI. By obtaining the necessary consents and identifying proper individuals, creating comprehensive policies and procedures, training staff, and performing audits, the organization may well remain in compliance.

Physician and Vendor Relationships

In 2009, the DHHS announced the creation of an interagency task force to address healthcare fraud and increase coordination among the various agencies, thereby optimizing criminal and civil enforcement of violations. The program, called the Health Care Fraud Prevention and Enforcement Action Team (HEAT), has yielded historic results and has recovered $14.5 billion in federal healthcare dollars. Most of these recoveries related to Medicare and Medicaid fraud (Office of Public Affairs, U.S. Department of Justice, 2014).

Physician Self-Referral Law (Stark)

The **Stark** law prohibits many physician relationships. Specifically, a physician who has direct or indirect ownership or a compensation relationship with a provider of certain "designated health services" (DHS) may not make referrals to that provider for the provision of DHS for Medicare residents unless an exception is available.

The recipient of a DHS referral may not bill the Medicare program, the resident, or anyone else for the DHS performed as a result of the prohibited referral. DHS includes clinical laboratory services; physical and occupational therapy services; radiology services, including MRI, CT scans, and ultrasound services; radiation therapy services and supplies; durable medical equipment and supplies; prosthetics, orthotics, and prosthetic devices and supplies; home health services; outpatient prescription drugs; and inpatient and outpatient hospital services. Thus, a physician who has a direct or indirect ownership or compensation relationship with a provider of clinical laboratory or radiology services may not refer Medicare residents to that provider unless an exception under the Stark laws exists.

For LTC communities, physicians determine the scope of services their patients receive. For instance, although nursing facility services are not designated health services, other services, such as laboratory and therapy, are.

LTC communities are in a difficult position in helping ensure that Stark is upheld. Specifically, resident/clients choose their physician. The community must respect that choice. The physician orders the care and services the resident/client is to receive (laboratory testing, radiology exams, medications, therapy services, hospice services, medical equipment, transfers to different level of care, etc.). To the extent that the physician has a financial relationship with these entities, the physician may be in violation of Stark. This, in turn, may subject the LTC community to investigation by government agencies for assisting the physician.

So how does the community maintain compliance? Initially, the community must have a general understanding of Stark and how it pertains to the LTC community. The community must have (and enforce) clear policies and procedures (P&P) (a CCP is strongly recommended). The physicians must be advised of the P&P/CCP wherein they are advised that the community intends to comply with state and federal laws and that violations of the same will be investigated and reported to the appropriate governmental agencies. Staff is provided general training on the scope of state and federal laws and how they impact the provision of LTC services. (This training is necessary because frontline staff are often the "eyes and ears" of the organization and potential problems may be identified more quickly.) Thereafter, audits are done concerning physician ordering practices. For example, if a treating physician in an LTC organization specifies which laboratory he wants all of his patients to use, a potential problem may exist that needs investigating. If a physician requires that all orders for durable medical equipment go through a particular supplier, the organization should review the scope of that relationship and speak with the physician, reporting this to the authorities if necessary.

Anti-Kickback Statute (AKS) and False Claims Act (FCA)

The AKS prohibits the exchange (or offer to exchange) of anything of value in an effort to induce (or reward) the referral of federal healthcare program business. The AKS seems similar to Stark, but AKS is much broader in scope. Figure 8.1 shows a comparison.

The FCA works with Stark and the AKS and is the government's primary civil remedy to recoup monies that it believes were submitted through improper/illegal means. So what are false claims? A false claim is a claim (bill) to the government (state or federal) for payment or reimbursement for services that were not provided, not provided in accordance with the contract, or unnecessary. The FCA attaches to virtually every government contract, including national security and defense, as well as under government programs as varied as Medicare, veterans' benefits, federally insured loans and mortgages, transportation and research grants, agricultural supports, school lunches, and disaster assistance. The FCA has been so successful that in 2014, the U.S. **Department of Justice** obtained a record $5.69 billion in settlements and judgments from civil cases involving fraud and false claims against the government. False claims against federal healthcare programs, such as Medicare and Medicaid, accounted for $2.3 billion of the total amount recovered (Office of Public Affairs, U.S. Department of Justice, 2014).

Some examples of the government's success against healthcare providers include a 2014 case against two hospital chains wherein the hospitals agreed to pay $333 million related to FCA violations. The actions against the entities arose because the entities billed the Medicare program for services deemed unnecessary and that could have been handled at a lower level of care (inpatient services that should have been provided in a less costly outpatient or observation setting).

For the LTC provider, an AKS/FCA violation may take many different forms. Specifically, the government has alleged overuse of therapy services, failure to discharge the patient from services in a timely manner, and exaggeration of complexity of the resident's medical condition (thereby increasing RUG scores and allowing overpayment), or even referring a resident for further services, such as hospice or home health, when the patient's condition does not warrant same.

More recently, two whistle-blowers argued that the nursing home where they had worked had submitted "thousands of false claims to the Medicare and Medicaid programs." At the crux of the allegations was that the nursing home provided substandard care and amounted to "worthless

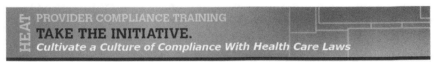

PROVIDER COMPLIANCE TRAINING
TAKE THE INITIATIVE.
Cultivate a Culture of Compliance With Health Care Laws

COMPARISON OF THE ANTI-KICKBACK STATUTE AND STARK LAW*

	THE ANTI-KICKBACK STATUTE (42 USC § 1320a-7b(b))	THE STARK LAW (42 USC § 1395nn)
Prohibition	Prohibits offering, paying, soliciting, or receiving anything of value to induce or reward referrals or generate federal healthcare program business	• Prohibits a physician from referring Medicare patients for designated health services to an entity with which the physician (or immediate family member) has a financial relationship, unless an exception applies • Prohibits the designated health services entity from submitting claims to Medicare for those services resulting from a prohibited referral
Referrals	Referrals from anyone	Referrals from a physician
Items/ Services	Any items or services	Designated health services
Intent	Intent must be proven (knowing and willful)	• No intent standard for overpayment (strict liability) • Intent required for civil monetary penalties for *knowing* violations
Penalties	Criminal: • Fines up to $25,000 per violation • Up to a 5 year prison term per violation Civil/Administrative: • False Claims Act liability • Civil monetary penalties and program exclusion • Potential $50,000 CMP per violation • Civil assessment of up to three times amount of kickback	Civil: • Overpayment/refund obligation • False Claims Act liability • Civil monetary penalties and program exclusion for *knowing* violations • Potential $15,000 CMP for each service • Civil assessment of up to three times the amount claimed
Exceptions	*Voluntary* safe harbors	*Mandatory* exceptions
Federal Healthcare Programs	All	Medicare/Medicaid

*This chart is for illustrative purposes only and is not a substitute for consulting the statutes and their regulations.

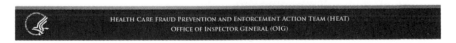

HEALTH CARE FRAUD PREVENTION AND ENFORCEMENT ACTION TEAM (HEAT)
OFFICE OF INSPECTOR GENERAL (OIG)

Figure 8.1 Comparison of the Anti-Kickback Statute and Stark Law (Office of Inspector General, U.S. Department of Health and Human Services & Health Care Prevention and Enforcement Team, 2014)

services" (i.e., services that were not provided in accordance with the contract/OBRA guidelines). Initially, a jury found in favor of the whistle-blowers, awarding $3 million to the United States to compensate it for the reimbursements (ultimately trebled to $9 million under the FCA) and $19 million in fines for the qui tam claims. Only after a lengthy legal battle did the court of appeal rule that the provision of services, even at a lesser value, does not equate to "worthless services"—that is, "Services that are 'worth less' are not 'worthless'" (*U.S. ex rel. Absher v. Momence Meadows Nursing Center*, 2014).

A more common example of AKS/FCA violations relates to the provision additional services. Assume a hospice agency offers to pay an SNF $100.00 for every patient that the SNF refers to the hospice agency. The hospice agency accepts the referral and submits a claim to the federal Medicare program. The hospice agency's offer to pay for referrals is a violation of the AKS—so too is the facility's acceptance of the payment. Also, the claims submitted by the hospice agency are considered false claims because they were a result of an illegal payment scheme.

The LTC provider, however, may face an ethical dilemma. Assume that the SNF is both Medicare- and Medicaid-certified, serving a low-income population. The extra money would be used to provide more services to the residents. Moreover, the SNF believes that the hospice company's services are of good quality.

From a legal point of view, the AKS and FCA do not consider the honorable intentions of the provider. An inducement for a referral payment by the federal government is considered illegal. By engaging in such actions, both organizations (SNF and hospice) are subject to civil and criminal prosecution.

Most states have enacted laws that either mimic or expand upon the federal AKS and FCA. This means that prosecution for violations may come from two different sources: federal and state. The penalties for violations are quite harsh and include repayment, with a double or treble multiplier; the government may seek to revoke the organization's license, place the provider on the Office of Inspector General's **excluded provider list**, mandate a corporate integrity agreement (see Chapter 7), and initiate criminal prosecution.

Qui Tam Actions

Qui tam litigation is sometimes referred to as whistle-blower actions. Such actions may arise when a private party, called a relator, brings an action against an organization on behalf of the government. The False Claims Act authorizes qui tam actions against parties who have defrauded the federal government. If a relator brings an action that is accepted by the government, the government, not the relator, is considered the real plaintiff. If the government succeeds, the relator receives a share of the award, often up to 30% (31 U.S.C. § 3279).

Qui tam actions have come to the forefront for many providers. The actions are often the result of disgruntled employees or former employees who are enticed by the financial benefits gained from exposing perceived violations.

In 1983, 30 qui tam actions were filed. Now, qui tam actions exceed 700 each year. The growing number of qui tam lawsuits has led to increased recoveries: $2 billion for the first time in fiscal year 2010, and approaching or exceeding $3 billion ever since. As recoveries have increased, so have whistle-blower awards.

Advance Care Planning

Defined

Advance care planning is the process wherein a person begins "end-of-life" planning. Specifically, the person decides the extent of medical intervention he wants as the end of life approaches; he may review who he would want to make/enforce his wishes (in case he became unable to do so); he may indicate how he wants his remains addressed. Once these advance care planning efforts are documented, they can be easily communicated to healthcare providers and family.

Advance care planning should be approached at any stage in life and reevaluated occasionally thereafter. For example, a young woman with small children may desire to have every life-sustaining measure taken and the legally responsible person may be her spouse. As she ages, her end-of-life decisions may also change—she may now want her legally responsible decision maker to be one of her children and minimal interventions taken to sustain life.

Advance Directives

The phrase "advance directives" (sometimes referred to as a living will) encompasses the bulk of documents and information that outline a person's end-of-life wishes. All of these documents, taken together, provide necessary information concerning decision-making authority and the scope of healthcare treatment options desired.

Often one of the first documents created is the **durable power of attorney (DPOA)** (sometimes referred to as a power of attorney or POA). Most individuals will create two DPOAs: one for healthcare decisions and one for other financial and/or legal matters. In essence, the DPOA sets forth the parameters of authority wherein the principal gives authority to another person, allowing the other person to make decisions on his behalf. A financial/legal DPOA is often limited to those matters that involve transactions, contracts, legal matters, and finances. A healthcare DPOA deals with medical decisions, including seeking/withdrawing treatment, admission to/from healthcare communities, and the ability to receive confidential healthcare information. Regardless of the type(s) of DPOA, there is usually a statement that dictates when the decision-making authority takes effect. Some DPOAs do not take effect until the principal is deemed incompetent. Other DPOAs take effect immediately, regardless of patient's level of competence/incompetence.

> The difference between a POA and a DPOA is subtle yet extremely important. A POA is created by the principal (the person who desires the advance care planning) to accomplish a task or tasks. The principal appoints a person to act in his capacity to complete a task or tasks. The POA expires when the task is complete *or* when the principal becomes incapacitated. With a DPOA, the principal outlines the tasks and appointment that can survive the completion of the tasks as well as the principal's incapacity. As such, for advance care planning, the DPOA is the most effective means of accomplishing the principal's purpose.

The DPOA should provide clarity. However, many times the healthcare provider fails to:

• Ask for a copy of the DPOA (and a copy placed in the resident's file)

• Review the DPOA to determine the scope of authority

• Identify when the DPOA takes effect

From a legal perspective, the DPOA is the only evidence setting forth the patient's wishes. It is the proof that would be submitted to court and would explain why a certain person signed the admissions agreement, signed the arbitration agreement, or was advised of the patient's progress. Absent the DPOA, the LTC provider may not have enforceable contracts and may well violate HIPAA, and the ethical challenges are far greater.

For example, a resident is admitted to an LTC community by her daughter for assisted living services due to progressive Alzheimer's disease. The daughter assures the community that her mother does have a DPOA and will bring it in "soon." The admissions paperwork is completed, including arbitration and financial agreements. All documents are signed by the daughter. The resident moves in and begins receiving care. The provider continues to remind the daughter to bring in the DPOA, the daughter continues to "forget," and the matter is delayed. Eventually, everyone forgets about the DPOA, the residency proceeds, and the daughter contacted as issues arise. Unfortunately, many of these issues relate to the resident attempting to leave the facility, asking to go home, and asking to speak to her son. The resident's behavior is attributed to her Alzheimer's diagnosis.

Three months later, the resident's son comes to visit. (Assume he had been stationed out of the country and had just returned.) The son is surprised to learn that his mother lives in an assisted living environment. He complains loudly that the mother was placed without his knowledge and consent and immediately produces a DPOA. The DPOA grants the son *all* powers to make all healthcare and financial decisions for the resident. Further, the DPOA states that only the son is to be consulted as healthcare issues arise and *not* the daughter.

The facility faces numerous issues:

• Providing care without consent and whether it amounts to abuse.

• Having invalid/unenforceable admissions, financial, and arbitration agreements.

• Potential violation of resident rights/confining a resident against her wishes.

• HIPAA violations for communicating with the wrong individual.

These problems could have been avoided if the community had received and reviewed the DPOA *before* admitting the resident and the documents were signed.

Taking this scenario one step further, assume the community is able to resolve the son's complaints. They assure him that his mother is well taken care of, she appears happy and healthy, and she is overjoyed to see him. The matter of the resident's Alzheimer's is addressed, and the son concedes that his mother is in the appropriate environment. The son executes the admission agreements, financial documents, consents for care, and arbitration agreement, and all are placed in the resident's file along with the DPOA.

The resident's medical condition deteriorates due to her age and medical comorbidities, and she requires a higher level of care. She is admitted to the skilled nursing section within the community. Again, the son executes all of the necessary paperwork. Shortly thereafter, the resident attempts to get out of bed unassisted, falls, and has to be rushed to the hospital, where she is diagnosed with a subdural hematoma and hip fracture. She is placed on hospice and passes away shortly thereafter.

The son is angry about his mother's death and wants to sue the community. He asks for a copy of the medical records, and the community immediately complies. The medical records are turned over to the son's lawyer, and the community is sued. The community attempts to enforce the arbitration agreement. During this process, the DPOA is again reviewed and reads *that it takes effect only when the resident is "deemed incompetent by two separate physicians."* After extensive review of the medical record, the community cannot locate in the medical record where two physicians have deemed the resident incompetent. Rather, the physicians note her cheerful disposition and her seeming ability to respond to questions.

Because the community failed to read/catch the phrase about when the DPOA took effect, they face many of the same problems as before. Moreover, in many states, a DPOA "dies" once the principal dies. As healthcare providers, giving out healthcare information on a deceased resident to the "former holder" of the DPOA may result in a HIPAA violation. With this in mind, the organization should not have released the resident's medical records to the son.

In sum, DPOAs are legally enforceable documents. They may be amended, modified, or revoked at any time by the principal, so long as the principal has the ability and mental capacity to do so. The community's obligation is to assure itself that the person purporting to be the holder of the DPOA is in fact the person identified in the DPOA document, the correct person is signing on behalf of the resident, and healthcare information is properly communicated.

If a community intends to rely upon on a DPOA, it must: (a) make sure it is relying upon the most recently executed DPOA; and (b) review the DPOA so that it can comply. Failure to do so may result in unwitting violations of numerous regulations.

Physician Orders for Life-Sustaining Treatment and Code Status

Other documents forming the advance directive relate to the scope of services a person wants to receive toward the end of his life. Occasionally this information is set forth in the healthcare DPOA, but more often than not, the scope of life-sustaining services is left for the family to decide. It is here that ethical dilemmas come to the forefront because absent instructions to the contrary, modern medicine will provide all lifesaving measures, and patients and their family members are often left to balance between what they consider to be life versus quality of life.

The phrase "quality of life" is individual to each person and often tied directly to religious beliefs and personal preferences. The dilemma is that individuals or organizations attempt to impose personal beliefs upon the patient or the family, or, in some very unethical organizations, push for providing extensive life-sustaining care so that they can bill for same.

Some states require that healthcare organizations implement **physician-ordered life-sustaining treatment (POLST)**. The POLST is a form signed by the patient (or his legally recognized decision maker) and the physician and is maintained in the patient's medical record to assist in the decision-making process. The form outlines end-of-life care, including medical treatment or extraordinary measures (e.g., a ventilator or feeding tube), CPR, and so forth. This may be referred to as "code status." Failure to maintain the POLST may amount to a regulatory violation, but, more importantly, it may create confusion and stress when the eventuality of the patient's death is imminent.

Absent the POLST (wherein care treatment options are outlined), the two most common code statuses are full code and no code. "Full code" means that *every* lifesaving measure will be implemented in order to stop the death—cardiopulmonary resuscitation (CPR), mechanical ventilation, dialysis, and artificial nutrition (feeding tubes and naso-gastric tubes). "No code" is the direct opposite. If a patient is "no code" and he experiences a significant change in condition, minimal if any intervention will be attempted.

The problems for the healthcare provider arise in the gray areas between "full code" and "no code." If the patient had no advance directive/no POLST, the patient/family must make these decisions under very stressful circumstances. Unfortunately, these decisions may create family conflict and trigger feelings of guilt.

Healthcare providers should not get involved in the family's decision-making process. Rather, they should be available to answer questions, and refer patients and their family members to the appropriate counseling agencies/individual available. LTC organizations may call upon the religious groups with whom the resident (or family member) affiliates, or call in grief counselors and specialists in end-of-life decision making. The bottom line for the organization is that whatever decision is made, it should be made by the patient or his legal representative.

Other Important Issues to Consider

More often than not, patients have no advance care planning in place and a guardianship or conservatorship should be considered. Such an appointment is done through the various state courts, and a judge will appoint a "guardian" to protect the "ward." (Wards may be minor children or incapacitated adults.) Guardians owe a fiduciary duty to their wards—that is, a duty to act solely in the ward's interests (*Neilson v. Colgate-Palmolive Co.*, 1999).

> In some jurisdictions, "custodial" or "conservator" is used instead of "guardian."

The scope of the guardian's power is delineated by court order. Some may be limited to addressing financial matters, while others may be limited to addressing healthcare matters. Oftentimes, two **conservators** will be appointed (much like having two DPOAs). In this way, an inherent conflict exists and the two conservators must work together for the benefit of the ward. It should be noted that there are often significant costs associated with creating/implementing a guardianship/conservator. As such, this avenue should be used only as a last resort.

No Advance Care Planning or Responsible Party

Unfortunately, there are some situations where the patient does not have any family or friend willing or legally able to make decisions. Although some states, such as Arizona, outline who may make decisions for a mentally/medically incapacitated person, the community must have a decision-making process in place that is consistent with state law. Communities should consider implementing a bioethics committee (see ahead).

Court-Appointed Treatment

Circumstances may arise when care and treatment are provided to a patient without his consent. However, such circumstances must be pursuant to court-granted authority. Usually these cases arise from a mental or psychiatric condition whereby the patient may pose a threat of immediate harm to himself or others and involuntary commitment is warranted. The laws for each state vary, and the LTC provider is recommended to seek legal counsel in the state where it operates.

Practical Solutions to Complicated Problems

Policies, Procedures, and Protocols

It is important for the community to have very clear P&P addressing different areas of patient care. P&P must cover all departments, including housekeeping, laundry, maintenance, social service, nursing, activities, and so forth (P&P should never eliminate the professional experience and good common sense of staff). P&P must be reviewed frequently. This review should evaluate the effectiveness of the protocol and modified to address changes in the regulations and best practices. Staff need to be frequently trained on the P&P to ensure that they are being followed (see training and disciplinary process ahead).

Bioethics Committee

A **bioethics committee** makes healthcare decisions for the individuals who can no longer make their own decisions and do not have anyone to make those decisions. The scope of the bioethics committee should be outlined in the community's P&P, and members should consist of at least two physicians, one of whom should be the community's medical director and the other the resident's physician (if different from the medical director and community staff, including the administrator and director of nurses/clinical care and social service). The community should also invite the ombudsman to attend the meeting. The ombudsman will act as an observer to guarantee that the resident's rights are not violated. (Often the ombudsman refuses to attend to eliminate any possible conflict or liability for the decisions made.)

Documentation of these meetings must be kept in the resident's clinical chart and include meeting minutes and attendance records. After the decisions are made, the administrator should sign consents "on behalf of the bioethics committee" and not as administrator of the community.

The committee's decision-making authority extends only to the care provided within the community. Once the resident is transferred to an acute hospital or any other community, the bioethics committee no longer has authority.

Training/Evaluation/Discipline

The community's success depends greatly on the quality of services provided. One manner of ensuring quality care is through regular staff training (sometimes referred to as an "in-service"). Unfortunately, some staff members may attempt to "multitask" during the training, completing other paperwork, responding to e-mails/texts, and so forth. This should not be allowed. Training is a time to learn and not just to be present.

Finally, employee evaluation is necessary. This ensures that the training was successful and the procedures implemented. Often, the evaluation reveals that the training was *not* effective, and further training is required.

Sadly, there are individuals who will disregard regulations, P&P, and best practices. Community staff must be held accountable for such actions, especially if patient care is affected. Therefore it is essential that the community have clear P&P regarding disciplinary actions (see Chapter 5 for further information).

Reporting Process

The community should have a process wherein residents, family members, visitors, and staff may report incidents, concerns, abuse, theft, and harassment. Such reporting may be done anonymously and without fear of retaliation.

In the past, communities had a "suggestion box" placed in a common area. Unfortunately, the "suggestion box" may create feelings of mistrust. Specifically, (a) most reports were handwritten and someone could recognize the handwriting; and (b) individuals could be observed depositing a suggestion into the box.

Today's technology has allowed alternative reporting mechanisms—for example:

• A toll-free hotline

• Website report

Both of these methods would need to be monitored 24 hours/day, 7 days/week, because if an allegation of abuse was received, obligations under the EJA and state reporting statutes would be triggered.

Audit

The community must implement an auditing program to help to verify legal and regulatory compliance as well as the quality of care being provided. These audits should be coordinated with the administrator, together with the corporate compliance committee, quality assurance performance improvement (QAPI)/quality assurance (QA) committee, and HIPAA committee. Some areas requiring regular audits include: privacy issues, billing, therapy over/underutilization, contracts, clinical care, personnel files, and OIG's excluded list.

Summary

The LTC provider has numerous legal and ethical responsibilities. Although the federal and state governments have attempted to legislate ethical conduct by prohibiting certain actions, this does not eliminate the community's obligation to "do what is right." In providing services to one of the very vulnerable segments of society, the LTC community must constantly consider its legal and ethical obligations, and especially the gray areas in between.

Key Terms

Adult protective services (APS): APS is typically administered by local or state health, aging, or regulatory departments and includes a multidisciplinary approach to helping older adults, and younger adults with disabilities, who are victims. Services range from the initial investigation of mistreatment, to health and supportive services and legal interventions, up to and including the appointment of surrogate decision makers, such as legal guardians.

Advance care planning: The process wherein a person evaluates LTC and treatment options. Through this process, the person decides, in advance, the extent of medical intervention they want as the end of life approaches.

Anti-Kickback Statute (AKS): A criminal statute that prohibits the exchange (or offer to exchange) of anything of value, in an effort to induce (or reward) the referral of federal healthcare program business.

Bioethics committee: A committee constructed by the community and composed of professionals covering the LTC continuum, including physicians, nursing, activities, social services, therapies, clergy, and ombudsman or APS. This committee addresses ethical concerns as they arise and may be needed to provide care planning for residents who do not have family or friends to assist in this process.

Breach: The acquisition, access use, or disclosure of protected health information in a manner that compromises the security or privacy of the protected information (45 CFR section 164.402).

Conservator: A legally appointed representative for the resident. The scope of the conservatorship is outlined in the court order.

Custodial care: Nonskilled, personal care, such as help with activities of daily living, like bathing, dressing, eating, getting in or out of a bed or chair, moving round, and using the bathroom. It may also include care that most people do themselves, like using eye drops.

Department of Justice (DOJ): The United States federal department responsible for enforcing federal laws (including the enforcement of all civil rights legislation).

Elder Justice Act (EJA): A law passed under the PPACA designed to "prevent, detect, treat, understand, intervene in and, where appropriate, prosecute elder abuse, neglect and exploitation." The EJA imposes reporting requirements upon "covered individuals" where there is a "reasonable suspicion of a crime" that is committed against any individual who is a resident of a long-term healthcare facility.

False Claims Act (FCA): A series of statutes that create liability for any person or organization who (1) knowingly submits a false claim to the government, (2) causes another to submit a false claim to the government, or (3) knowingly makes a false record or statement to get a false claim paid by the government.

Health Insurance Portability and Accountability Act (HIPAA): Addresses the access and disclosure of protected health information (PHI). PHI is defined as "individually identifiable health information" held or transmitted by a covered entity. HIPAA applies to health plans, healthcare clearinghouses, and to any healthcare provider who transmits health information in electronic form.

Health maintenance organization (HMO): A type of Medicare managed care plan where a group of doctors, hospitals, and other healthcare providers agree to give health care to Medicare beneficiaries for a set amount of money from Medicare every month. You usually must get your care from the providers in the plan.

Mandated reporters: Any person who has assumed full or intermittent responsibility for care or custody of an elder or dependent adult, regardless of whether that person receives compensation, including administrators, supervisors, and any licensed staff of a public or private facility that provides care or services for elder or dependent adults, or any elder or dependent adult care custodian, health practitioner, or employee of a county adult protective services agency or local law enforcement agency.

Office of Civil Rights (OCR): This office is part of HHS. Its HIPAA responsibilities include oversight of the privacy requirements.

OIG excluded provider list: The OIG has the authority to exclude individuals and entities from federally funded healthcare programs pursuant to sections 1128 and 1156 of the Social Security Act and maintains a list of all currently excluded individuals and entities, called the List of Excluded Individuals and Entities (LEIE). Anyone who hires an individual or entity on the LEIE may be subject to civil monetary penalties (CMP).

Ombudsman: An advocate (supporter) who works to solve problems between residents and nursing homes, as well as assisted living facilities. Also called "long-term care ombudsman."

Omnibus Budget Reconciliation Act (OBRA): A series of regulations that govern skilled nursing facilities accepting Medicare.

Physician-ordered life-sustaining treatment (POLST): This document outlines the amount of medical intervention the resident wants to receive in the event there is a change in condition.

Qui tam: Sometimes referred to as a whistle-blower action, such an action may arise when a private party, called a relator, brings an action against an organization on behalf of the government, so long as the statute authorizes the relator to bring the action. A successful qui tam action may bring significant monetary awards for the relator(s).

Resident rights: A series of statutes that outline the specific rights of each resident in an LTC community. Depending upon the type of community, these rights may be federally based, state-based, or both.

Skilled nursing facility: A facility (which meets specific regulatory certification requirements) that primarily provides inpatient skilled nursing care and related services to patients who require medical, nursing, or rehabilitative services but does not provide the level of care or treatment available in a hospital. It is a nursing facility with the staff and equipment to give skilled nursing care and/or skilled rehabilitation services and other related health services.

Social media: Social media is defined as: forms of electronic communication, such as web sites for social networking and micro blogging through which users create online communities to share information, ideas, personal messages, and other content (e.g., videos). Some social media samples include, but are not limited to:

- Facebook • Personal Blogs • LinkedIn • YouTube • Twitter • Foursquare • MySpace

Stark I and II: Federal self-referral statute that prohibits physicians from referring Medicare patients for designated health services to entities with which the physician (or an immediate family member) has a financial relationship, unless an exception applies.

Survey: The activity conducted by state survey agencies or other CMS agents under the direction of CMS whereby surveyors determine compliance or non-compliance with requirements for participation.

Review Questions

1. Why do the payer sources (e.g., Medicare and Medicaid) care about the long-term care community's compliance with the laws governing the delivery of healthcare services?

2. Why is it important for residents in long-term care communities to have "resident rights"? And why must the long-term care community respect those rights?

3. Name some of the laws that govern long-term care community relationships with vendors. Why must the community monitor its vendor relationships?

4. What is advance care planning and why is it important?

5. Please list five things that a long-term community can do to promote compliance with its legal and ethical obligations.

Case Studies

Case #1

The community has an inquiry for a male resident to be admitted. However, the only available beds are for female residents (i.e., the other residents in the room are female). The admission's director asks a resident to move to another room, with a roommate, to accommodate the possible male resident, but the resident refuses to do so.

- Is the community able to move the resident, regardless of her refusal?

- If the resident goes to the hospital, will that be enough to relocate the resident during her absence?

- If the resident gets moved against her will, will that action be:

- A violation of the resident's right
- Treating the resident without dignity
- Abuse
- All the above

Case #2

Mary is a staff member at the ZAB skilled nursing facility. During her weekend shift she noticed something that might be considered resident abuse. She promptly wrote a note for her director of nursing (DON) and slid it under her door.

- Under the Elder Justice Act, when does the timely reporting start—at the time she observed the alleged abuse, or when the DON reads the note? Even though Mary is not sure if what she observed was abuse, was reporting the incident to the DON consistent with regulations and the facility policy?

- Did Mary fulfill her reporting duty by reporting the alleged abuse to the DON?

References

California Department of Aging. (2012). *Long-term care ombudsman program.* Retrieved from http://www.aging.ca.gov/Programs/LTCOP/

Elder Abuse Exposed.com. (2013). *US Attorney, FBI urged to investigate CA AG Kamala Harris' Elder Abuse Unit.* Retrieved from http://elderabuseexposed.com/us-attorney-fbi-urged-to-investigate-ca-ag-kamala-harris-elder-abuse-unit/

Francine M. Neilson v. Colgate-Palmolive Co., 199 f.3d 642 (2d Cir) (1999).

Haverhill Care Center v. HCFA, DAB NO. CR-522 (1998).

Medicare.gov (n.d.a). *What Part A covers.* Retrieved from http://medicare.gov/what-medicare-covers/part-a/what-part-a-covers.html

Medicare.gov. (n.d.b). *What Part B covers.* Retrieved from http://medicare.gov/what-medicare-covers/part-b/what-medicare-part-b-covers.html

Office of the Assistant Secretary for Planning and Evaluation. (2015). *Federal financial participation in state assistance expenditures; Federal matching shares for Medicaid, the children's health insurance program, and aid to needy aged, blind, or disabled persons for October 1, 2014 through September 30, 2015.* Retrieved from http://aspe.hhs.gov/basic-report/fy2015-federal-medical-assistance-percentages

Office of Inspector General, U.S. Department of Health and Human Services & Health Care Prevention and Enforcement Team. (2014). *Provider compliance training: Take the initiative—Cultivate a culture of compliance with health care laws.* Retrieved from http://www.oig.hhs.gov/compliance/provider-compliance-training/index.asp

Office of Public Affairs, U.S. Department of Justice. (2014). Justice department recovers nearly $6 billion from false claims act cases in fiscal year 2014. Retrieved from http://www.justice.gov/opa/pr/justice-department-recovers-nearly-6-billion-false-claims-act-cases-fiscal-year-2014

Stiegel, L. A. (2010). Elder abuse prevention: Elder Justice Act becomes law, but victory is only partial. *Biofocal, 31*(Mar–Apr), No. 4. Retrieved from http://www.americanbar.org/content/dam/aba/administrative/law_aging/elder_abuse_eja_act_art_prtl.authcheckdam.pdf

U.S. Department of Health & Human Services. (n.d.). *U.S. Office for Civil Rights.* Retrieved from http://www.hhs.gov/ocr/office/index.html

U.S. ex rel. Absher v. Momence Meadows Nursing Center, Nos. 13-1886 & 13-1936 (2014, Aug 20).

CHAPTER 9

MARKETING AND PUBLIC RELATIONS

Janice Frates
Susie Mix

Most people who become senior citizens will need long-term care services at some point, and anyone can suddenly become seriously disabled. However, few people plan ahead for it, mostly for emotional and financial reasons. All types of long-term care services present a common marketing challenge: how to promote a service that customers don't want, are highly reluctant to use, or, in many cases, do not recognize as a need. A further complication is that while the service user is the frail elderly or disabled individual, often the decision maker is a family member and the purchase decision is driven by what financial resources are available. Each type of long-term care service has its unique marketing challenges, as shown in Table 9.1.

Assessing Local Demand for Long-Term Care Services

A critical success factor for long-term care communities is the number of people in the area who will be attracted to the type of housing that a community offers (Ehlers, 2010). Are there enough seniors and disabled individuals with the characteristics of your **target market**? What are

LEARNING OBJECTIVES

- Assess the demand for long-term care in a given service area.

- Identify long-term care customers and define their service needs.

- Analyze competitors in the various long-term care service market sectors.

- Recognize the principal distribution channels for long-term care service providers.

- Explain the influence of regulatory agencies for long-term services marketing.

- Articulate the basic tenets of long-term care customer service and retention.

- Prepare a basic marketing plan for long-term care services.

Table 9.1   Marketing Challenges for Different Types of Long-Term Care Services

Service type	Target customer	Benefits and features	Objections/fears	Key marketing messages
Home care	Hospital discharge planners, skilled nursing facilities, physicians, families of frail elderly and disabled	Patient able to receive care in the comfort of his own home	Stranger in the home; limited treatment by paraprofessional caregivers; transportation needed for more complex care; agencies are 30% to 50% more expensive than privately hired caregivers	Allows aging in place safely with agency personnel; hard to find qualified and trustworthy caregivers on your own
Adult day services	Families of frail elderly and disabled, senior housing communities, skilled nursing facilities	Social interaction with others, gives respite to primary caregiver	Can be costly if current benefits do not cover this service; patient may not fit in the environment	Allows clients to remain at home with supervised care, meals, and social contact during the day
Assisted living	Frail elders and their families, physicians, skilled nursing facilities, senior housing communities	Social interaction and activities, different levels of service accommodations available	Difficulty giving up home, can be costly; not a health insurance benefit; all private pay; resident must be ambulatory	Assisted living is *not* a nursing home; assisted living is living well
Board and care	Frail elders and their families, hospital discharge planners, skilled nursing facilities, home health agencies, assisted living facilities, physicians	Homelike environment, usually smaller and more intimate setting than skilled nursing facility, less costly residential alternative	Difficulty leaving current living situation; quality of care varies greatly	If you can't live at home, at least you can live in a homelike setting
Nursing home (skilled nursing facility or SNF)	Hospital discharge planners, physicians, assisted living facilities, managed care discharge planners, board and care facilities	Intensive rehabilitation services and 24-hour nursing available	Somewhat similar to a hospital environment; stigma of nursing home; privacy can be limited if you share a room	Nursing homes are not what they used to be; new rehabilitation therapies for stroke, fractures
Continuing care retirement communities (CCRCs)	Senior housing communities, estate planners, financial advisors	Many different levels of care offered, transition in levels made very easy, social interaction	Can be very costly; large initial investment required to purchase living unit	Range of services to meet your varying care needs no matter how ill you become or how long you live

the population growth projections? Data sources to answer these questions include the following:

- Number of seniors and disabled individuals in the market service area: These data (current and projected) are available from the U.S. Census, some state and county agencies, and the local governmental unit for the federal Area Agency on Aging.

- Hospital payer mix: This critical variable determines to which hospitals you want to market. For nearly all hospitals, as shown in Figure 9.1, Medicare accounts for the largest share of both patients and revenues; however, within a service area the **hospital payer mix** reflects patient demographics and managed care penetration. The availability of these data varies greatly by state. For example, the California Office of Statewide Health Planning and Development (OSHPD) collects and compiles quarterly utilization and financial data from almost all hospitals. The OSHPD web page includes an interactive set of Excel pivot tables that provide market share and patient origin data by payer and geographic area, down to the zip code level (California OSHPD, 2013).

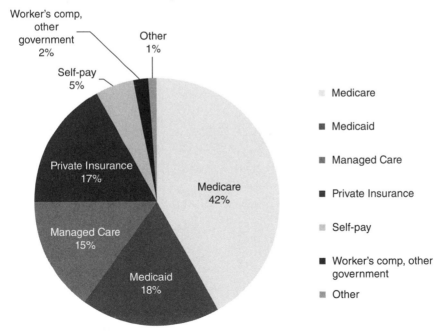

Hospital Revenue Share

Figure 9.1 National Average Hospital Payer Mix, 2009
Source: Adapted from Gamble (2012).

Public Perceptions and Public Relations

Given that public perceptions of long-term services are poorly informed and for the most part highly negative, what can be done to improve consumer knowledge and attitudes?

Naming and Vocabulary

What's in a name? Many associations and emotions, which create perceptions and hugely influence service purchase decisions. Depending on the target market, the community's promotional emphasis can be on independence (freedom from home maintenance chores, cooking, etc.), companionship, socialization, recreation opportunities, caring, and/or comfort.

Janis Ehlers (2010) notes the importance of language that connotes a homelike atmosphere for seniors and recommends specific words and communication behaviors to avoid, as shown in Table 9.2. She also reminds us that:

• People typically think of themselves as 20 years younger than their chronological ages.

• It is often the subliminal messages that attract or repel prospective residents and their families.

• The marketing focus must always be on dignity.

Table 9.2   Words and Terms to Lose and Use

Lose	Use
Unit	Apartment, room
Patient	Resident
Facility	Community
Leasing, sales center	Welcome center
Salesman, saleswoman, sales agent	Sales counselor
Your mother, father, aunt/uncle	Mom, Dad, Aunt Betty, Uncle Bob
Colloquialisms, such as sweetie, bud, honey	Person's preferred name
Three meals a day	Breakfast, lunch, dinner
Industry acronyms (ADLs, AL, CCRC, SNF)	Correct or commonly used name
Alzheimer's, dementia	Memory care

Source: Adapted from Ehlers (2010).

Addressing Suspicions and Fears

Long-term care services, especially nursing homes, have received a lot of bad press over the years, some of which was well deserved. The broader consumer demand for transparency, facilitated by the availability of information through the Internet and social media, has influenced both consumers and regulators to become better educated and more discerning purchasers and users. Online information and tools, such as the Medicare Nursing Home Compare website (http://www.medicare.gov/nursinghomecompare/About/What-Is-NHC.html), present some marketing challenges but even greater advantages for long-term care service providers. The challenges involve monitoring the information sources; developing strategies and allocating resources to manage them; and ensuring that marketing communications are consistent with external reviews and reports about your industry sector in general and your organization in particular. These online tools, provided by ostensibly neutral third-party nonprofits or government agencies, offer the consumer accurate and unbiased information. And informed consumers (or their family members or agents) who know what services they need and what they can reasonably expect to receive are far more likely to be satisfied customers than those who are misinformed, which can often lead to unrealistic or unreasonable expectations.

Table 9.3, from the Commonwealth Fund, addressing common misperceptions about nursing homes, is an example of consumer information resources available from government and nonprofit sources (Eisner & Lorber, 2006).

Customers and Their Needs

While the end user of long-term care services is the elderly or disabled individual, the purchaser or decision maker is more likely to be a family member, healthcare professional, or an organizational representative, such as a health plan case manager or hospital discharge planner.

Families

Families are the most important influencers of long-term care service use decisions. They make the initial suggestion, begin exploring options, and encourage discussion and ultimately a decision. In the best-case scenarios, the family is available to help with the transition into the new living environment. However, the dynamics vary considerably according to the nature and quality of the relationship between the individual needing the

Table 9.3   Nursing Home Myths and Realities

Myth	Reality
Medicaid does not pay for the service you want.	Medicaid residents are entitled to the same service as other residents.
Only staff can determine the care you receive.	Residents and family have the right to participate in developing a care plan.
Staff cannot accommodate individual schedules.	A nursing home must make reasonable adjustments to honor residents' needs and preferences.
You need to hire private help.	A nursing home must provide all necessary care.
Restraints are required to prevent the resident from wandering away.	Restraints cannot be used for the nursing home's convenience or as a form of discipline.
Family visiting hours are restricted.	Family members can visit at any time of day or night.
Therapy must be discontinued because the resident is not progressing.	Therapy may be appropriate, and Medicare may pay even without current progress.
You must pay any amount set by the nursing home for extra charges.	A nursing home may require only extra charges authorized in the admission agreement.
The nursing home has no available space for residents or family members to meet.	A nursing home must provide a private space for resident or family councils.
The resident can be evicted because he is difficult or refuses medical treatment.	Being difficult or refusing treatment does not justify eviction.

Source: Adapted from Carlson (2006).

service and the family member. The loving husband of a woman with dementia who can no longer care for herself must not only deal with feelings of guilt for perceived abandonment of his lifelong companion but also face a painful separation and loneliness when his life partner is no longer physically present in his home.

Overwhelmed adult children who are caregivers for their elderly parents must deal with similar issues of guilt and abandonment, often complicated by pressures to fulfill other family responsibilities to their spouses and children. If there are several adult child siblings and/or a spouse involved in the decision, they may have conflicting opinions about the preferred alternative, or varying degrees of resolve about implementing a care decision.

Whatever the family dynamics are, it is vital for long-term care marketing professionals to tune into them, and to listen empathically in order to allay concerns, correct misperceptions, and assist the family to obtain the services that their loved one needs. Establishing a positive relationship with the family encourages them to become partners in care with the service provider, working together to ensure their loved one feels valued and is well cared for by both the professional caregiving staff and the family. This is especially important for families of residents in long-term care residential facilities.

TIPS FOR WORKING WITH FAMILIES IN LTC RESIDENTIAL FACILITIES

- Ask the family to designate one member as the primary or lead contact, and a second as the backup, responsible for communicating with other members.

- Provide regular updates on the resident's status, services received, and activities. If the resident agrees, health providers may share or discuss his information with family members—but only what the person involved needs to know about the resident's care or payment for such care. If the resident is incapacitated, the provider may share information with the power-of-attorney holder or appropriate surrogate decision maker. If using e-mail or text messaging, be aware that the 1996 **Health Information Portability and Accountability Act (HIPAA)** regulations require encryption of electronic communications containing patient information (iHealthBeat, 2011).

- Invite family members to participate in social and recreational activities; let them know they are always welcome and make it easy for them to do so (e.g., no advance RSVP requirements).

- Create special events to honor families, while also ensuring that residents without family visitors do not feel left out. Volunteers, such as high school students earning community service hours, can participate in these events as surrogate families for isolated residents. A "guardian angel" program whereby each department manager is assigned a certain number of residents, checks in regularly with the resident, and provides additional support can also ameliorate the lack of family involvement.

- Establish a family advisory board that can function as a support group as well as provide feedback on their perceptions of service quality. Partner with families to establish how they can continue to assist their loved one in the caring relationship.

- Make referrals to outside resources, support groups, and websites.

- Help family members have successful visits, especially for residents with dementia. Often family members just don't know what to talk about or how to start a conversation.

Third-Party Payers

Because they control financial resources, third-party payers play a key role in long-term care service purchasing decisions. This category includes public insurance and benefit programs, such as Medicare, Medicaid, and the Veterans Health Administration, private health and long-term care insurers, and **managed care organizations**. These payers follow a set of criteria and rules for service use eligibility and for provider participation. It's up to them what services a client may receive and where. All have definitions of **medical necessity**; either the client's physician or the payer's designated medical professional (sometimes both) must describe and document in the acceptable terminology that the prospective service recipient is sufficiently disabled or unable to perform specified **activities of daily living (ADLs)**.

Payer criteria for provider payment begin with requirements for satisfactory compliance with state licensing and quality standards and can include more specific certifications, accreditations, ratings by consumer groups, and scores on patient satisfaction surveys. In general, the higher the reimbursement and the larger the proportion of privately funded patients, the more stringent the requirements are for provider participation.

Managed care organizations (MCOs), a category that includes health maintenance organization (HMO) and preferred provider organization (PPO) health plans, are the dominant payers in many areas of the United States. They are increasingly important long-term care service payers because approximately 13.5 million people or 27% of Medicare beneficiaries are enrolled in some type of managed care health plan (Kaiser Family Foundation [KFF], 2012). Some 9.4 million low-income elderly and/or disabled individuals are "**dual eligibles**" or "**Medi-Medis**" who receive benefits from both Medicare and the Medicaid program for low-income (KFF, 2013).

As a long-term care administrator, it is imperative to know the MCOs that have members in your area because these organizations determine where their members may receive care. In addition to the MCOs, some states have **independent practice associations (IPAs)** that also drive the managed care business into skilled nursing facilities. A few key resources for researching this information are the following:

- Centers for Medicare and Medicaid Services (CMS): This federal agency publishes monthly reports of enrollment in Medicare managed care and drug plans by county (CMS, n.d.). The availability of Medicaid enrollee data varies by state, and will not be useful unless it is broken out by age or disability status.

- Facility medical director: He may have knowledge of which medical practices are affiliated with the various MCOs and IPAs in the community.

- Hospital discharge planners and case managers: What health plan members do they see most often being admitted to the hospital?

- MCO websites: Most plans have websites that list membership service areas and often the affiliated IPAs and hospitals.

- Insurance brokers and benefits consultants: Most are aware of the main MCOs in a given area.

- Business journals: Most of these city or regional publications publish an annual "Book of Lists" with the largest businesses in each category, including hospitals and health plans (American City Business Journals, 2012).

Once the MCOs and IPAs have been identified, contracts should be obtained with health plans in your facility's service area that hold financial risk for skilled nursing facility services. These contracts will be the first step in creating access to managed care admissions to your facility.

Marketing efforts to increase managed care census in the facility are usually done at the local level. Most health plans and IPAs have case managers and discharge planners who either work at the local hospitals or work closely with the hospital discharge planners to move patients to a lower level of care. Developing relationships with these key decision makers is vital to increase the managed care census in your facility.

Understanding the expectations of the MCOs and being familiar with the key quality care measures and statistics that drive performance for them are also important to the growth of the managed care member census in your facility. Here are the key utilization management protocols for MCOs:

1. Acceptance of admissions 24/7 to the facility, from home or hospital emergency room

2. Short length of stay

3. A discharge plan within 24 to 48 hours of admission

4. A single point of contact to provide updates

5. Low percentage of hospital readmissions

6. Monthly reports on individual patient and average length of stay, number and percentage of hospital readmissions

7. Facility survey outcomes that measure quality of care, and skilled nursing facility star ratings

With the healthcare industry moving more and more into managed care as opposed to fee-for-service reimbursement, it is vital to understand the importance of developing solid relations with managed care organizations.

Identifying Customer Needs

Long-term care marketing professionals must understand what customers want in order to assist them to obtain the services they need. The frail elder wants to maintain her independence, and either does not realize or refuses to acknowledge that she needs help with activities of daily living. Her children want peace of mind and to know that their mother is safe, and realize that she needs some form of supervised care. However, they do not know the types of services that are available, how to assess their quality, what they cost, or how to access them. Often a specific event sparks a senior's or a family member's decision to use long-term care services, especially residential placement.

TRIGGER EVENTS FOR USE OF LONG-TERM CARE SERVICES

Declining health

- Gradual

    Physical: loss of flexibility, difficulty getting out of chair or bed, toileting independently

    Memory loss, confusion, uncertainty about decisions or actions, unpaid bills

    Repeated hospitalizations or trips to the emergency room

- Sudden

    Physical: slips, falls, dizziness

    Mental: unable to find parked car, find one's way home, getting lost

    Health crisis: broken hip, stroke

Spouse's death or loss of another primary caregiver

Failure to pass driver's license examination or suspension of driver's license after an accident

Deciding they have had enough cooking, cleaning, yard work, home repairs, and so forth

Market Segmentation

The essential foundation of an organization's marketing program is the target market, or the customers the organization seeks to serve. **Market segmentation** is the first step in developing a viable targeted marketing strategy. It involves grouping customers into clusters who have similar needs and wants, and then tailoring marketing program elements for that cluster. For long-term care services, the major **market segment** categories are as follows:

- Age: There are several generational senior cohorts. Recent retirees have vastly different needs and wants than the "oldest old." Key attractions for this younger customer segment are affordable housing costs in areas with a high cost of living, extensive and affordable recreational opportunities, and socialization offered by clubs and scheduled activities.

- Abilities, physical and mental: Consider the vastly different needs of active baby boomers compared with extremely frail elders or those with dementia.

- Income, education: While closely linked, not all affluent customers are highly educated and vice versa. Affluent customers will expect a wide range of food choices and well-appointed individual and common living areas. Highly educated customers may want more intellectually oriented activities, such as trips to museums, plays, and symphony concerts. Others will prefer simpler food, less fancy furnishings, and more middlebrow activities.

- Ethnicity: Most long-term care services are oriented to serving Caucasians, while the U.S. population is increasingly ethnically diverse, particularly in major metropolitan areas. Areas with large minority communities often make up an underserved niche market, especially for people with limited English proficiency.

- Religion: While long-term care communities cannot exclude applicants on the grounds of race or religion, under state regulations for restricted occupancy they can offer services to meet the specific needs of a particular population, such as a Jewish home for the aged that observes Kosher dietary laws and adheres to other tenets of the religion. However, if the facility allows any exceptions to the qualifying criteria, it must have an open admission policy.

The demographics of the surrounding community determine the size of the various market segments for long-term care services. These market segments are the primary source of prospective residents, who generally want to continue to live in their home communities even when they can no longer live in their own homes. The typical prospect for a retirement community is female, 80 or older, who needs assistance with two or more activities of daily living (ADLs); she or her family lives within 10 miles of the community; there is a 50% chance she is a homeowner and if so, over an 80% probability that she has no mortgage (Pearce, 2007). There are also market segments of adult children who will relocate their aging relatives to live with or near them. In this case, the elder is a prospective customer for home healthcare or adult day services or a potential resident in an assisted living or skilled nursing community.

Competition

If the market is deep enough to support a retirement community or other long-term care service, what organizations currently serve this market? Consider as your competitors not just organizations that offer the same services but also those that offer alternative services all along the continuum of long-term care—especially those that provide less intensive and less expensive care.

Positioning

Positioning a community so that it stands out from competitors in a positive way involves research, analysis, and creativity:

- Analyze the competition: Identify the market leaders and your organization's market position. Create a spreadsheet with key data, such as location, size, services offered, pricing, amenities, buyer profile, unit mix, promotional methods, incentives, future community expansion plans, and a worksheet for each competitor that includes pictures (Ehlers, 2010).

- Visit competitor facilities and note:

  - First impressions: How do the public and private spaces look and smell?

  - Customer service: How friendly and informed was the marketing representative? How easy was it to arrange the visit?

  - Truth in advertising: Do the marketing materials accurately reflect the appearance and style of the community?

  - Shared decision making: Is there evidence that residents can direct their care, and that families are included as care partners (Loughney, 2005)?

Marketing Approaches

After assessing the market and your competition, market the benefits of your community service compared to the alternatives. Lee Duffey (2002) offers several tips for achieving this objective:

- Consider a non-traditional marketing segmentation approach, such as by medical conditions rather than location or age. Memory care is one such approach; another could be the 25% of people over 65 with diabetes, a population cohort that the federal Centers for Disease Control and Prevention (CDC) project will increase to 33% by 2050 (Landro, 2013).

- Establish recognition through branding—what will consumers think when they hear your company name?

- Create and strengthen relationships to securely bond with customers—and their families. Encourage them to be advocates, proud to be a part of your community or a user of your services. Customer advocates are especially important when the decision to use the service is a reluctant one.

- Look for and create new referral relationships by emphasizing attributes that are important to various stakeholders. Investors and bankers will welcome information attesting to your organization's financial stability; physicians and other clinicians will be concerned about quality of care metrics and ratings; insurers' decisions are based on price, quality, and the facility's ability and willingness to accommodate MCO utilization management protocols.

Collaboration

Working with competitors is not only possible but also a wise marketing strategy. Customers will comparison shop on their own to find and select the type of long-term care service that offers the most value in relation to what they want and think they need. However, these preferences and needs will change over time. Organizations along the long-term care service continuum will establish systems of cross-referrals for their mutual benefit and to most effectively serve their shared clientele (Brandenburger & Nalebuff, 1996).

Referral Agents

Long-term care service organizations are embedded in a larger community, where there are many types of individuals and organizations that can influence and direct prospective customers to your door. **Referral agents** include but are not limited to: physicians and their medical staff, nurses, hospital discharge planners, hospital and community-based social workers, pharmacists, community health and social service agencies (especially those specifically serving seniors), clergy and faith-based organizations, funeral home directors, fiduciaries, trustees, attorneys, health plan case managers, geriatric care managers, real estate agents, state and local department of aging and adult services, transportation service providers, and members of advocacy and professional organizations. Professional organizations, such as the local medical society and hospital association, can help you reach professionals in the leading organizations and meet individual service providers.

Referral relationships are based on trust and knowledge. Because the referring agent is putting his credibility or reputation on the line when making a referral, he has a professional and personal obligation to verify the quality of the service. Just being listed in a directory is insufficient, as the referral will be tepid and qualified. There are referral registries that charge fees for listing a facility and for an executed placement. As the federal Stark laws have strict prohibitions against providers receiving or paying any type of "kickback" fee for serving Medicare and Medicaid beneficiaries, these agencies limit their placement activities to private pay patients, and in some states they are illegal.

An important first step in obtaining referrals of Medicare post-acute care and rehabilitation patients is learning who determines discharges from hospitals. It varies by community and by hospital. The decision driver can be the physician, the case manager, or the discharge planner. Furthermore, each hospital operates differently. In some hospitals the decision depends on the payer; in others it varies by unit or floor.

Networking

There is no substitute for personal connections to key influencers in the community. Cultivating and managing relationships are both a science and an art. The science involves collecting and organizing information about the services available for your target market customers, and developing a variety of informational packets for the various types of referral agents. The art involves making contact with them to establish and nurture a relationship that will produce referrals. Pearce (1998) suggests that the initial marketing contact be a request to learn about their services rather than to tell them about yours, with follow-up to thank them for their time and inform them that they have been designated a referral resource for the community's residents; he also advises to always give residents a choice of at least two different resources to minimize perceptions of favoritism and the risk of providing inappropriate direction or advice.

USEFUL TOOLS

- **Nursing home checklists.** The CMS have a downloadable form for consumers to use when visiting a facility; see http://www.medicare.gov/files/nursing-home-checklist.pdf. Another more detailed version, with additional questions on clinical quality of care measures, is available at: http://www.medicare.gov/nursing/checklist.asp.

- **Competitor assessments.** Authors Janis Ehlers (2010) and Benjamin Pearce (2007) each provide helpful instruments for evaluating what a competitor residential facility has to offer. Ehlers's tool (Figure 5-1 in her book) offers a comprehensive list of questions to answer about the facility and staff. Pearce has developed a three-page form for a confidential **mystery shopper** analysis, presumably to be used by someone posing as a prospective resident or family member. While the use of mystery shoppers is common in some industries, it is not recommended for long-term care service providers. There are plenty of opportunities to openly visit competitor communities, such as open houses, or a straightforward visit with a reciprocal invitation to visit your community.

- **Prospect registration form.** Ehlers (2010) has also designed a useful prospect registration form (Figure 18-1) on which to record information about a potential future customer, including contact information for future follow-up communications.

Public and Private Oversight of Long-Term Care Services Providers

Public concern about care for vulnerable elderly and disabled individuals and media reports of abuses have resulted in heavy regulation of all types of long-term care services, with regulatory oversight increasing proportionately to service level intensity. Public reporting mechanisms include report cards, the federal "Nursing Home Compare" website, and various state rating systems. There are also private efforts, such as the National Consumer Voice for Quality Long-Term Care, a national advocacy or consumer watchdog organization. Some states also have public rating systems.

The **Medicare Five-Star Quality Rating** system (CMS, 2013) appears on the CMS Nursing Home Compare website. Health plans are starting to focus on these star ratings as a criterion for contracting. Users can download detailed quarterly reports that give each nursing home a rating of between one and five stars, overall and on three factors:

1. Health inspections for the past 3 years

2. Staffing—average number of hours per day of nursing care provided to each resident

3. Quality measures—nine different clinical measures for nursing home residents, such as pressure sores and mobility changes

The federal government has delegated oversight responsibility for hospitals and nursing homes to state licensing agencies. These agencies conduct on-site inspections, and document and report their findings on **Form 2567** state inspection reports, which the nursing homes must make available to the public within 14 days after receipt. The facility must post the notice in a prominent location accessible to the public. The form lists deficiencies cited by the survey team to which the facility must submit a plan of correction.

While regulation can be onerous, it can be a useful marketing element. Since the results are readily available to the public, it is advisable to capitalize on strong survey ratings and correct deficiencies as soon as possible. High ratings, with a short and simple explanation of what they mean, are a vital element to include in all promotional materials. If there are deficiencies, it's important for the administrative staff to: (a) communicate with all staff about the deficiencies and what to say if someone questions them about a deficiency; and (b) respond to inquiries with specific information about what corrective actions will be taken and when.

Customer Services and Retention

Long-term care is an intensely personal service, so attentive, personalized customer service is the critical success factor in customer retention. Excellent customer service begins with the first contact. It continues after the placement ends, with attention to the family to ensure either a smooth transition to another care setting or a comforting closure in the event of a resident's death.

Preplacement Evaluation

Preadmission assessment is a prerequisite for satisfaction, to ensure a good fit between the resident and the community and establish realistic expectations for the resident and family. If the resident has little hope of becoming a satisfied customer, his negative experience will negatively impact resident relations, staff morale, and the organization's reputation in the community service area.

Customer Service

Customer service is everyone's job, because all aspects of a resident's experience in a senior living community influence satisfaction, which in turn impacts the community's reputation and referrals to it. Ehlers (2010) offers these tips to demonstrate a caring attitude, according to which residents come first:

- Offer reassurance and assistance with moving in.
  - Designate a move-in coordinator if possible.
  - Prepare instructions, including a checklist and timetable.
  - Provide a welcome basket and/or stock refrigerators in an assisted living community.
  - For skilled nursing facilities, ask resident or family to bring a few family photos and treasured keepsakes for placement where resident can easily see them. For assisted living communities, offer staff assistance or provide information about a reliable service to help unpack, arrange furniture, hook up televisions/computers, hang pictures, and so forth.
- Establish a comprehensive welcome program involving staff, family, and residents, with particular attention to:
  - Making introductions and arrangements for dining companionship.
  - Encouraging new residents to participate in social activities.
  - Informing families about how the resident is settling in.
  - Providing very clear, accurate, and up-to-date information about the community's services, how to access them, and when they are available.
- Provide appropriate assistance to surviving residents and family when a resident dies or leaves the community for whatever reasons.

Resident Ambassadors

While some residents are naturally sociable and gracious and will reach out to new arrivals, having a formal program in place recognizes and rewards their efforts and encourages a culture of inclusion that makes a huge impact on customer satisfaction and retention. If done well, participating in such a program will be an honor for residents and generate strong interest—even competition—to become a resident ambassador. Satisfied and enthusiastic residents can help generate the best possible type of promotion and referrals, which is word-of-mouth.

While it is inappropriate—and under Medicare and Medicaid rules, illegal—to offer resident ambassadors any form of financial compensation or payment discounts, it is both permissible and advisable to acknowledge their contributions to the community with such things as badges, business cards, door plaques, or distinctive pieces of clothing, and to recognize them publicly with various types of appreciation ceremonial activities.

Monitoring Customer Satisfaction

Keeping track of this important metric is a sound marketing practice. As well, long-term care service providers that receive federal funds (Medicare or Medicaid) must keep records of patient/resident grievances and how they were resolved. Facilities must establish a residents' council, hold meetings at least monthly, and make records of these meetings available to regulators. If residents raise concerns or make complaints, the facility must respond and document its actions to address the complaint or concern.

Because of the importance of this metric, many skilled nursing firms work with a third-party vendor who specializes in gathering customer satisfaction data, usually by phone, after the patient is discharged from the facility. Facilities use this information to follow up with the patient as well as to improve internal systems.

Marketing Plan

The purpose of a marketing plan is to establish business growth objectives and develop strategies and tactics to achieve them. Objectives, strategies, and tactics are the building blocks of market planning. **Objectives** are measurable and time-specific statements of what is to be accomplished. **Strategies** are the means to achieve marketing objectives. **Tactics** are specific actions to implement a strategy—the nuts and bolts of the plan. The plan for a skilled nursing facility in Exhibit 9.1 and Exhibit 9.2 illustrates the relationship among these three foundational elements of a marketing plan.

Exhibit 9.1   Sample Marketing Plan Objectives, Strategies, and Tactics

Topanga Park Marketing Plan

OBJECTIVE: To achieve 100% occupancy with a combination of general Skilled Nursing and Special Care Dementia units.

STRATEGIES AND TACTICS

1. Broaden Topanga Park's visibility in the Canoga Park civic community.
    a. Join community organizations including Chamber of Commerce, Rotary Club.
    b. Participate in and sponsor local community events.
    c. Strengthen relationships with political leaders.
    d. Develop a partnership with CSUN Gerontology Program.

2. Strengthen outreach to the healthcare community.
    a. Continue to work with area hospitals' discharge planners.
    b. Develop relationships with assisted living communities, adult day health centers, and home health agencies..
    c. Strengthen relationships with leading referral doctors and residents' personal physicians through office visits. Provide office managers with literature on aging and SNF services.
    d. Plan events at Topanga Park for doctors' office staff and representatives of other referral agent organizations.

3. Target the caregiver market.
    a. Participate in community programs for caregivers.
    b. Present quarterly caregiver educational program on aging parents.
    c. Contact, provide literature to Employee Assistance Programs.

4. Develop relationships with churches and pastoral contacts.
    a. Continue to develop and update religious organization database.
    b. Present workshop on aging issues for pastoral community.
    c. Give church communities caregiver information and literature.

5. Increase visibility within the general community as a referral base.
    a. Establish relationship with local banks.
    b. Expand referral base of financial planners, attorneys and trust officers.
    c. Develop plan for financial lecture series co-sponsored by Topanga Park and Conservators & Fiduciary Association.

6. Maintain a competitive package of services and fee structure.
    a. Establish comprehensive pricing structure with fees for special services.
    b. Institute a comprehensive Dementia Program.
    c. Continually update competitive pricing and program information.

7. Continue a systematic, effective procedure for follow-up and tracking inquiries from first contact through move-in.
    a. Hire a marketing representative.
    b. Introduce a computer tracking system to record inquiries and sources, schedule follow-up calls, and produce required correspondence.
    c. Track residents who are hospitalized for proper follow-up and communication with the hospital discharge planners.

Exhibit 9.2   Marketing Plan Outline

Note: This is a generic plan that will need customization for the specific service or facility

   I.   Introduction: <u>Brief</u> description of service, customers, market service area

      A.   Features and corresponding benefits

      B.   Key attributes of the market environment

  II.   Demand Analysis

      A.   Geographic service area demographics

      B.   Market size (total potential users)

      C.   Demand estimates—calculate/estimate number of likely potential customers

      D.   Payers and payer mix

 III.   Competitor Analysis

      A.   Identify market leaders

      B.   Compare strengths and weaknesses of your and competitor organizations (chart)

      C.   Differentiation: State why and how your organization is different and better than competitors

      D.   Articulate your organization's sustainable competitive advantage

 IV.   Distribution Channel Analysis

      A.   Identify and define the role of your partners, if intermediaries are involved

      B.   Research distribution channel demographics—how many of each type of distributor are there in your service area?

  V.   Implementation of Marketing Plan

      A.   Marketing objectives—must be measurable and time-specific

      B.   Strategies—how to achieve objectives; link each strategy to an objective

      C.   Tactics—specific actions to carry out strategies; link each tactic to a strategy

 VI.   Promotional Mix—discuss all that apply, omit if not applicable

      A.   Advertising

      B.   Personal selling

      C.   Publicity and public/government relations

      D.   Sales promotion

      E.   Social media

      F.   Other (specify)

Exhibit 9.2 *(Continued)*

VII. Budget (for all marketing, promotion, PR, advertising—not program operations); use line item format and document data sources for all figures

    A. Staff

    B. Materials

    C. Equipment

    D. Media

    E. Entertainment

    F. Vendors/consultants

    G. Other (specify)

VIII. Time line (1 year): Quarterly or monthly sequence of action steps (tactics) to implement strategies and achieve objectives

IX. Performance assessment: How will you track and measure marketing plan results to ensure that you achieve your marketing objectives?

Return on Marketing Investment (ROI)

Spending money on marketing is easy; measuring the results is more complex. Matthieson and Whitehurst (2010) offer several practical suggestions for measuring how marketing efforts result in referrals.

- Track leads (names and contact information) obtained for each marketing activity, event, advertisement, or mailer

- Key metrics

  - Number (census) and occupancy/vacancy ratios (percentage of filled or empty units) are the primary indicators of success for residential facilities

  - For skilled nursing facilities
    - Conversion rates: Contacts→inquiries→referrals→admissions
    - Cost per contact, inquiry, referral, admission

  - For assisted living facilities
    - Conversion rates: Leads→visits→deposits→move-ins
    - Cost per lead, visit, move-in

  - Length of time to fill vacancies

Customer Buying Behavior

A study of generational differences among healthcare consumers in the United States found that older people seldom buy on impulse; comparison shop carefully; appreciate detailed brochures and other printed materials; are loyal to brands and stores; respond to direct mail invitations and call toll-free numbers; value service over price; and dislike products that are too clearly targeted to seniors (Berkowitz & Schewe, 2011). Mindful of these facts, long-term care service marketing professionals developing marketing communication programs and pieces are well advised to:

• Remember that you are marketing to a dual audience, elders and their adult children—and to a broader audience of current and potential referral agents in the professional arena and the general public.

• Avoid stereotypes of the elderly.

• Accentuate the positive: Emphasize services and benefits instead of the need for care (Adkins, 2000).

Branding

Duffey (2002, p. 1) describes branding as "creating identification of a company or product in consumers' minds when they see or hear the company's name," and notes the importance of establishing recognition through branding so that consumers connect the company name to the services offered. Ehlers (2010) suggests researching local history to find ideas that reflect the area and have not been used by others.

An essential but often overlooked aspect of branding is the internal marketing that employees can and should do for the organization—if they are proud of what they do and where they work. If they are dissatisfied or unenthusiastic about the company, what they say about it will undermine marketing efforts. Make sure that employees understand the service offerings and have positive things to say about them. Including employees in identifying service outcomes and new service offerings is one example of how to engage staff in marketing efforts.

Ethical Marketing

Truth in advertising, and all marketing activities, is a critical success factor. Adkins (2000) cites research showing that elders, especially those born before 1925, tend to be more trusting than younger generations, and thus are more vulnerable to inflated claims. Regulatory agencies and consumer watchdog organizations are on the lookout for deceptive practices, and there are strict penalties for organizations that violate regulatory guidelines or abuse the public trust. When this happens, it can result in not just a dissatisfied consumer but a public relations disaster, as well as severe financial sanctions. Sins of omission also count, as, for example, the nursing home that fails to note on any of its printed materials nor in any discussion with the family that the facility does not accept Medicaid patients, so residents who exhaust their financial resources would have to leave when they could no longer pay for their care.

False Promises

The federal Merchandising Practices Statute or Little FTC (Federal Trade Commission) Act establishes that statements made in marketing materials that are false, deceptive, or create false promises may be legally actionable. States each have their own standards for advertising, but a crucial consideration is that any statement that could create a false impression, mislead, or deceive often violates the state law. And some aggressive attorneys are filing class-action lawsuits based on one resident's complaint to allege that other residents are suffering from the same abuse and winning very large settlements for their clients (Dewitt, 2008). To minimize legal exposure and maximize trust and confidence:

- Make sure that marketing materials claims are realistic and verifiable.
- Make promises and promotional statements based on facts, not predictions.
- Instead of making promises when families express concerns, address the issue and discuss the treatment plan.
- Consider including a disclaimer approved by an attorney in the admissions contract.

Advertising and Promotional Activities

An organization's objectives and strategies and its financial resources will determine the marketing mix of activities. Table 9.4 lists the most common elements for long-term care service marketing.

Social Media

Just as an Internet website presence is now essential for any business, social media is an integral element of the marketing mix. Seniors are increasingly using social media as a communication tool and to evaluate products and services, including over 34 million caregivers in the United States (Stern, 2009). However, it's crucial to create the right message and tone of caring.

Table 9.4 Marketing Activities for Long-Term Services

Activity	Definition/examples	Comments
Advertising	Paid promotional messages Examples: - Print, TV spots, radio ads - Billboards - Telephone directory ads (Yellow Pages) - Direct mail - Public transportation vehicles, waiting spot ads	Media purchases are complex and expensive Consider local cable channels
Events	Educational or social purpose Examples: - Seminars and forums - Open house - Special events (seasonal and holiday celebrations, senior proms, honoring events for veterans, Holocaust survivors, volunteers)	Creativity is key; possibilities are endless Tie into publicity Use to establish, strengthen brand
Public relations -Publicity -Community relations (CR)	Nonpaid promotional message - Publicity: Media stories about your facility Examples: - Human interest stories - Event promotion, coverage CR: Positive relationships with service area organizations and individuals Examples: - Organizational memberships (chamber of commerce, service clubs, United Way, interfaith coalitions, nonprofit boards) - Facility advisory councils - Electronic newsletters - Support of, service purchases from relevant community service organizations	Publicity: Prepare media kit Plan well ahead for event promotion Cultivate relationships with reporters, other media people Send press releases selectively CR: Seek/create co-op efforts with hospitals, senior service agencies, relevant community service agencies

Table 9.4 (*Continued*)

Activity	Definition/examples	Comments
Referral relationship management	Activities to establish and nurture relationships with organizations and individuals that can direct customers to your organization Examples: - Continuing education seminars for clinicians, with educational credits - Resident/family referral incentive programs*	*No financial compensation for Medicare/Medicaid beneficiary referrals
Visits/tours	Activities designed to generate foot traffic to your office or community Examples: - Meals or food events (ice cream socials, healthy eating) to showcase food service - Scavenger hunts with prizes - Respite care - Holiday youth group carols - Surrogate grandparent program	Specifically scheduled or ongoing Walk-in or appointment Have large print materials, not too lavish
Prospect/waiting list groups	Establishes a pool of potential future residents to maximize occupancy ratio, minimize vacancy fill time	Requires periodic communication and cultivation to retain interest and commitment; importance of reassessment prior to admission as status may change
Social media	Methods for interactive electronic communication with target audience(s) Examples: - Interactive website - Yelp and other review sites	Requires both technical and marketing communication skill, as well as regular attention to maintain fresh content

Marsha Freidman (2012) warns that done poorly, social media wastes time, energy, and money and can alienate potential customers and referral agents; her guidelines are listed here.

- Be sure to monitor communications and respond to inquiries in a professional manner.

- Technical proficiency is a necessary but not sufficient qualification for a social media manager.

- Establish policies to screen and add qualified social media contacts that will exclude spammers and people who indiscriminately add others to their networks.

Pam Lontos (2010) offers several practical tips for social media communications:

- Choose sites carefully, where they will be seen by your target customers; check and recheck periodically to be sure you are where your market is.

- Understand the purpose of each site—for business networking (LinkedIn), personal communications (Facebook), and real-time messaging (Twitter).

- Don't post too often and craft the message carefully.

- Think in sound bites, especially for Twitter.

As with all marketing activities, it is important and challenging to evaluate the return on investment (ROI). The use of online service providers depends on the business model—advertising, professional referral, and placement services are most common. Be aware, however, of Medicare/Medicaid anti-kickback rules prohibiting payment to placement coordinators. Look at how referral agents use online services and how their consumers find them online. Examine website traffic statistics and insist that the service provide performance metrics and reports to document qualified leads. Also, ask for client references and ask the service provider for data to document performance claims (Stern, 2009).

Crisis Management

Crisis consultant Jonathan Bernstein (n.d.) defines a crisis as "Any situation that is threatening or could threaten to harm people or property, seriously interrupt business, damage reputation and/or negatively impact the bottom line." Handling crisis communications when things go wrong is an unpleasant but necessary aspect of marketing. Controversial events attract media attention, which can escalate with amazing rapidity via electronic communication and social media.

Proactive planning. Thinking ahead and preparing for what could go wrong is the best way to prevent avoidable workplace crises. This preparation involves developing both prevention strategies and an action plan to respond to crises when they arise. In a worst-case scenario exercise, team members articulate their worst nightmares (wandering or lost residents, deaths or injuries under suspicious/unexplained circumstances, a regulatory agency deficiency, or poor "report card" rating to name a few) and then make specific plans to both prevent and handle them.

Disaster recovery. When a controversial event occurs, the following techniques can help mitigate its impact:

- Do
  - Talk to the media, stakeholders, employees, and so forth.
  - Tell the truth.
  - Designate a single spokesperson (chief executive officer is best).
- Don't
  - Lie or mislead.
  - Say "No comment" (what people imagine can be worse than the facts).
  - Hide from the media.

Summary

Marketing long-term care services is challenging because most people hope they won't ever need them, and because there are many negative perceptions of long-term facilities. Deciding to use long-term services is almost always difficult, particularly when the decision is made under pressure or when family members disagree about the need and type of care that the client requires. There is a wide range of long-term care services available, depending on the individual's needs and resources. The emphasis in this chapter is on marketing long-term care residential services in either assisted living or skilled nursing facilities. Because these facilities serve individuals (primarily but not exclusively older adults) who are mostly frail and impaired, and thus vulnerable to abuse and exploitation, they are highly regulated by government as well as the focus of considerable consumer advocacy.

For nursing facility providers, marketing is an ongoing management function and responsibility—*not* a response to a drop in census. All staff must be considered a part of the marketing team, as everyone plays a part in making a good impression on prospective customers and ensuring that current customers remain satisfied and loyal. The target market includes not only residents but also their families. The community's promotional emphasis will vary for each market segment. For the prospective resident, major factors include independence, companionship, socialization, and recreation opportunities; for families, the emphasis is more on safety, caring, and/or comfort for their loved one, and freedom from worry for themselves.

Third-party payers (insurers and managed care organizations) also play an important role in long-term care service purchasing decisions. Thus, it is important to know and meet their criteria for service use eligibility and provider participation. At a minimum, a facility must demonstrate satisfactory compliance with state licensing and quality standards; private payers with higher reimbursement rates will usually require more specific certifications, accreditations, and above average ratings by consumer groups and on patient satisfaction surveys. In most metropolitan areas it is important for the facility to obtain contracts with managed care health plans.

In most regions, there is intense competition among long-term care facilities for privately insured or self-pay clients for whom reimbursement rates are higher, so a key responsibility of marketing staff is to assess and monitor the competition. Another key responsibility is to develop and nurture relationships with referral agents who can influence and direct prospective customers to the facility. Increasingly, consumers and referral agents rely on public and private oversight agencies and reporting mechanisms for information on long-term care facility service quality and patient satisfaction. A strong marketing plan will include research on the target population, analysis of the competition's strengths and weaknesses, identification of principal referral agents, recommendations, and a budget for promotional activities and advertising. Effective public relations planning also includes steps to prevent and handle an adverse event.

Key Terms

Activities of daily living (ADLs): Indicators of an individual's ability to perform basic self-care tasks, such as walking, bathing, toileting, dressing, and eating.

Dual eligible: Also known as "Medi-Medis," people who are eligible for both Medicare and Medicaid insurance coverage because they are both poor and either elderly and/or disabled.

Form 2567: Federally mandated, publicly available reports by state licensing agencies of nursing home deficiencies.

Health Information Portability and Accountability Act (HIPAA): 1996 federal law with provisions for protection of patient medical information.

Hospital payer mix: Proportion of revenue that a hospital receives from Medicare, Medicaid, private insurance, self-pay, and charity care patients.

Independent practice association (IPA): Organization made up of physician practices and medical groups that contracts with managed care organizations to provide medical care to the MCO members.

Managed care organizations (MCOs): Health insurance plans, such as health maintenance organizations (HMOs) and preferred provider organizations (PPOs), that use financial incentives for both providers and patients to control costs.

Market segment: Section of a market; for example, the frail elderly segment of the senior market.

Market segmentation: Dividing a market into distinct segments for which different marketing approaches are appropriate.

Medicare Five-Star Quality Rating: System established by CMS for members of the public to compare nursing home quality.

Mystery shopper: Person who poses as a new or prospective customer, observes, and reports on his experience.

Objectives: Measurable statements of what marketing activities are designed to accomplish.

Referral agent: Individuals and organizational representatives who can influence prospective customers to use a particular service or product.

Strategies: Means to achieve marketing objectives.

Tactics: Specific actions to implement marketing strategies.

Target market: Customers whom the organization wants to serve.

Review Questions

1. What are the principal types of research needed to assess local market demand for residential facility long-term care services?

2. How do family members influence the decision to use long-term care facility services?

3. What do managed care organizations expect of long-term care facilities in terms of quality and utilization care management?

4. Discuss the role of referral agents in marketing long-term care services.

5. How do government agencies regulate long-term care facilities and inform the public about them?

6. Discuss the role of objectives, strategies, and tactics in developing a long-term care facility marketing plan.

7. Imagine you are a nursing home administrator. What is the worst thing that could happen at your facility? What actions would you take to prevent this event from occurring and to deal with it if the worst-case scenario became a reality?

Case Studies

Case Study #1: SNF Marketing in a Post-ACA World: Memorial Hospital of Gardena (California)

Memorial Hospital of Gardena (MHG) in Southern Los Angeles County is a 177-bed acute hospital, which includes a 69-bed subacute unit. In 2014 MHG developed the South Bay Care Collaborative (SBCC), which focuses on population management and patient-centered care as opposed to simply providing care in a hospital setting. This shift in focus has dramatically changed the way MHG works with skilled nursing facilities (SNFs) in the community, and how these SNFs market to MHG as well.

The key program developed by the SBCC is a post-acute network (PAN) made up of SNFs in communities surrounding the hospital. Participating SNFs agree to:

- Exceed a benchmark quality standard on an ongoing basis

- Host transition team members for a weekly meeting to update patient disposition in the SNF and discuss discharge plans

- Contact the hospital each time a patient is transferred to the emergency department

- Implement and utilize the following quality and readmission prevention tools
  - POLST form (physician orders for life-sustaining treatment)
  - COMS brand interactive predictive software
  - INTERACT tools (http://www.interact2.net/tools.html):
    - Stop and Watch protocols
    - Return to Acute Log
    - Return to Acute Root Cause Analysis
    - SBAR (Situation, Background, Assessment, Recommendation) communication protocol (Safer Healthcare, 2014)

SNFs in the SBCC network have also been asked to work with the same home health providers that the hospital includes in its narrow network.

SBCC is managed by the MHG director of case management, in collaboration with hospital administration and the chief medical officer. Participating SNFs will see an increased level of care and a more cohesive relationship with the hospital and its affiliated physicians. While traditional SNF marketing relied heavily on outreach to physicians, case managers, and health plans to increase awareness of an individual facility and drive admissions, that outreach has become less relevant as these groups have begun to integrate. Thus, there is likely one case manager working together on behalf of all three of these groups to efficiently manage costs.

Case Study #2: Skilled Nursing Facility Marketing in the Future

As a result of national health reform initiatives, SNFs must position themselves as part of the population health system, and focus more on delivering quality data that makes your facility stand out as a quality leader, and the facility with the lowest readmission rate. Position yourself to be included as a preferred provider by demonstrating quality care results consistently through quantitative data. Provide referral sources with these data monthly, and show them how you are helping them to accomplish their goals, improve care, and save money.

- Illustrate your commitment to a seamless transition between levels of care by utilizing the SNF tools offered by your state's quality improvement organization (QIO) and other organizations. For example, send discharge reports to both the MCO and the primary care physician so that all parties are aware of the patient's condition and location.

- Promote your facility's 24/7 accessibility and rapid response to referrals. Consider a "20-minute response guarantee," implement it 24/7, and train your staff to live up to it!

- Start marketing in the emergency department (ED) and on observation floors (where patients stay longer for additional testing and are closely monitored to assess the results of initial treatment) in acute hospitals. Reform initiatives have incentivized the health plans and hospitals not to admit patients who can be cared for at lower levels of care, and who don't meet acute criteria. This spells opportunity for SNFs—and that opportunity lies in the ED and on observation floors.

- Some hospitals don't have observation floors, but simply mix observation status patients among the inpatients. If this is the case, simply identify who the observation status case manager is for the day, and market to them.

Adjusting to reform initiatives is no longer optional for SNFs—it is necessary to ensure continued census stability and financial growth. In many cases formal alignment and acquisition between acute and post-acute providers are not an option, so a partnership approach may be the best option. For freestanding providers in both the acute and post-acute sector, this requires a significant change in how care is delivered and how facilities market themselves.

Case Study Review Questions

1. How would you evaluate the requirement to use a specific software program as a condition for participation in a regional post-acute provider network?

2. What quantitative data are essential for marketing SNFs to hospitals in your service area?

References

Adkins, C. (2000, May 1). *Ethical marketing.* Retrieved from http://long-term-care.advanceweb.com/Article/Ethical-Marketing.aspx

American City Business Journals. (2012). *Market info.* Retrieved from http://thebusinessjournals.squarespace.com/markets

Berkowitz, E. N., & Schewe, C. D. (2011). Generational cohorts hold the key to understanding patients and health care providers: Coming-of-age experiences influence health care behaviors for a lifetime. *Health Marketing Quarterly, 28,* 190–204.

Bernstein, J. (n.d.). *The 10 steps of crisis communication.* Retrieved from http://www.bernsteincrisismanagement.com/articles/10-steps-of-crisis-communications.html

Brandenburger, A. M., & Nalebuff, B. J. (1996). *Co-opetition.* New York, NY: Doubleday.

California Office of Statewide Health Planning and Development. (2013, February 8). Healthcare Information Division, patient origin & market share pivot profiles. Retrieved from http://www.oshpd.ca.gov/HID/Products/PatDischargeData/PivotTables/PatOrginMkt/default.asp

Carlson, E. (2006). Twenty common nursing home problems and the laws to resolve them. *Clearinghouse Review Journal of Poverty Law and Policy, 39*(9–10), 519–533.

Centers for Medicare and Medicaid Services. (n.d.). *Medicare/Part D enrollment contract and enrollment data.* Retrieved from https://www.cms.gov/Research-Statistics-Data-and-Systems/Statistics-Trends-and-Reports/MCRAdvPartDEnrolData/Monthly-Enrollment-by-Contract-Plan-State-County.html

Centers for Medicare and Medicaid Services. (2013, April 18). *Medicare Five-Star Quality Rating System.* Retrieved from http://www.cms.gov/Medicare/Provider-Enrollment-and-Certification/CertificationandComplianc/FSQRS.html

Dewitt, A. L. (2008, May 1). What you say can be used against you. *Advance for Long-Term Care Management, 16,* 24–28.

Duffey, L. (2002, September 1). Outshine the competition. *Advance for Long-Term Care Management, 5,* 29–30.

Ehlers, J. R. (2010). *Marketing senior housing.* Bloomington, IN: AuthorHouse.

Eisner, R., & Lorber, D. (2006, April 7). *Twenty common nursing home problems and the laws to resolve them.* The Commonwealth Fund. Retrieved from http://www.commonwealthfund.org/Publications/In-the-Literature/2006/Apr/Twenty-Common-Nursing-Home-Problems-and-the-Laws-to-Resolve-Them.aspx?view=print&page=all

Freidman, M. (2012, March 14). *Social media is serious business: Tips to make sure you are taking the right approach with this marketing tool.* Retrieved from http://long-term-care.advanceweb.com/Features/Articles/Social-Media-Is-Serious-Business.aspx

Gamble, M. (2012, April 9). America's payor mix by region. *Becker's Hospital Review.* Retrieved from http://www.beckershospitalreview.com/racs-/-icd-9-/-icd-10/americas-payor-mix-by-region.html

iHealthBeat. (2011, October 21). *Physicians' use of text messages sparks HIPAA compliance concerns.* Retrieved from http://www.ihealthbeat.org/articles/2011/10/21/physicians-use-of-text-messages-sparks-hipaa-compliance-concerns

Kaiser Family Foundation. (2012, December). *Medicare Advantage fact sheet.* Retrieved from http://www.kff.org/medicare/upload/2052-16.pdf

Landro, L. (2013, April 15). In diabetes care, a push to simplify. *Wall Street Journal.* Retrieved from http://online.wsj.com/article/SB10001424127887324030704578424734246102490.html?mod=WSJ_article_RecentColumns_TheInformed Patient

Lontos, P. (2010, January 13). *Keys to social media marketing success: Combine SMM with traditional media for profitable results.* Retrieved from http://long-term-care.advanceweb.com/Editorial/Search/SearchResult.aspx?KW=keys+to+social+media+marketing+success

Loughney, L. (2005, March 1). Master your market. *Advance for Long-Term Care Management, 8,* 38–43.

Matthieson, S., & Whitehurst, A. (2010, December 16). Targeted marketing. *Advance for Long-Term Care Management, 13,* 37–40.

Pearce, B. W. (1998). *Senior living communities.* Baltimore, MD: Johns Hopkins University Press.

Pearce, B. W. (2007). *Senior living communities* (2nd ed.). Baltimore, MD: Johns Hopkins University Press.

Safer Healthcare. (2014). *Why is SBAR communication so critical?* Retrieved from http://www.saferhealthcare.com/sbar/what-is-sbar/

Stern, E. M. (2009). Marketing your facility online: Long-term management care. *Long-Term Living, 58,* 27–29.

Acknowledgments

Sincere thanks to Josh Luke, PhD, and Courtney Downey, BS, for writing the case study in the Marketing and Public Relations chapter, and to Editor Rebecca Perley, MSHCA, for her leadership developing this book.

CHAPTER 10

HEALTH INFORMATION SYSTEMS

Abby Swanson Kazley

Information technology (IT), or the use of software and hardware to automate a system, has been used in industries from banking to the military to airlines. In fact, most banks have interoperability that allows access to accounts from non-affiliated banks and ATMs throughout the world. While hospitals and other healthcare organizations, such as skilled nursing facilities (nursing facilities), have been using IT for administrative and financial purposes for many decades, the use of **health information technology (HIT)** for clinical purposes is a fairly new practice. Health information technology refers to software and hardware applications that seek to improve the quality, coordination, and efficiency of care. These applications are intended to automate the processes of care, reduce or eliminate errors, increase efficiency, decrease duplication of tests, improve the coordination of care with better follow-up and information sharing, and increase adherence to best clinical practices through support applications. Until recently, most clinical resident information has been recorded and stored in paper medical records. Paper medical records have several weaknesses. First, they can be lost or misplaced, or destroyed in a natural disaster; second, they can be illegible; third, they are expensive to store and maintain, often requiring transcription charges; fourth, for residents with complex medical conditions, they can be very large, which makes transferring them to other providers difficult and thus leads to fragmented care; and fifth, they can be incomplete due to filing errors.

It is believed that using HIT, including **electronic health records (EHRs)**, could improve the delivery and

LEARNING OBJECTIVES

- **Understand the benefits and costs of using health information technology in nursing facilities.**

- **List and define HIT applications.**

- **Recognize the prevalence of HIT use in nursing facilities.**

- **Describe the challenges of HIT use.**

- **Describe steps to adopt and use electronic health records (EHRs) in nursing facilities.**

documentation of care. EHRs are fully automated systems that contain documentation of resident medical history and care. The **Institute of Medicine (IOM)**, a nonprofit, private organization that provides unbiased information on health care, recommended the development of a national technology infrastructure to eliminate most handwritten clinical data by the end of the decade (Committee on Quality of Health Care in America). Thus, there has been increasing interest in and pressure for healthcare organizations to adopt and use HIT. In 2004, President George W. Bush signed Executive Order 13335, *Incentives for the Use of Health Information Technology and Establishing the Position of the National Health Information Technology Coordinator*, to develop a federal and national focus on the use of HIT to improve care. Building upon this, in 2009, the American Recovery and Reinvestment Act (ARRA) provided $2 billion in incentives for implementing HIT to improve healthcare efficiency and resident safety and approximately $17 billion in Medicare and Medicaid payments to promote **meaningful use** of certified EHRs (Blumenthal, 2009).

Prevalence of Use

HIT describes a wide array of computer applications, from administrative (e.g., census management, billing) to management (e.g., staffing and scheduling modules), to direct care (e.g., EHRs, telemedicine), and even to residents (e.g., personal health records [PHRs], text message reminders of care) (Kramer, Richard, Epstein, Winn, & May, 2009). These applications are intended to automate the processes of care, reduce or eliminate errors, increase efficiency, decrease duplication of tests, improve the coordination of care with better follow-up and information sharing, and increase adherence to best clinical practices through support applications. Despite the potential benefits of HIT, long-term care settings, such as nursing facilities, continuing care retirement communities, assisted living, specialty units, and independent living facilities have been slow to adopt HIT. Slow HIT adoption rates have been attributed to several factors, including the costs of acquiring, implementing, and maintaining HIT/EHRs, uncertainty about the benefits, delay in adoption of national standards for HIT functionality and interoperability, lack of time, lack of technical support staff and knowledge, and a history of instability and lack of customization or suitability in the vendor market (Ash & Bates, 2005; Booz Allen Hamilton, 2008; Middleton, Hammond, Brennan, & Cooper, 2005; Poon et al., 2006; Sidorov, 2006). Estimates of HIT adoption rates vary widely, in part due to problems defining application terms, and in part due to a lack of reliable national data measures of use (Wang & Biederman, 2012). Estimates of EHR adoption in skilled nursing facilities range from approximately 1% to 42% (Kaushal et al., 2005; Centers for Disease Control and Prevention, 2008). However, adoption and use of EHRs with broad functionality are likely at the low end of this range. In the state of California, nearly half of long-term care facilities with more than one facility report using some form of HIT, but fewer freestanding long-term care facilities reported such progress (California HealthCare Foundation, 2008). In Texas, a survey found that 39.5% of all long-term care facilities have fully or partially implemented EHRs, and 15% have no plans to adopt EHRs (Wang & Biederman, 2012). This same survey in Texas revealed that rural long-term care facilities are significantly less likely to adopt and use EHRs than facilities in more urban or suburban locations, indicating possible barriers to adoption and use of EHRs.

Despite the slow adoption and use of EHRs and other HIT applications, policy makers, and payer groups such as Leapfrog, have been encouraging providers and healthcare organizations to adopt and use the systems to improve the quality and efficiency of care. This encouragement comes in the form of payments and regulations. Payments include incentive sums of money or higher levels of reimbursement for organizations that use HIT, while Leapfrog, a group of purchasers and employers from across the country that aims to increase public knowledge of healthcare quality and promote use of practices that improve health care, will contract for care only with healthcare organizations that use certain practices. One such practice required by Leapfrog is **computerized provider order entry (CPOE)**, an application that requires all orders to be typed into a computer in order to be completed.

Regulations, Laws, and Standards

Several laws and regulations are promoting the use of HIT in long-term care facilities and will guide and govern its use. The first is the Health Information Portability and Accountability Act (HIPAA), which seeks to protect sensitive resident information and allows for the provision of transfer of such information between providers. Since resident records can contain sensitive resident information, such as diagnoses and prescriptions, protecting such information is essential. While paper records are also subject to such regulations, the ease with which EHRs or other electronic documentation of sensitive medical information can be transferred or shared between providers and patients has highlighted this need and increased concern over exposing sensitive health information. As EHRs are increasing in use, there is also increasing concern from residents about the privacy and security of their medical information. Ensuring that EHRs and the processes of care comply with HIPAA regulations requires work with experts and legal advisors in some cases. However, in some ways, EHRs are more likely to protect sensitive health information since the systems are generally password-protected, and users leave electronic trails of where they have logged in to ensure they are accessing only information that they need to provide care and complete their job duties. Providers, such as long-term care facilities, are required to comply with HIPAA regardless of what type of resident medical records they have, and they must also inform residents of their rights related to their **personal health information (PHI)** through HIPAA.

Other laws also provide regulation and guidance to long-term care facilities related to HIT. The **Health Information Technology for Economic and Clinical Health (HITECH) Act**, a federal law to change health care, was enacted as part of the American Recovery and Reinvestment Act of 2009, and provides incentives for organizations and individual practitioners to use EHRs in a meaningful way and builds upon HIPAA (Buntin, Burke, Hoaglin, & Blumenthal, 2011). The HITECH Act modifies the existing HIPAA privacy and security requirements by providing additional privacy and security rights and requirements that benefit individual residents, such as allowing providers to enter into confidentiality agreements with third parties, including EHR vendors or consultants. This means that third parties are subject to HIPAA privacy requirements. The HITECH Act also attempts to increase information security by creating new standards. These new standards include a breach notification requirement, guidelines for disclosing only the minimum necessary for an intended purpose, providing disclosure of information from the EHR upon request of the resident, a request that information be withheld from a health plan payer if the resident pays for medical care in full, and prohibits the sale of personal health information (PHI) (Sanger, 2009). PHI includes sensitive and identifying information about residents, such as test results, diagnoses, birthdate, or treatment. These new regulations mean that business associates could face increased liability and nursing facilities more risk, and they may require updated vendor lists and negotiation of business associate agreements to comply with HIPAA requirements (Sanger, 2009). One example of this is the case of compromised PHI. If such an incident happened at an SNF as the result of a vendor's representative losing a computer with sensitive information, both organizations must notify individuals affected of when, how, and why the event happened, what information was breached, things a resident could do to protect himself, what corrective actions the organization is taking to prevent a future incident, and contact information if there are any questions. Violations of such breaches of PHI can carry penalties of $25,000 to $1,500,000 per person. On the other hand, trails of exposed PHI through paper records were difficult to track in some instances. EHRs allow for better tracking and documentation of data breaches, and employers have used EHRs to identify and punish employees who have used systems inappropriately to access information that they did not need to complete their job duties. Such features of an EHR system demonstrate the power EHRs hold to protect PHI. Administrators of long-term care facilities can prevent data breaches by ensuring computers with PHI are stored in secure locations and that the systems are encrypted and password-protected so that only authorized individuals may access the information. Administrators should also consider providing thorough and regular education regarding HIPAA and related processes and procedures to staff to ensure compliance and prevent loss of PHI.

The Office of the National Coordinator for Health Information Technology was created by an executive order from President Bush in 2004 to oversee and promote the use of HIT, including EHRs, in healthcare organizations throughout the country (http://www.healthit.gov/newsroom/about-onc). This office is part of the federal government in Washington, DC, and is charged with overseeing the implementation and use of HIT throughout the country. The creation of this office demonstrated the federal government's interest in promoting and supporting an infrastructure for HIT use, and President Bush set a goal for all or nearly all Americans (i.e., individual citizens) to have an EHR by 2014. The **Office of the National Coordinator for Health Information Technology (ONCHIT)** received a large increase in funding under the American Reinvestment and Recovery Act of 2009 (Blumenthal, 2010). The office has been tasked with coordinating the implementation and use of health information technology under HITECH. The HITECH Act specifically provides a $19 billion program to encourage the adoption and use of HIT, especially EHRs (Blumenthal, 2009). Of this money $17 billion is specifically earmarked to encourage and reward physicians and other healthcare organizations to adopt and use EHRs (Blumenthal, 2009; Burke, 2010). Physicians who do so may be eligible for $44,000 over a 5-year period that began in 2011 (Blumenthal & Tavenner, 2010). The requirements of meaningful use are listed in Table 10.1. The HITECH Act also has penalties in place for physicians and organizations that are not using EHRs in 2015. These physicians and organizations who do not adopt and use EHRs in a meaningful way will lose 1% to 3% of their Medicare fees, beginning in 2015 and continuing through 2017 (Blumenthal, 2009). As of May 2012, more than 60,000 eligible providers had attested to meaningful use of EHRs under the Medicare

Table 10.1   EHRs Record Requirements for Meaningful Use

Electronic prescribing
Health information exchange with other providers
Automated reporting of quality data
At least one clinical decision support tool
Created care summary documents
Electronic recording of residents' history (demographics, vital signs, medication and diagnosis lists, and smoking status)

program, representing 12.2% of those eligible (Wright, Henkin, McCoy, Bates, & Sittig, 2013). The popularity of the program and the volume of the applications for the incentives demonstrate that providers and organizations are succumbing to the pressure to adopt and use EHRs and that they recognize the potential impact such systems may have on improving the quality and efficiency of care.

Organizations of all types are eligible for the HITECH incentives. These include hospitals, skilled nursing facilities, nursing facilities, home health agencies, long-term care facilities, clinics, mental health centers, dialysis centers, blood centers, ambulatory surgery centers, emergency medicine providers, federally qualified health centers, physician practices, laboratories, rural health clinics, and Indian health service providers (www.arrahitechsolutions.com/ARRA_HITECH_Act_FAQ_s.html#who_ Qualifies_for_HITECH?). They also include clinician providers, such as pharmacists, physicians, practitioners, and therapists. The inclusion of all types of organizations and providers in the HITECH meaningful use incentives program will hopefully promote use throughout all types of providers since the greatest benefits of EHR use will occur when a resident's medical information can travel with him on a single record throughout the entire continuum of care, from primary care to acute care and rehabilitation. The thought behind the legislation is that the incentives could help healthcare organizations, such as nursing facilities and other providers, defray the up-front costs of purchasing and implementing an EHR system, which represents one of the greatest barriers of EHR use for healthcare providers and organizations.

Record Retention Requirements

Requirements for information systems standards have begun to be more regulated. In fact, standards for EHR systems designed for hospitals and physicians have been established over the past 5 years, and about 75% of the EHR systems are certified by the Certification Commission for Health Information Technology (CCHIT), an organization that helps promote the use of EHRs across the nation. There is less regulation for EHRs in long-term care facilities as the practice has not yet become widespread. The HITECH Act requirements for meaningful use incentives provide clear standards and requirements that are set up by Medicare. To qualify as a meaningful user and for the related incentives, EHR systems must include electronic prescribing, health information exchange with other providers, automated reporting of quality data, electronic recording of residents' history (demographics, vital signs, medication and diagnosis lists, and smoking status), created care summary documents, and at least one clinical decision support tool (Blumenthal & Tavenner, 2010; Burke, 2010; Jha, 2010). Such meaningful use requirements are believed to improve the legibility of records, reduce prescription errors, improve adherence to best clinical practice guidelines, improve resident and clinician access to records, and allow exchange of health information (Jha, 2010). However, given that organizations are adopting and using varying systems of EHRs, the interoperability or communication between such systems is limited. The requirements for certified meaningful use status of an EHR system are listed in Table 10.1.

Health Information Technology Applications

HIT refers in general to software and hardware applications that seek to improve the quality, coordination, and efficiency of care. In this section, we will outline several specific applications that are considered HIT applications and are currently being used in healthcare organizations, such as long-term care facilities. These applications and the associated benefits are listed in Table 10.2.

Electronic health records (EHRs) are one of the most prominent HIT applications that also hold the greatest promise for improving. EHRs are also referred to as electronic medical records (EMRs), computerized patient records (CPRs), and personal health records (PHRs). In essence, EHRs are fully automated systems that contain documentation of resident medical history and care, including observations, diagnosis, history, prescriptions, and lab results, and may work with other HIT applications described ahead. Implementation of EHRs in the long-term care setting is still in its infancy since current implementation and use are limited and vary among institutions. EHRs are accessed and maintained using computers, and may be backed up remotely to protect and preserve clinical data. EHRs hold great potential to improve quality, improve coordination of care, and decrease

Table 10.2   Applications and Potential Benefits of HIT

Benefit	HIT application associated
Ease of access to information	HIE, EHRs
Time-saving	EHRs, CPOE, telemedicine, CPA
Better coordination of care	HIE, EHRs, CPA, CDSS
Access to making orders for care from multiple locations	EHRs, telemedicine, CPOE, CPA
Increasing efficiency	CPOE, CDSS, CPA
Improved quality management through reports, alerts	CDSS, EHRs, CPA
Health information exchange between providers	HIE, EHRs
Improve resident safety	EHRs, CPOE, CPA, CDSS
Support delivery of effective resident care	Telemedicine
Facilitate management of chronic conditions	CDSS, EHRs, HIE, CPA
Improve efficiency across all care settings	EHRs

costs and inefficiencies by making current resident information and clinical decision-making tools accessible to clinicians in an easily readable format (Bates & Gawande, 2003; Booz Allen Hamilton, 2008; Kaushal, Shojania, & Bates, 2003; Shekelle, Morton, & Keeler, 2006). Currently, residents may see various providers throughout the continuum of care. For long-term care residents, these can include primary and specialty physicians, a variety of therapists, including physical, occupational, and respiratory, pharmacists, social workers, dietitians, and nurses. Coordinating care and communication among these providers, many of whom may be in different locations or never meet face to face, can be a challenge. Thus, a centralized location and storage place for information related to the resident through an EHR is an important tool to inform these providers of other aspects of the resident's care. Likewise, a resident with a complex medical condition or multiple chronic conditions, as often seen in long-term care residents, may have a difficult time transporting a large, heavy paper medical record from one provider to the next. In fact, there is a high probability that pieces of the record may become lost or are never added to the record. Such omissions from the record may negatively impact the quality of care for the resident or result in the duplication of tests or services. On the other hand, a transportable EHR can serve as a secure repository for information and can be updated from multiple locations at the same time. Long-term care facilities, where physicians may work only part-time, may require that a great deal of consultation and orders happen over the phone. An EHR could allow providers to access the record from multiple locations so long as Internet access was present.

Conversion to an EHR system is not currently a requirement for long-term care facilities, and the conversion to such records can be complex, time-consuming, and costly. Thus, the HITECH incentives for providers, as previously discussed, are intended to increase conversion to EHRs for organizations such as long-term care facilities. EHRs can also assist in automating the process of closing records when residents leave the facility, using a developed algorithm, but this would be at the administration's discretion. The benefit would be that the closed records would not take up space at the facility, and the system could be customized to ensure that a consistent practice is followed when residents are transferred elsewhere.

CPOE has the potential to reduce or eliminate handwriting errors. CPOE is a component of some EHR systems, and it can also be a stand-alone application. CPOE is an electronic application that allows clinicians to directly enter orders into a computer for resident prescriptions, diagnostic tests, and requests for consultation (Rochon et al., 2005). Specifically in nursing facilities, it is believed that CPOE could be an important systems-based approach to reduce medication errors or drug-related injuries (Subramanian et al., 2007). In fact, residents of long-term care and nursing facilities are especially susceptible to adverse drug events (ADEs) because they are often high users of prescription drugs overall, including psychoactive medications, anticoagulant therapy, and diuretics, due to having multiple chronic conditions (Rochon et al., 2005). In fact, on average, SNF residents are prescribed more than six concurrent medications, and in a 100-bed SNF two ADEs could be expected per month given national estimates (Gurwitz et al., 2000; Rochon et al., 2006). In a national context of all U.S. nursing homes, 1.9 million ADEs occur each year, 40% of these are preventable, and 86,000 of the ADEs may be fatal or life-threatening (Subramanian et al., 2007). By using a CPOE system, any errors that occur through faulty or unclear communication between providers can be eliminated. For example, with paper records, if a physician orders a diagnostic test for a resident by telling a nurse, there is a possibility that the nurse may not correctly hear the physician, that the nurse may become distracted and forget to order the test, or that the nurse may write the orders illegibly. Each of these scenarios would likely cause the diagnostic test to not be completed as ordered, thus reducing the quality of care.

A **clinical decision support system (CDSS)** supports EHRs and CPOE by offering a variety of aids for clinicians, including computerized reminders, prompts, and advice regarding issues such as drug selection, doses, interactions, drug allergies, and the need for corollary orders (e.g. prompting the ordering of a follow-up international normalized ratio level in a resident on warfarin therapy who is prescribed an interacting medication). (Rochon et al., 2005, p. 1780)

You can imagine a resident ordering a diagnostic test for a resident with a paper record, but the results never arrive. If the order is just listed in the paper record, the provider with a heavy caseload of residents may fail to recall that the test was ordered and not investigate further as to why the results were not received. It could be that the resident did not get the test or that the diagnostic center did not send the results. Without CDDS, this test may be completely forgotten until the next visit, when the test results may show a more advanced stage of disease. However, with CDDS, a reminder will appear on the provider's screen to let him know that a test was ordered, but results weren't received. Then, the provider can investigate further as to why the test results are missing and fix the problem. The potential for CDDS to improve care is great.

Another application for EHRs is **computerized pharmacy administration (CPA)**. CPA can improve accuracy and timeliness of medication administration. It can be integrated into EHRs and reduce waste, adverse drug events, and medication delivery time errors. CPA often uses bar coding to ensure that residents are given the correct medication since a code on their bracelet must match the code on the medication given. Since SNF residents are often on many medications, such an application has great potential to ensure that medication is administered properly and reduce any medication errors.

Telemedicine is a tool that is being used with increasing frequency and allows greater access to care. Telemedicine can be delivered in a number of ways, including telephone, e-mail, or two-way video camera. Telemedicine use has been especially prevalent for stroke and psychiatric conditions since it can connect specialized providers with residents at remote conditions. Several small hospitals have connected to stroke experts via telemedicine to assess and treat residents with acute stroke, since there are treatments that are very time-sensitive, and it would be impossible for residents to travel to the experts in the limited window of time. In nursing facilities, the use of telemedicine could reduce the burden of travel for residents who need specialist care if the physician can assess and treat the resident via telephone or remote two-way video. It is also possible for telemedicine to connect providers to other providers who are caring for the resident and request specialist advice. In the SNF setting, it is easy to imagine a resident with Alzheimer's disease who has an unusual rash that may need a dermatologist consult. Rather than transport the resident to the specialist or the specialist to the resident, the two could be connected through telemedicine. The disadvantages of telemedicine are that it does not allow for physical contact or examination between the provider and the resident and that some residents may not feel like they can connect with a provider who is not in the same room. The advantages are that it can increase resident access to emergency or specialty care and reduce the burden and expense of traveling to another provider. Unfortunately, reimbursement for telemedicine is lagging and stalling use of telemedicine since most payers will not pay for telemedicine consultations. Thus, its use has not met its full potential.

Health information exchange (HIE) refers to the electronic sharing of resident health information between providers in the same state or region. Such sharing has been limited to date, but the creation of HIEs, through public or private partnerships, encourages organizations to create a standardized way of sharing resident medical information to improve the quality of care and reduce duplication of services. Such sharing has been difficult in the past given that healthcare providers in the same area have viewed other organizations as competitors and have thus been hesitant to share anything with them, and the HIT systems in place have not always communicated with other systems. However, when a resident is seen by multiple providers that may be independent or part of a different system, sharing resident medical history, diagnoses, laboratory results, or diagnostic results can greatly illuminate the picture of the resident's experience for a clinician, possibly leading to better understanding, diagnosis, and outcomes.

Advantages of Health Information Technology Use in Long-Term Care

There have been several anticipated benefits of HIT use in long-term care facilities, and though many of these have not necessarily been realized yet, there continues to be anticipation for positive changes in the areas of quality, access to care, cost containment, and efficiency related to HIT. Specifically, it is believed that HIT can provide benefits in nursing facilities, including ease of access to information, including resident medical history and diagnosis, diagnostic and laboratory results, and more complete documentation. The more complete documentation in electronic format will allow for queries to easily identify residents who meet criteria if needed for identifying public health concerns or recalls of medications.

One example may be a breakout in a skilled nursing facility of a contagious illness, such as tuberculosis. An EHR system with reporting capabilities may make it easier for administrators and public health professionals to identify and track such a breakout. Similarly, in a very large long-term care facility with varying levels of care, a paper record review to identify those impacted could be very slow, while an EHR system would allow for daily automated reports to allow for quicker response. Another benefit is that HIT, and EHRs specifically, will allow providers to see the notes that other providers make about the same resident and connect them when needed to collaborate on a care plan. In a long-term care facility where a resident with diabetes and a history of stroke may see a gerontologist, an endocrinologist, and a neurologist along with an occupational therapist and dietitian, the providers will be able to see notes and care plans for each of the conditions, whereas with paper records, the notes may have been maintained on different paper medical records in each practice and would never be seen by the resident's other providers. The potential benefits and the corresponding HIT applications associated with the benefit are listed in Table 10.2.

Proponents of HIT also believe that it will be time-saving for providers and residents, allow for better coordination of care between providers as illustrated earlier, and increase access by allowing orders for care from multiple locations, which could be especially beneficial for a provider who cares for residents of an SNF but is on-site only for limited periods of time. Many believe that HIT will increase efficiency by providing electronic reminders in the EHR of abnormal test results or upcoming requirements for resident care. It is also believed that if providers enter their notes and orders into the EHR themselves, it will save the time and cost of transcription and storage of bulky paper records. If physicians can access records of results about acute resident conditions from anywhere, including their homes, they can more quickly respond with orders. This is illustrated when you imagine an SNF resident with an infection. If the individual is regularly being tested for infection levels, a provider could access the results from anywhere, even at home, and respond quickly with a prescription order if the results indicate need for intervention. Without such a system, the results may wait until the provider is next on-site for a visit with the resident or when the resident next has a visit at the provider's office.

Perhaps the greatest area of potential impact for HIT is in the improvement of quality. Improved quality management is expected from EHRs through reports, alerts, and CDDS, which can identify errors, prevent harmful drug interactions, ensure regular monitoring of residents with chronic conditions, and ease any errors that might occur through verbal communication of orders between providers. It is not uncommon for a physician to see a resident and then give the orders for care to a nurse or medical assistant who may be in the middle of completing orders for another resident. The potential for misunderstanding, forgetting, or error when the orders are given informally and verbally is great, while a physician entering orders into a CPOE system leaves little room for error, and the system could then provide reminders to ensure the orders are correct and completed. Such systems are intended to improve resident safety and support delivery of effective resident care. Errors can be related to medication or the coordination of care of follow-up, and CPOE can prevent them. The most often cited keys to gaining the full benefit of technology in health care are interoperability and integration among clinical systems, decision support, and physician usage. The anticipated benefits and the applications that are expected to contribute in each corresponding area are shown in Table 10.2.

Also related to quality specifically in long-term care facilities, EHRs have been used to collect data on the activities of daily living (ADLs) in SNF residents. The data can then be collected and aggregated to create predictive models for proactive care. The models can also help providers to anticipate upcoming needs and necessary services and accommodations for individual residents. Essentially, EHR use can make resident information and data much more readily available and allow it to be used to improve the overall quality of care for residents by identifying trends in the progression of illness.

Cherry and Owen (2008) found specific anticipated benefits of EHR use in nursing facilities to be electronic communication between healthcare providers across multiple care settings, electronic reports of laboratory results and radiology procedures with automated display of previous results, reminders about preventive practices, such as immunizations, dosing and drug interactions, administrative functions, such as scheduling systems, billing, and claims management, insurance eligibility, inventory management, and public and private sector reporting (minimum data set; MDS) requirements. In a subsequent study, Cherry, Ford, and Peterson (2011) name numerous benefits of EHRs:

• Making up-to-date resident information available instantly wherever it is needed

• Avoiding costly duplicate tests and hospitalizations that are not necessary

• Providing the best and latest treatment options for residents

• Eliminating medical records

- Streamlining the public health information reporting for early detection and response in the cases of disease outbreaks

- Creating opportunities to gather protected private health information and outcomes for research to identify best practices

- Better, more current medical records at a lower cost

- Protecting privacy

In addition, the same study found that administrators reported savings of $3,000 to $4,000 per month based on reductions in pharmacy expenditures with EHRs. Such savings can be significant for nursing facilities and other health providers who may distribute many expensive medications to residents on a regular basis, especially given the fact that many residents are on multiple medications. Nursing facilities may also see financial benefit in the increase charge capture made possible by EHRs for both RUGS and MDS. This increased financial capture will be the result of automation and more clear and legible notes of procedures and care allowed through EHR use.

EHRs may also hold important information about residents' preferences for care, including advanced directives. Nursing facilities can work with EHR system providers to ensure that systems collect information about advanced directive wishes. Nursing facility staff can then gather information about residents' advanced directives to enter into the EHR system, which will ensure that such wishes can be honored.

Disadvantages of Health Information Technology Use in Long-Term Care

Despite the many anticipated benefits of HIT use in quality, efficiency, access, and cost containment, adoption and use of applications have been slow, especially in long-term care facilities. There are several barriers to adoption, but the greatest barrier seems to be cost of implementation and maintenance. Purchasing a system involves great up-front costs in the range of hundreds of thousands to millions of dollars, depending on the system, features, support, customization, and volume of anticipated use. An initial purchase includes software, support, and computer stations (hardware) to allow providers access to use the system. It may also include personal handheld devices that allow providers to take the system with them from one resident room to another. Costs associated with an HIT adoption include hardware and software, maintaining duplicate paper and electronic records, labor costs for maintenance, and physician or provider time spent learning the system. Purchasing an HIT system will include acquisition costs and annual costs that range from the hundreds of thousands to millions of dollars. Acquisition costs include the initial purchase, hardware or other infrastructure requirements, hiring additional staff (IT), implementation of systems, integration with CPOE or CDS systems, initial training of staff, and lost productivity while becoming familiar with the system (Subramanian et al., 2007). Annual costs include maintenance, annual license fees, upgrades, monitoring systems, update of clinical and pharmaceutical information, ongoing staff training and support, increased laboratory costs due to more tests (if suggested by CDDS), and increases in physician time by an average of 238% (Subramanian et al., 2007). One estimate puts the cost at $30,000 to $50,000 to purchase and install a basic system for a 100-bed skilled nursing facility, with annual maintenance costs of $25,000 to $40,000, but this is a low estimate for a system that likely wouldn't meet meaningful use criteria (http://www.leadingage.org/Whats_Keeping_Some_Nursing_Homes_from_Adopting_Electronic_Health_Records.aspx). Physician time may be increased because the providers are not yet used to the system and may work slower as they navigate through the EHR while providing care to residents. One challenge to the adoption, implementation, and use of HIT is that the costs incurred are not aligned with the benefits (Subramanian et al., 2007). The meaningful use incentive payments are intended to overcome this challenge.

Other barriers to HIT implementation and use include physician acceptance and security concerns. Some physicians and other providers have resisted the adoption and use of HIT for fear that it would change the way they practice medicine and that the automation and focus on a computer screen may detract from the art of medicine and the relationship between a provider and physician. Although the risk for such security breaches of information existed with paper records, the benefit of having EHRs is that such breaches could potentially be more easily identified and tracked since they would leave an electronic trail. Finally, there is great concern over the initial investment in time needed to adopt and use EHRs or other HIT applications. The time required includes training, troubleshooting, and adjustment, and many organizations have found that they are initially less efficient and slower immediately after adoption of an application. There is also the challenge of whether to add previous medical information from the paper record(s) to the new EHR system. Given the length and volume of the medical records of older individuals, especially those with chronic medical conditions, the time and manpower required to enter the information into electronic format, either through data entry or through the scanning of documents, are significant and would likely require additional hired personnel for a period of time until all such information could be entered. The challenge of not entering the historical resident medical information is that the system is unlikely to yield benefits if it does not include all or most pertinent information.

Beyond these listed barriers, a study by Cherry and Owen (2008) shows that human factors are the third most common barrier for nonusers of EHRs. Human factors can include staff resistance to change, unfamiliarity with computers, fear, and lower education levels of certain positions (Cherry & Owen, 2008). This same survey found that decision makers were concerned about choosing the right system that was not too complex and user-friendly as well as converting paper records to electronic data. According to Rochon et al. (2005), the ideal implementation team will include all key participants, such as physicians, providers, pharmacy, nursing, and information technology. A team that is planning on implementing an HIT application, such as EHRs or CPOE, should plan to meet often to create criteria for the system (a wish list), review and select available systems, and anticipate the communication flow and documentation requirements. Often nursing facilities will issue a request for proposals (RFP) to solicit vendors who may wish to create and implement a system that meets the SNF's requirements.

Electronic Devices

Electronic devices, such as smart phones, computers, and tablets, such as iPads, can help to improve the delivery and documentation of resident care. Smart phones and tablets can be used to connect residents to providers, using FaceTime or other applications for consultation or check-in; however, caution should be exercised. Nurses or other health aides should be present during any such interactions with physicians or other providers to ensure that information from the consultation is recorded, understood, and followed. The smart devices can also be useful for reminding residents to do things to improve their own health, such as taking medicine at the correct time by setting a timer or receiving a text message. Staff and providers might also talk by phone or text about questions that arise or to provide information, such as how a new medication is being tolerated or recent blood sugar levels for a diabetic resident. Staff must be trained to use these devices, and caution must be used to ensure that the use of such devices does not infringe upon the personal time of providers when they are not at work. If staff members engage in any type of electronic communication with residents or family members, there must be a policy and procedure in place to guide this interaction and to ensure that it upholds HIPAA regulations and is defensible from a risk management perspective. Staff must be instructed to communicate with residents in an appropriate way as a representative of the organization, and care must be taken to ensure that staff are not expected to be "on-call" 24 hours a day, 7 days a week.

Another risk with the use of electronic devices is that the devices may be lost or stolen. Such instances have occurred in long-term care facilities, including the Michigan Long-Term Care Ombudsman's office on January 30, 2014 (Ellison, 2014). In this instance, the records of more than 2,500 residents were compromised when a laptop and flash drive were stolen. Notification of data breaches to residents and state regulators is required, and residents may be concerned that their information will put their privacy at risk. Such incidents are costly for organizations both in terms of monetary fines and lawsuits as well as the loss of trust that residents might feel following a notification of a data breach (McMillan & Cerrato, 2010). Thus, encryption of PHI should be encouraged for mobile devices to protect the loss of PHI from residents. Administrators should also work with IT professionals to ensure that safeguards, such as encrypted data and firewalls, are used throughout the facility to prevent data from being compromised or accessed inappropriately.

Implementation and Conversion to Health Information Technology

The process from RFP to implementation can span from several months to years, depending upon the complexity of project and the decision-making speed at the SNF. Once a system has been selected, the transition to use of an EHR requires organizations to select the right system for their practice, develop an implementation plan, install the system, and connect to other networks and providers. Administrators must be sure to include the right people in decision making regarding the selection and adoption to increase the likelihood of selecting a system that is accepted by frontline staff and meets the unique needs of the organization, or the system may not be designed with the user in mind or it may be rejected by clinicians and other users if it is perceived to be not user-friendly or technical support and training are not provided. The demand to install systems may outweigh the number of HIT software vendors and consulting professionals to supply the products and services in the current environment.

EHRs can be either hardware-based or web-based. A web-based system is maintained electronically at a remote location. An advantage of using a web-based system is data are stored and backed up remotely through a vendor. While this is often a more expensive option, it also provides additional security in the event of a natural disaster, such as a flood or fire. In such an instance, EHRs stored on-site would likely be lost, leaving residents and providers without important information, such as resident prescriptions or diagnosis. For residents with Alzheimer's or memory loss or those with many prescriptions, there is likely heavy reliance on the EHR, and such a loss would put a resident at risk of missing important medication administration or follow-up diagnostic tests.

Given the variance in size for long-term care facilities, it is often a question of how large should a long-term care facility be to make various technologies cost-effective? What can be done for smaller homes interested in technology but unable to invest as much as larger operations? The answer to these questions is that it depends on size, where the long-term care facility is in the process of adoption and use, infrastructure available (IT support, computers in place), system affiliation, management support, and potential return on investment (Alwan, 2008). Nursing facilities that are less profitable can take adoption and implementation in stages, taking into account the organization's leadership, financial resources, and tolerance for change. Limited resources may equate to a SNF starting with a smaller application and continue adding applications as possible (http://www.fortherecordmag .com/archives/092809p28.shtml). Such systems may first wish to start with CPA, and then consider CPOE and, eventually, an EHR. Economies of scale, whereby larger nursing facilities by bed size will be better suited to justify the cost, are present, and thus a system-affiliated SNF may also be better equipped to make the large investment.

When selecting an EHR system, administrators must think of the goal of use of the EHR and select a system that will allow them to meet the goal. If the goal is to meet meaningful use criteria, the system may need to be more advanced than if the goal is to simply move from paper to electronic medical records. When selecting a vendor, administrators will want to take cost, interoperability, customization, and ability to work with other vendor applications into account. It is not unusual for an organization to select one system and then be committed to that system, as adding on another feature from another vendor is not possible or is cost-prohibitive. Administrators will also want to ensure that the agreement for training and technical support from the vendor is part of the initial agreement with a vendor.

Nursing home owners and administrators must be prepared to undertake a major change, requiring many months of planning, to successfully implement an HIT application, such EHR, CPOE, or telemedicine. Administrators are advised to designate a committee with representatives from all potentially impacted areas and users, and to also participate themselves.

The committee should begin by clearly identifying what is hoped to be gained through use of a new HIT application. Certain HIT applications, such as HIE and telemedicine, require partnerships with outside entities, and identifying trustworthy and similar partners in such endeavors will increase the likelihood of success.

Related to the benefits of EHRs, SNF administrators reported advantages in immediate access to medical records for all staff, improving consistency, accuracy, and quality of documentation, and improved employee satisfaction and retention (Cherry, Ford, & Peterson, 2009). These same administrators identified the disadvantages of HIT use as being technology problems, maintenance, and Internet outages. Additionally, surveyors may ask for reports that can more easily be accessed through the use of EHRs, or surveyors may be granted access to the EHR system. In such instances, administrators must be sure that HIPAA standards are upheld to protect resident information.

Staff Training

As with any major transformation, it will take nurses, physicians, administrators, and residents to truly make these types of tools work in an SNF. Cherry and Owen (2008), two researchers of HIT use in skilled nursing facilities, found this to be a top concern for nonusers of EHRs who worried about the cost and time involved for training staff, ongoing training, and quality of training programs. This time will involve adjustment to the systems themselves and will also require that old habits or practices (e.g., documenting in a paper record or giving verbal orders) be broken to make way for the new ones. Often, new policies and procedures for the expectation of use of such systems as well as immediate abandon of old practices will increase the likelihood of success. Training sessions on how to use the software and to document in a computer during a resident interaction can increase provider skill and ease with the new system. In an SNF, it is also important to provide information about the new system to residents who can understand and anticipate changes and feel comfortable with new equipment. This may be especially true in nursing facilities where the residents have little to no experience with computers or other forms of information technology. Demonstrations of telemedicine or explanations of the benefits of EHRs may encourage buy-in and support from both providers and residents or family members. Family members who participate in the care of residents may also be present during telemedicine visits. Because the practice of telemedicine is still in its infancy, it is likely that residents and providers will need strong technological and other support during use.

Since nurses play an important role in the development of workflow automation and resident-monitoring tools that work to integrate technology and resident interaction, they will be paramount to developing and enforcing new policies and practices. Steps to successful implementation of any HIT application include setting realistic goals, involving users early in the process, determining how workflows will be impacted, and entering historic data into the system (Cherry & Owen, 2008).

After initial training, direct care staff will need support to learn to use the equipment, especially for the first 6 to 12 months after implementation. There should be a careful plan for continuing education opportunities so that staff learn to properly use the software and can benefit from the technology. This may require the addition of IT staff to answer questions and troubleshoot problems. Nursing facilities may also choose to train a number of "super-users," who are clinicians who receive intensive up-front training and can then assist their colleagues and peers in questions and problems that arise during shifts. Given the high rate of staff turnover in nursing facilities, the need for repeated and ongoing training presents an additional expense and challenge. Thus, EHR training should be part of orientation, and "super-users" or EHR "champions" (staff who are advanced in use and knowledgeable) can help train new employees on use. Additional training and support may be needed when there are software changes or updates.

HIT in nursing facilities must have built-in flexibility to accommodate different workflows related to residents' needs. SNF caregivers must adopt this same flexibility when it comes to utilizing HIT tools to meet residents' needs. This is especially pronounced since nursing facilities provide care through interdisciplinary teams of clinicians who all have to share the same record in order to coordinate care. One of the greatest related challenges is interoperability. Interoperability refers to the ability of EHR systems to communicate with one another within and across organizations, such as nursing facilities. In nursing facilities, many providers need to work together to treat residents—thus the greater the interoperability the better (Subramanian et al., 2007). SNF administrators may wish to examine the options for interoperability with other area providers, such as local and regional hospitals, prior to selecting and implementing an EHR or telemedicine system. This becomes increasingly important as the profession continues to move toward value-based purchasing and the reduction of readmissions. The benefits of collaboration and these HIT applications are unlikely to be realized if the systems cannot communicate with one another.

Summary

In summary, the literature review does not support the fact that HIT applications, such as EHRs, are currently being effectively and widely used in the long-term care settings (Phillips, Wheeler, Campbell, & Coustasse, 2010). However, federal policies, such as the HITECH Act, are intended to increase use of HIT since they provide incentives for organizations that use EHRs in a meaningful way. Other HIT applications include CPOE, telemedicine, CPA, CDDS, and HIE. HIT applications have the potential to improve care in the areas of cost, quality, access, and efficiency. Specific anticipated benefits include ease of access to information, time-saving, better coordination of care, access to making orders for care from multiple locations, increasing efficiency, improved quality management through reports, alerts, health information exchange between providers, improved resident safety, supported delivery of effective resident care, facilitated management of chronic conditions, and improved efficiency across all care settings. Despite these possible benefits, the financial cost of adopting and using HIT applications, along with physician and staff resistance, and security concerns have caused adoption and use of HIT to lag. Long-term care facilities that wish to adopt HIT applications should be thoughtful in doing so and consider the perspectives of all users of the system in the selection and design of an EHR.

Key Terms

Clinical decision support system (CDSS): Supports EHRs and CPOE by offering a variety of aids for clinicians, such as computerized reminders, prompts, and advice regarding issues such as drug selection, doses, interactions, drug allergies, and the need for corollary orders.

Computerized pharmacy administration (CPA): Can be integrated into EHRs and reduce waste, adverse drug events, and medication delivery time errors. CPA often uses bar coding to ensure that residents are given the correct medication since a code on their bracelet must match the code on the medication given.

Computerized provider order entry (CPOE): An electronic application that allows clinicians to directly enter orders into a computer for resident prescriptions, diagnostic tests, and requests for consultation.

Electronic health records (EHRs): Fully automated systems that contain documentation of resident medical history and care, including observations, diagnosis, history, prescriptions, and lab results, and may work with other HIT applications.

Health information exchange (HIE): Organizations, usually existing in states or regions, that facilitate the sharing of medical information between providers.

Health information technology (HIT): Software and hardware applications that seek to improve the quality, coordination, and efficiency of care. These applications are intended to automate the processes of care, reduce or eliminate errors, increase efficiency, decrease duplication of tests, improve the coordination of care with better follow-up and information sharing, and increase adherence to best clinical practices through support applications.

The Health Information Technology for Economic and Clinical Health (HITECH) Act: Enacted as part of the American Recovery and Reinvestment Act of 2009, provides incentives for organizations and individual practitioners to use EHRs in a meaningful way, and builds upon HIPAA.

Information technology (IT): The use of software and hardware to automate a system.

Institute of Medicine (IOM): An independent, nonprofit organization that was established in 1970 to provide unbiased advice on health care to the public and decision makers.

Meaningful use: A set of requirements mandated by the federal government and the Office of the National Coordinator for Health Information Technology (ONCHIT).

Office of the National Coordinator for Health Information Technology (ONCHIT): Created by an executive order from President Bush in 2004 and intended to oversee and promote the use of HIT, including EHRs in healthcare organizations throughout the country.

Personal health information (PHI): Information that is sensitive in nature, must be protected for resident security, and is guarded through HIPAA standards. May include diagnoses, treatment, age, or other identifying resident information.

Telemedicine: Can be delivered in a number of ways, including telephone, e-mail, or two-way video camera. Telemedicine can connect specialized providers with residents at remote conditions.

Review Questions

1. What HIT applications can be used in long-term care facilities?

2. What federal policies support the adoption and use of HIT in long-term care facilities?

3. What are the expected benefits and barriers to using HIT in long-term care facilities?

4. How prevalent is HIT use in long-term care facilities? What are the barriers to use?

5. How should long-term care facilities implement EHRs?

Case Studies

Case Study #1

Imagine you are the administrator of a small SNF in rural Iowa. Several of your residents have complex neurological conditions that require regular and intermittent intervention from a specialist located in Des Moines, which is located 2 hours away by car. The residents typically do not have appointments on the same day, but they do see specialists at the same practice. What are three alternatives for making sure your residents are seen by the neurologist? What are the benefits and challenges of each alternative? Which alternative do you recommend and how will you implement it?

Case Study #2

You are the brand-new incoming administrator at Franky Bishop Gardens, a large, privately held, independent SNF. When you were selected for the position by the board, they indicated that they would like to see the SNF adopt and use electronic health records, as several of the local competitors have done so. They would like to meet with you as soon as possible to hear updates and your plans for the SNF in the upcoming year, including the EHR use. Create an outline of the EHR plans to share with the board. Speak specifically to the benefits and challenges, the steps you will take to implement, who will be involved in selecting the system, the time line for adoption and use, and the ways that using an EHR will change the care, including how the change will be introduced to residents who may resist it.

References

Alwan, M. (2008). State of technology in aging services according to field experts and thought leaders. Retrieved from http://www.leadingage.org/State_of_

Technology_in_Aging_Services_According_to_Field_Experts_and_Thought_Leaders.aspx

Ash, J. S., & Bates, D. W. (2005). Factors and forces affecting EHR system adoption: Report of a 2004 ACMI discussion. *Jamia, 12*(1), 8–12.

Bates, D. W., & Gawande, A. A. (2003). Improving safety with information technology. *New England Journal of Medicine, 348*, 2526–2534.

Blumenthal, D. (2009). Stimulating the adoption of health information technology. *New England Journal of Medicine, 360*(15), 1477–1479.

Blumenthal, D. (2010). Launching HITECH. Retrieved from http://www.nejm.org/doi/full/10.1056/NEJMp0912825

Blumenthal, D., & Tavenner, M. (2010). The "meaningful use" regulation for electronic health records. *New England Journal of Medicine, 6*(363), 501–504. Retrieved from http://www.nejm.org/doi/pdf/10.1056/NEJMp1006114

Booz Allen Hamilton. (2008). *Toward health information liquidity: Realization of better, more efficient care from the free flow of health information.* Retrieved from http://www.boozallen.com/media/file/Toward_Health_Information_Liquidity.pdf

Buntin, M. B., Burke, M. F., Hoaglin, M. C., & Blumenthal, D. (2011). The benefits of health information technology: A review of the recent literature shows predominately positive results. *Health Affairs, 30*(3), 464–471.

Burke, T. (2010). Law and the public's health: The health information technology provisions in the American Recovery and Reinvestment Act of 2009. *Public Health Reports, 125*(1), 141–145. Retrieved from http://www.publichealthreports.org/issuecontents.cfm?Volume=125&Issue=1

California HealthCare Foundation. (2008). *The state of health information technology in California. Use among hospitals and long-term care facilities.* Retrieved from http://www.chcf.org/˜/media/MEDIA%20LIBRARY%20Files/PDF/H/PDF%20HITHospitalsAndLONG TERM CARESnapshot2.pdf

Centers for Disease Control and Prevention. (2008). *Adoption of health information technology among U.S. ambulatory and long-term care providers.* Retrieved from http://www.cdc.gov/nchs/ppt/nchs2012/SS-03_HSIAO.pdf

Cherry, B., Ford, E., & Peterson, L. (2009). *Long-term care facilities adoption of electronic health record technology: A qualitative assessment of early adopters' experiences* (Final report submitted to the Texas Department of Aging and Disability Service.). Texas Tech University, Lubbock, TX.

Cherry, B., Ford, E., & Peterson, L. (2011). Experiences with electronic health records: Early adopters in long-term care facilities. *Health Care Management Review, 36*(3), 265–274.

Cherry, B., & Owen, D. (2008, September 28). *Determining factors or organizational readiness for technology adoption in long-term care facilities: Final Report.* Texas Tech University Health Sciences Center, Lubbock, TX.

Committee on Quality of Health Care in America. (2001). *Crossing the quality chasm: A new health system for the 21st century.* Washington, DC: National Academies Press.

Ellison, A. (2014). *Michigan long-term care security breach affects 2,595 patients. Becker's Hospital CIO.* Retrieved from http://www.beckershospitalreview .com/healthcare-information-technology/michigan-long-term-care-security-breach-affects-2-595-patients.html

Gurwitz, J. H., Field, T. S., Avorn, J., McCormick, D., Jain, S., Eckler, M., . . . Bates, D. (2000). Incidence and preventability of adverse drug events in nursing homes. *American Journal of Medicine, 109,* 87–94.

Jha, A. K. (2010). Meaningful use of electronic health records: The road ahead. *JAMA, 304*(15), 1709–1710. doi:10.1001/jama.2010.1497

Kaushal, R., Blumenthal, D., Poon, E. G., Jha, A. K., Franz, C., Middleton, B., . . . Bates, D. W. (2005). The costs of a national health information infrastructure. *Annals of Internal Medicine, 143*(3), 165–173.

Kaushal, S., Shojania, K. G., & Bates, D. W. (2003). Effects of computerized physician order entry and clinical decision support systems on medication safety: A systematic review. *Archives of Internal Medicine, 163*(12), 1409–1416.

Kramer, A., Richard, A. A., Epstein, A., Winn, D., & May, K. (2009). *Understanding the costs and benefits of health information technology in nursing homes and home health agencies: Case study findings.* Retrieved from http://aspe .hhs.gov/basic-report/understanding-costs-and-benefits-health-information-technology-nursing-homes-and-home-health-agencies-case-study-findings

McMillan, M., & Cerrato, P. (2013). Healthcare data breaches cost more than you think. *Information Week.* Retrieved from http://reports.informationweek.com/ abstract/105/11839/Healthcare/Healthcare-Data-Breaches-Cost-More-Than-You-Think.html

Middleton, B., Hammond, W., Brennan, P.F., & Cooper, G.F. (2005). Accelerating U.S. EHR adoption: How to get there from here. Recommendations based on the 2004 ACMI retreat. *Journal of the American Medical Informatics Association, 12*(1), 13–19.

Phillips, K., Wheeler, C., Campbell, J., & Coustasse, A. (2010). Electronic medical records in long-term care. *Journal of Hospital Marketing and Public Relations, 20*(2), 131–142.

Poon, E. G., Jha, A. K., Christino, M., Honour, M. M., Fernandopulle, R., Middleton, B., . . . Kaushal, R. (2006). Assessing the level of healthcare information technology adoption in the United States: A snapshot. *BMC Medical Informatics and Decision Making, 6,* 1. doi: 10.1186/1472694761

Rochon, P., Field, T., Bates, D., Lee, M., Gavendo, L., Erramuspe-Mainard, J., . . . Gurwitz, J. (2005). Computerized physician order entry with clinical decision support in the long-term care setting: Insights from the Baycrest Centre for geriatric care. *Journal of the American Geriatric Society, 53*(10), 1780–1789. doi:10.1111/j.1532-5415.2005.53515.x

Rochon, P., Field, T., Bates, D., Lee, M., Gavendo, L., Erramuspe-Mainard, J., . . . Gurwitz, J. (2006). Clinical application of a computerized system for physician order entry with clinical decision support to prevent adverse drug events in long- term care. *Canadian Medical Association Journal, 174*(1), 52–54. doi:10.1503/cmaj.050099

Sanger, L. F. (2009, August). HIPAA goes HITECH. *Health Law Perspectives.* Retrieved from www.law.uh.edu/healthlaw/perspectives/homepage.asp

Shekelle, P. G., Morton, S. C., & Keeler, E. B. (2006). *Costs and benefits of health information technology.* Rockville, MD: Agency for Healthcare Research and Quality.

Sidorov, J. (2006). Computer-assisted technology: Not if, not when, but how. A systematic review of interactive computer-assisted technology in diabetes care. *JGIM, 21*(2), 201–202.

Subramanian, S., Hoover, S., Gilman, B., Field, T. S., Mutter, R., & Gurwitz, J. H. (2007). Computerized physician order entry with clinical decision support in long-term care facilities: Costs and benefits to stakeholders. *Journal of the American Geriatrics Society, 55,* 1451–1457. doi:10.1111/j.1532-5415.2007.01304.x

Wang, T., & Biedermann, S. (2012). Adoption and utilization of electronic health record systems by long-term care facilities in Texas. *Perspectives in Health Information Management.* 9:1g.

Wright, A., Henkin, S., McCoy, A., Bates, D., & Sittig, D. (2013). Early results of the meaningful use program for electronic health records. *New England Journal of Medicine, 368,* 779–780. doi: 10.1056/NEJMc1213481

Acknowledgment

Dr. Kazley is grateful for the contribution of Taylor Lawrence who provided assistance with the literature search in this chapter.

CHAPTER 11

BIOLOGICAL AND PSYCHOSOCIAL ASPECTS OF AGING

Implications for Long-Term Care

Barbara White

According to the National Center for Health Statistics (NCHS) (Harris-Kojetin, Sengupta, Park-Lee, & Valverde, 2013) the majority of users of long-term care in the United States are 65 years of age and older and 50.5% are 85 or older. Older adults, including residents in these long-term care communities, have specific **biological**, **psychological**, and **social** needs related not only to specific **acute illnesses** (rapid-onset, short-course, such as a common cold) and **chronic illnesses** (long-course, continuing-process, such as diabetes mellitus) but also to expected changes that occur with normal aging. These changes must be considered in the design of a well-run long-term care community, in services and supplies, and in personnel training, in order to meet the demands of regulatory agencies as well as the ethical and moral obligations to residents. This requires knowledge of **gerontology** (the study of aging) and of **geriatrics** (the study of illnesses commonly experienced by older adults).

Normal Physical Changes With Aging

Common **physical changes with aging** involve the **skin**, **immune**, **gastrointestinal**, **musculoskeletal**, **respiratory**, **circulatory**, **genitourinary**, and **nervous systems**. Normal changes with aging in these systems have implications for

LEARNING OBJECTIVES

- Describe the normal/expected physical, psychological, and social changes with aging.

- Identify common illness presentations in the older adult.

- Discuss reasons for possible adverse responses to medications in older adults.

- Discuss the impact of a move into long-term care on the older adult and family caregivers.

- Design staff and management interventions to provide resident-centered care to enhance quality of life.

care that older adults receive in the long-term care continuum. While normal changes with aging occur at an individual rate, most residents of long-term care communities will likely experience changes in most of these systems because of their advanced age and medical conditions.

Skin Changes

Skin is composed of three layers: **epidermis** (the outer layer), **dermis** (the middle layer), and **subcutaneous** (the inner layer, largely made up of fat cells) (Figure 11.1). Skin is the first line of defense against the environment, and undergoes normal changes with advancing age. Skin changes are influenced by genetics, nutrition, environment, sun exposure history, smoking history, side effects of treatments (e.g., radiation therapy), and medications. With aging, skin may become pale and almost transparent in color.

Dry skin. With aging the **sebaceous** (oil) **glands** in the dermis produce less lubrication, and the skin becomes drier (**xerosis**). Dry skin is, initially, most prominent on arms and legs, but may become generalized. This dry skin can cause the resident to scratch, which increases the danger of secondary infection. Keeping skin well lubricated with lotions, creams, or emollients, applied especially after bathing, while the skin is moist, can improve comfort and prevent complications.

Senile lentigo. It is common for pigment cells on previously sun-exposed areas to become larger with age. These are called liver spots, age spots, solar

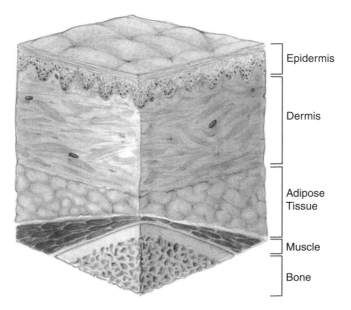

Figure 11.1   Normal Skin
Source: Used with permission of the National Pressure Ulcer Advisory Panel (2007).

lentigo, or **senile lentigo**. These are flat, tan to brown, pigmented areas that look like large freckles. They do not represent any pathology.

Seborrheic keratoses. **Seborrheic keratoses** are raised, wart-like lesions that are tan, brown-black, or gray in color. They appear to be greasy and to be stuck on the skin. Lesions with these characteristics are benign and do not need to be referred for evaluation. However, if there is a rapid appearance and growth of such lesions, if they change colors, or if they bleed, they should be reviewed for possible malignancy.

Senile purpura. Fragile **capillaries** (small blood vessels) in the skin may produce a **hemorrhage** (bleed), especially in previously sun-exposed areas of the body. These purple patches on the skin, called **senile purpura**, can appear with any minor injury, gripping, or shearing motion. Residents who take aspirin or other anticoagulation (blood thinning) drugs may bruise more easily and more extensively. Unlike the common bruise, these lesions may not go through the expected color changes and may remain as purple patches for long periods of time. The skin of older adults prone to developing purpura should be handled gently.

Temperature control. Various protective mechanisms help to maintain normal body temperature. With normal age changes in skin structures, some of these mechanisms may be compromised. **Sudoriferous glands** (sweat glands) provide evaporative cooling of body surfaces when the internal or external temperatures rise above normal. With aging these glands produce less sweat. Exposure to elevated internal or external temperatures may then cause **hyperthermia** or overheating. This can cause heat stroke, collapse, and death if gone unnoticed or unattended.

Conversely, subcutaneous fat decreases with age, initially in the extremities. Among its other functions, fat acts as insulation, keeping the body warm when external temperatures are low. Older residents exposed to cold temperatures for prolonged periods of time may become hypothermic, with core body temperature falling below 95 degrees (**hypothermia**). This can lead to weakness, confusion, coma, and even death. National regulations for nursing homes are identified as F-Tags. F-Tag 257 requires that long-term care communities maintain a comfortable and safe ambient temperature within the range of 71°F to 81°F.

Pressure ulcers. Pressure ulcers, also known as pressure sores, bed sores, or decubitus ulcers, are breaks in the integrity of the skin that occur due to persistent pressure of a bony prominence against a bed, chair, or a medical device, or with the shearing force of pulling the body over sheets or sheets out from under the body. A resident who is poorly hydrated or undernourished, or who is diagnosed with a heart/circulation condition or diabetes, is at increased risk for the formation of a pressure ulcer. While not an expected occurrence with aging, these ulcers may be more easily formed because of skin changes with aging and illness.

Pressure ulcers form in stages (National Pressure Ulcer Advisory Panel, 2007):

*   Stage I: A reddened area of intact skin, usually over a bony prominence, that does not **blanch** (turn pale) when digital pressure is applied (Figure 11.2). If pressure is not relieved, ulceration will occur.

*   Stage II: Blistering or abrasion of the skin or formation of a shallow ulcer with a pink or red base that exposes the dermal layers (Figure 11.3).

*   Stage III: Full skin thickness ulceration with exposure of fatty tissue. **Slough** (light-colored, soft, moist tissue remnants in the process of separating from healthier tissue) may be present (Figure 11.4).

*   Stage IV: Full thickness tissue loss with exposure of muscle, tendon, and even bone. Thick, leathery, dark-colored **necrotic** (dead) tissue may be present (**eschar**) (Figure 11.5). In the latter stages bacterial infection can occur, and prolonged treatment is required in an attempt to heal the ulceration.

*   Unstageable/unclassified: Full thickness skin/tissue loss with actual depth obscured by slough or eschar (Figure 11.6).

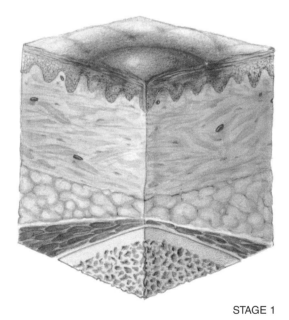

STAGE 1

Figure 11.2   Stage I

Source: Used with permission of the National Pressure Ulcer Advisory Panel (2007).

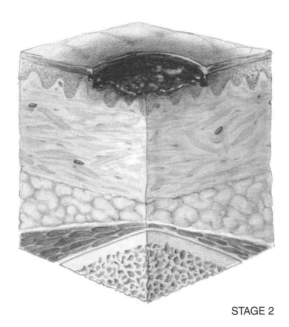

STAGE 2

Figure 11.3   Stage II
Source: Used with permission of the National Pressure Ulcer Advisory Panel (2007).

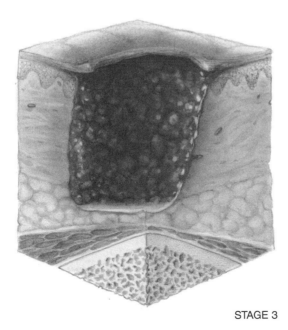

STAGE 3

Figure 11.4   Stage III
Source: Used with permission of the National Pressure Ulcer Advisory Panel (2007).

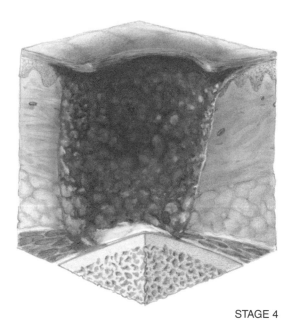

STAGE 4

Figure 11.5   Stage IV
Source: Used with permission of the National Pressure Ulcer Advisory Panel (2007).

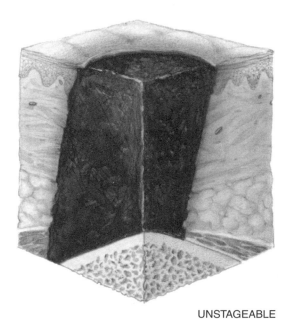

UNSTAGEABLE

Figure 11.6   Unstageable/Unclassified
Source: Used with permission of the National Pressure Ulcer Advisory Panel (2007).

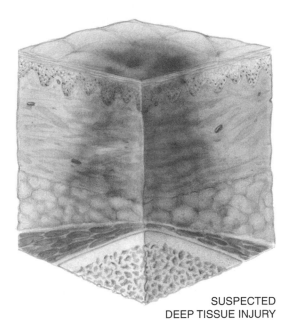

SUSPECTED
DEEP TISSUE INJURY

Figure 11.7   Suspected Deep Tissue Injury
Source: Used with permission of the National Pressure Ulcer Advisory Panel (2007).

- Suspected deep tissue injury: Intact skin that is purple or maroon or appears as a large, blood-filled blister that may be painful, firm, or mushy, and warmer or cooler than surrounding skin; this signifies tissue injury that is as yet unstageable (Figure 11.7).

Bedridden and chair-ridden residents are at the highest risk for pressure sore formation. They need to be repositioned at regular intervals—even hourly—if necessary. Skin breakdown can be further accelerated if the skin is moist, which may occur when the resident is perspiring or incontinent of urine or feces and allowed to sit/lie in wet clothing. Dark-skinned residents are at increased risk for unrecognized Stage I and suspected deep tissue injury pressure sores because of the difficulty in assessing changes in skin color. Careful attention to changes in skin temperature and firmness is required in order to identify developing problems in this population.

Quality of care regulations for nursing homes include F-tag 314, Pressure Ulcers. This regulations states that

Based on the Comprehensive Assessment of a resident, the facility must ensure that (a) a resident who enters the facility without pressure sores does not develop pressure sores unless the individual's clinical condition demonstrates that they were unavoidable; and (b) a resident having pressure sores receives necessary treatment and services to promote healing, prevent infection, and prevent new sores from developing. (National Pressure Ulcer Advisory Panel, 2014, p. 8)

The Minimum Data Set 3.0 Resident Assessment Instrument provides the long-term care community with tools for initial and ongoing assessment of risk and actual pressure ulcer progression (Section M).

Nails. The nail is a hardened extension of the epidermis. Nails provide support for the finger and toe pads, and allow improved sensation in the tips of fingers and toes (Danon, 2007). Thickening (**hypertrophy**) and discoloration of toenails may result from decreased peripheral circulation associated with normal aging, repeated trauma, nutritional deficiencies and metabolic diseases, drug reactions, degenerative diseases, or **peripheral vascular disease** (Hefland, 2003). Nail color may also change to yellow, gray, or opaque and may become ridged, brittle, and easily split.

Exposure to persistent moisture, poor hygiene, circulatory disorders, and/or immunocompromise increases the risk for fungal infections (**onychomycoses**) of the nails. Untreated, this may progress to infection of skinfolds (**paronychia**) surrounding the nail. These infections are difficult to treat, require prolonged treatment regimens, and are usually chronic. Nails should be cleaned, dried, trimmed, and inspected regularly in association with bathing. Proper nail care enhances the fit of footwear and pain-free ambulation. Residents with extremely thick nails, diabetes, or peripheral vascular disease should have nail care provided by a licensed foot care professional, such as a **podiatrist**.

Sensory Changes

Senses provide a mechanism to gather information and communicate with the outside world. Unrecognized changes in key senses can affect health and quality of life for the long-term care resident.

Eyes/vision. The most common vision change with aging is the need to wear eyeglasses due to alterations in the ability to see near or distant objects. According to the National Eye Institute survey in 2005, 94% of adults 65 years of age and older reported using eyewear related to **refractive errors** (National Eye Institute, n.d.). The problems that may occur when an older adult does not have eyeglasses available include compromised mobility, risk for falls, changes in appetite, and behavioral changes, including confusion, withdrawal, depression, anger, and paranoia. Overlooking the need for eyewear may contribute to misdiagnosis of symptoms.

Another change with aging is the development of **cataracts**, a yellowing, clouding, and, eventually, an opacity of the lens of the eye. Because of expanded life expectancy, cataracts are now considered a normal change with advanced age. Untreated cataracts may result in similar problems as those associated with lack/loss of eyeglasses. Early cataracts may blur vision and distort colors, making it difficult to distinguish colors because of the yellowing lens. If a resident self-administers pills by color, this can cause medication errors.

Age-related **macular degeneration** also affects vision and usually begins with a blurred area in the center of vision. It can progress slowly and affect either one or both eyes. It can also occur rapidly, and in either case has the potential to cause total blindness.

The use of high-contrast colors to signal changes in the environment, for example, on the first and last stair of a flight of stairs may prevent injury due to vision loss. This may also assist with any loss of depth perception due to aging or eye disease.

Peripheral vision can also be affected by eyelid drooping related to loss of elasticity of eyelid tissue. This can cause the older adult to be unaware of surroundings and subject to injury.

Hearing. Loss of the ability to hear high-frequency sounds (**presbycusis**) is a normal change with aging. There is often confusion in distinguishing **sibilant sounds**, such as *s, f, sh, th, z, ch*, which may cause an individual to misinterpret what is said, or to require frequent repetitions in order to understand the spoken word. The tendency of the person attempting to communicate with someone who is hard of hearing is to shout. Shouting is a high-frequency sound that will only exacerbate the problem. Speaking in a low pitch, slowly, and facing the resident will enhance communication with the hearing-impaired. Conditions other than presbycusis, such as lifelong exposure to loud noises, may also affect hearing not only for high-frequency but also for low-frequency sound.

Similar to not being able to access eyeglasses, inaccessibility or loss of a hearing aid may be misdiagnosed as confusion, withdrawal, depression, anger, or paranoia. It is imperative that any resident with a hearing aid has it cleaned, with charged batteries, and placed in the outer ear correctly. Since most hearing aids amplify *all* sounds, communication will be more effective if background noise is kept to a minimum. Uncorrected communication difficulties can lead to both resident and staff frustration and affect quality of life for both.

Another normal change with aging that can affect hearing is excessive **cerumen** (wax) in the ear canal. This can also cause **tinnitus** (ringing in the ears), and in extreme cases can affect verbal communication and balance. Staff can remove soft earwax with a washcloth during bathing. Dark, hard (impacted) wax should be removed by professional staff, using commercial softeners and low-pressure irrigation. Persistent tinnitus should be referred to a medical professional for evaluation.

Taste and smell. Taste and smell sensations remain intact well into the late 60s and 70s, unless the person has smoked or is taking medications that cause dry mouth or abnormal taste sensations. Aging may bring a diminished sense of taste, especially true for salty and sweet foods. Any of these losses can negatively affect appetite. Simple interventions, such as routine oral care, serving liquids with meals, and enhancing flavors with salt and sugar substitutes or various flavoring agents, consistent with dietary restrictions, can enhance appetite and promote adequate nutrition. Resident food preferences can also be respected with a **liberalized diet**, consistent with F-Tag 325. Consultation with the facility dietitian is recommended in these instances.

Both senses—taste and smell—can be further compromised by a history of smoking, by medications, and by certain diseases, such as Alzheimer's and Parkinson's disease. Additional concerns with loss of sense of smell are the inability to detect a gas leak, a fire, or odors associated with poor personal hygiene.

Thirst. Thirst sensation is also diminished with age. **Dehydration** can have deleterious effects, including **hypotension** (low blood pressure), lightheadedness, falls, and fainting. Poor hydration can also increase the concentration of drugs absorbed into the bloodstream and produce concentrated and stagnant urine that may contribute to **urinary tract infections**. Staff must ensure that water is readily accessible and that each resident receives 6 to 10 glasses of fluids each day, unless fluid restriction is in place related to a medical condition.

Immune System

Healthcare facilities, including long-term care communities, are a major source for outbreaks of infections, including those caused by viruses, bacteria, and multidrug resistant organisms. These organisms can affect respiratory, gastrointestinal, skin/wound, and **urinary tract** function. The Centers for Disease Control (CDC) (2015) estimated that 1 million to 3 million such infections occur in long-term care communities each year. Such infections are a major cause of hospitalizations, and an estimated 380,000 deaths per year.

Older adults are especially vulnerable to such infections because of changes in the immune system that may occur with normal aging. This **immuno-senescence** may include changes in the **white blood cells** (T and B lymphocyte cells) and in the **thymus gland**; weakening of **antibodies** (proteins produced by the body to neutralize harmful substances) developed in response to specific **antigens** (foreign substances toxic to the human body); and dangerous susceptibility to new **pathogens** in the environment. Overprescribing of antibiotics leads to antibiotic resistance that can increase a resident's vulnerability to pathogens, such as *Clostridium.difficile* (C.diff), methicillin-resistant *Staphylococcus aureus* (MRSA), vancomycin-resistant *enterococcus* (VRE), and carbapenem-resistant *Enterobacteriaceae* (CRE). Susceptibility to such hard-to-treat infections is highest in communal living situations, such as long-term care communities. The first line of defense against the spread of these infections is attention to thorough hand cleansing before and after contact with each resident, and careful observance of all required isolation precautions by all staff, healthcare providers, and visitors (CDC, n.d.).

Skin testing. **Tuberculosis** (TB) is an easily transmitted bacterial infection commonly tested for on admission to a long-term care community and annually. Because of the problem of immuno-senescence in vulnerable residents it is recommended, and in many states required, that the tuberculin skin test (PPD) be administered to residents in a two-step process. If the first test is negative, a second test is performed 1 to 3 weeks later. If the second test is negative, it usually indicates that the resident does not have TB, or in rare and obvious cases is **anergic** (unable to react to the PPD antigen) due to immune-suppression, poor nutrition, or acute illness. If the second test is positive, it indicates a boosted reaction to an infection that may have occurred several years before and warrants a follow-up chest x-ray to assess possible new disease activity.

Vaccinations. In order to protect long-term care residents from common infections, immunizations should be current. Standard recommendations for all who are not immunocompromised due to disease or prescribed immune-modifying drugs include administration of the following vaccines—with the concurrence of the primary healthcare provider and/or long-term care community medical director:

- Influenza vaccine, annually.

- Tetanus/diphtheria/pertussis series (if not previously vaccinated) followed by tetanus/diphtheria booster every 7 to 10 years.

- Pneumonia vaccine at age 65 with at least 23-valent vaccine. If vaccine was received before age 65, repeat at age 65 or later, so that 5 years have elapsed since the first dose.

- Herpes zoster vaccine at age 60 or later to prevent or decrease the severity of shingles and possible post-herpetic pain.

It is also vitally important that employees are current on these same recommended immunizations *and are provided sick time when acutely ill,* to prevent transmission of infections to vulnerable residents.

Fever response. An additional consequence of immuno-senescence is an altered fever response to infection. This requires vigilance on the part of both nursing assistants and licensed personnel in interpreting body temperature and evaluating fever in a resident. Criteria for defining fever in an older adult include (High et al., 2009) the following:

*   A single oral temperature of >100F (>37.8C), or

*   Repeated oral temperatures >99F (>37.2C), or

*   Rectal temperatures > 99.5F (>37.5C), or

*   An increase in temperature of >2 degrees F (>1.1C) over the baseline temperature

Because disease prevention is of paramount importance in a well-run long-term care community, attention must always be paid to hand washing, gloving, disinfection of equipment, and **aseptic techniques** in providing urinary catheter and wound care to a resident, and after resident and employee toileting.

Gastrointestinal System

The gastrointestinal system begins at the mouth and ends at the anus. Common changes in this system with aging may have profound consequences for nutrition and quality of life. Inadequate dental care prior to or after LTC admission may present problems with chewing and require nutritional or dental consults for dietary management. Long-term care communities are required to provide access to dental care.

Swallowing and normal gag reflexes may be compromised due to age and/or disease. Rapid feeding by untrained staff/caregivers or inadequate chewing of foods risks choking, or **aspiration** of foods/fluid into the lungs, creating a "chemical" aspiration pneumonia, often complicated by associated aspiration of bacteria. Modification of food texture and consistency may reduce aspiration risk. F-Tag 325 also states that liberalized diets are encouraged and appropriate for person-directed care. Many older adults' difficulty in swallowing may be due to a narrowing or **dysmotility of the esophagus** secondary to aging or disease. Such conditions should trigger evaluation by a speech pathologist.

A **hiatal hernia** (stomach pushing upward into the chest, above the diaphragm) causes indigestion and regurgitation of stomach contents secondary to a weak lower **esophageal sphincter** and/or a weakened diaphragm. It is often the result of pressure on abdominal muscles secondary to overweight/obesity, and causes symptoms of pain and indigestion. It can be exacerbated by eating certain foods and by lying down during or immediately after a meal. Slowed emptying of contents in the stomach (**gastroparesis**) is often a discomforting side effect of diabetes (or it may have no known cause), with complaints of nausea, bloating, pain, and loss of appetite. Non-medication management of these conditions may include raising the head of the bed 4 to 6 inches, smaller more frequent meals, not lying down for 1 to 2 hours after a meal, avoidance of caffeine, chocolate, alcohol, and fatty foods, and weight loss.

Diverticulosis is a condition of the large intestine, said to occur in 50% of the older adult population. The musculature in the colon causes pockets to form that can collect undigested food particles. This can produce pain in the lower left abdomen and an infection known as **diverticulitis**, which requires medical attention. A diet high in fiber and fluids is recommended to control and prevent diverticulosis and, ultimately, diverticulitis.

Likely the most common change with aging in the gastrointestinal system is **constipation**. Decline in physical activity, low-fiber diet, limited fluid/water intake, and certain medications cause stool to harden during its transit through the intestines. This may require softening with stool softeners, enema, or laxatives, and may potentiate dependence on these aids. Regular activity and attention to diet and fluid intake may prevent constipation. Many residents, however, enter a long-term care community already laxative-dependent and may be resistant to modifying lifelong habits.

Diarrhea (loose/liquid stool) is not a normal change with aging, and other causes should be investigated, including medication side effects, stool impaction, food or milk intolerances, irritable bowel syndrome, gastrointestinal infection, or stress response.

Musculoskeletal System

Falls are a leading cause of injury in the elderly population in long-term care. According to the CDC (2015) from 50% to 75% of residents fall each year, and many do so multiple times. Normal changes in the musculoskeletal system may account for some of these falls. Residents who are bedridden or who come to the facility after a prolonged period of inactivity lose muscle mass and experience muscle weakness (**sarcopenia**). Deconditioning happens more quickly in older than in younger adults, and recovery takes longer. Pain associated with arthritic conditions may also affect **gait** stability. Additionally, older women following **menopause** may experience **osteopenia** or **osteoporosis** that causes bones, especially in spine and hips, to become honey-combed and structurally unsound. In this instance, a fall may cause a hip fracture, or vice versa. Men are also susceptible to osteoporosis, usually about a decade older than their female counterparts. Limited food intake and weight loss (markers for malnutrition and osteopenia) also put the resident at risk for falls.

Environmental obstacles (poor lighting, wet floors, incorrect bed height, improperly fitted durable medical equipment and shoes, furniture, rugs), and poor eyesight and hearing may further potentiate falls. Other causes include confusion, depression, impatience, poor judgment capabilities, and use of physical restraints. **Chemical restraints** in the form of medications that affect orientation and control mood and behavior (**psychotropic drugs**) may also affect balance and contribute to falls (see ahead). Forgetting simple safety steps, such as locking a wheelchair, are also risk factors for falls, as are a resident's actions to meet a need that the staff has overlooked, such as not leaving eyeglasses or water within reach, or not answering a call light promptly. Some residents place themselves at risk for falls by refusing to use mobility aids for ambulation. This may be due to embarrassment or a false sense by the resident of his capabilities.

Respiratory and Cardiovascular Systems

The lungs provide for the exchange of oxygen and carbon dioxide. With inhalation, oxygen enters the lungs and is absorbed into the bloodstream. Oxygen is essential for the **metabolic processes** of every body cell, and to meet the energy requirements to carry out daily activities. With exhalation, carbon dioxide, a waste product of those metabolic processes, is eliminated from the body. With normal aging, lung capacity diminishes as lung tissue becomes less elastic, the respiratory muscles become weaker (sarcopenia), and the ribs and spine change shape. This decreases the amount of oxygen available to body cells and increases the amount of carbon dioxide left in the body.

The amount of oxygen delivered to cells is also affected by the circulatory system. Oxygen is transported through the body by red blood cells in the arteries of the circulatory system. Carbon dioxide is transported back to the lungs in veins. Movement of blood through arteries and veins is controlled in large part by the efficiency of the pumping action of the heart and the elasticity and patency of the blood vessels.

In addition to oxygen and carbon dioxide, blood carries nutrients, such as proteins, sugar, and fats, to cells for energy production or storage. Diminished nutrient (food) intake further slows the metabolic processes needed for daily activities, and the availability of stored energy needed in times of stress or illness.

Frailty Syndrome

With age energy may diminish and there is less reserve capacity to deal with everyday and stressful situations. Musculoskeletal, respiratory, circulatory, nutritional, and psychosocial changes with aging and disease may contribute to what has become known as the frailty syndrome, a collection of signs and symptoms that include weight loss of 10 pounds or more within a year, being easily fatigued, low activity level, slowed walking speed, and diminished grip strength. This may lead to slow recovery from even minor illnesses, increased risk for falls, increasing dependency, and even death (Xue, 2011). Early evaluation and treatment of acute and chronic health conditions and nutritional deficiencies, evaluation for polypharmacy and pain, depression management, and interventions to improve muscle strength and physical activity may prevent or slow the progression of frailty.

Urinary Tract

With advancing age weakness extends to the muscles that control urination. Older women are especially prone to **urinary incontinence** secondary to childbirth, the loss of **estrogen** following menopause, and overweight/obesity. Men can experience urinary incontinence from the results of **benign prostatic hyperplasia** (BPH), **malignancy**, and **obesity**. While women, due to the anatomical proximity of urinary, vaginal, and rectal outlets, are subject to urinary tract infections (UTIs) throughout life, men's anatomy is protective until later in life. **Urinary retention**, **dehydration**, use of incontinence products, and **urinary catheters** increase the risk of UTIs. Urinary samples frequently demonstrate the presence of bacteria that do not require treatment if there are no associated symptoms (asymptomatic bacteria), due to the risk of medication side effects or unintended consequences (e.g., C.diff infections), and decisions are made on an individual basis. For this reason, risk factor reduction and preventive measures need to be consistently applied. These include preventing cross contamination of urinary and fecal materials, and providing opportunities for regularly scheduled urination for those without urinary catheters. Residents who do not get 6 to 10 glasses of liquid per day (unless the resident is on fluid restriction) will produce concentrated urine that is a medium for the growth of urinary pathogens. Routinely encouraging fluid intake is a simple measure that is essential to prevent **nosocomial** (facility-caused) infections that can lead to hospitalization, sepsis, and death.

Neurological Changes

The nervous system is composed of the brain, spinal cord, and peripheral nervous system, composed of the **somatic** and **autonomic nervous systems**. The brain regulates thinking, reasoning, and emotions, as well as interprets sensory information (vision, hearing, touch, taste, and smell) and regulates balance and movement. The spinal cord is the conduit to the brain from the peripheral nervous system. If it is damaged, information between the brain and peripheral nervous system is compromised. The peripheral nerves provide information from skin and muscles (somatic nerves) that allows the brain to regulate voluntary movements and responses to touch, pain, and temperature. The autonomic nervous system regulates involuntary activities, such as heart rate, blood pressure, breathing rate, digestion, body temperature, urination, defecation, and sexual arousal. It responds to environmental stimuli and internal body signals.

As previously discussed, physical changes in skin and other organ systems with age may compromise the body's voluntary and involuntary responses. Drying and compression of the discs in the spinal cord, with advancing age, may injure sensory and motor nerve fibers and result in decreased sensation, movement, and balance. Residents with compromised sensation may experience numbness and tingling of affected body areas and may not respond appropriately to painful stimuli. This may cause injuries to go unnoticed, including scalding injuries from bath water that is too hot and pain associated with an evolving pressure sore or other injury.

Some changes in memory can be expected with advancing age. The brain's volume and number of nerve cells decline gradually, and noticeable changes in memory begin to occur in the fourth decade of life, such as difficulty remembering new names and in multitasking. With advancing age individuals may also experience a decline in the ability to find the right word in conversation and more difficulty in organizing activities, thinking flexibly, and making new long-term memories. Researchers feel this is more an issue with the way an individual processes information (e.g., being distracted and thus encoding information poorly), or possibly the increased amount of information an older brain has to sort through, than an actual pathology (American Psychological Association, 2006).

Problem-solving ability, or **fluid intelligence**, begins to decline in middle age. **Crystallized intelligence** or the font of knowledge from past learning and experience may become better with age. Crystallized intelligence can be measured by vocabulary, language, cultural experiences, and general intellectual achievements of the individual.

These normal changes are recognized in a small number of residents in long-term care facilities. The majority of residents, however, may be diagnosed with **dementia**, which, though not a normal change with aging, has an increased incidence and prevalence as the population ages. It is estimated that 5 million Americans have been diagnosed with dementia (Zimmerman et al., 2012). Because of the cognitive, memory, and behavioral symptoms associated with this diagnosis, it has been estimated that at least 1 million of these individuals reside in long-term care (Zimmerman et al., 2012). Many of those are in advanced stages of the disease and require extensive care, such as bed bathing, feeding, and frequent repositioning in bed. Those with milder disease may require less physical care, but more staff time and attention to keep them as independent as possible in **basic activities of daily living**, such as dressing, bathing, and eating.

Dementia, whether due to **Alzheimer's disease**, multiple strokes, **Parkinson's disease**, **Lewy body dementia**, or other causes, is progressive, and to date, not reversible. However, there are preventable and curable conditions that may *mimic* dementia and that should be recognized and treated in long-term care settings. These include: depression, **delirium**, medication side effects, thyroid gland disease, vitamin deficiencies, overuse of alcohol (Alzheimer's Association, 2013), and sleep deprivation.

Health Promotion, Disease Prevention

Residing in a long-term care community does not preclude continued attention to routine screenings for treatable diseases. In collaboration with the medical director or personal physician, all residents should have an annual wellness examination, including routine blood tests. Residents with a life expectancy of 5 years or longer should be routinely screened for tuberculosis, and considered for screening for colon, breast, cervical, vaginal, and/or prostate cancers, as well as bone density testing, each according to age-specific guidelines and overall medical relevance. Functional ability and the existence of comorbidities must also be taken into consideration, as well as the wishes of the resident. Disease prevention also includes ensuring that immunizations (discussed earlier) are up to date. The older resident should also be considered for appropriate programs for smoking cessation, nutrition counseling, and drug and alcohol misuse treatment at any age.

Common Psychosocial Changes With Aging

In addition to the physical changes that occur naturally with aging, older adults are confronted with psychological and social changes. Some of these changes are exacerbated by moving to a long-term care setting.

Losses and Isolation

With aging comes loss: loss of employment; death of family, friends, and pets; and loss of health. With a move to long-term care, additional losses include a loss of home and belongings, mobility restriction and a loss of independence, and the loss of privacy from living in a communal situation with a group of strangers. For those with intact cognitive abilities and memory, the world as they know it may "become smaller." It may become physically defined by a bed, a nightstand, a small closet, perhaps a sitting area, and some pictures and photos. Residents' needs are now met by strangers, who may not speak the resident's language, or who may be difficult to understand for the untrained ear or for the hearing-impaired. This can result in feelings of depression, anxiety, isolation and withdrawal, and self-imposed isolation.

Depression

Estimates of **depression** (a persistent mood of sadness and loss of interest) in long-term care vary. Major depression is thought to occur in between 6% and 24% of residents, while minor depression is estimated to occur in 30% to 50% of residents. Depression can be a long-standing diagnosis or it can be provoked by the changes and losses with aging. Depression is a significant cause of **morbidity** (illness) and **mortality** (death) in the older adult population, including worsening of chronic disease, increased susceptibility to acute illness, increased dependence in activities of daily living, and increased fall risk. Depression often goes as unrecognized and undertreated in long-term care as it may in ordinary life (Gellis & McCracken, 2008).

Symptoms of depression may include:

- Disturbed sleep (sleeping too much or too little)
- Changes in appetite (weight loss or gain)
- Physical aches and pains
- Lack of energy or motivation
- Irritability and intolerance of people and situations
- Loss of interest or pleasure in daily life
- Feelings of worthlessness or guilt
- Difficulties with concentration or decision making
- Noticeable restlessness or slow movement
- Recurring thoughts of death or suicide
- Changed sex drive (Geriatric Mental Health Foundation, n.d.)

Treatment recommendations encourage behavioral therapies and group therapy before, or in concert with, the introduction of antidepressant and antianxiety medications. Medication management of depression must be carefully monitored and discontinued when feasible. Depending on the cause of the depression, simple interventions, such as providing the resident with small responsibilities and opportunities to contribute to the setting in a useful way, and involvement in communal activities, may be helpful. It is important that these activities and responsibilities be meaningful to the individual and enhance his interaction and feelings of self-worth.

Anxiety

Depression and **anxiety** are often found together. Feeling anxious or nervous can be a long-standing mental disorder or a response of an older adult to recent stress or trauma. Common changes with aging, including poor health, fear of falling, losses of family and friends, transition to a new living arrangement, and fear of abandonment and death, can cause acute anxiety. According to the Geriatric Mental Health Foundation (n.d.), symptoms of an anxiety disorder may include:

• Excessive worry or fear

• Refusing to do routine activities or being overly preoccupied with routine

• Avoiding social situations

• Being overly concerned about safety

• Racing heart, shallow breathing, trembling, nausea, sweating

• Poor sleep pattern

• Muscle tension or feeling weak and shaky

• Hoarding and collecting things

• Depression

Such behaviors need to be evaluated by both the primary healthcare provider and a mental healthcare professional. Treatment may include behavioral therapies, stress reduction strategies, coaching new coping skills, family or other social support, and medications. Medication treatment for anxiety disorders must be carefully monitored and discontinued when feasible.

Sleep Pattern

Older adults, like younger counterparts, need 7 to 8 hours of sleep per night. With aging, however, there is usually a change in sleep patterns. These include taking a longer time to transition into sleep, with easy arousability during this initial sleep phase. Deep and dream sleep phases are shorter and more fragmented, with frequent awakenings. Research suggests that many of these changes are due to physical conditions, such as pain, psychological/psychiatric illness (depression, anxiety, dementia), **sleep apnea** (interrupted breathing periods during sleep), environmental factors (noise, lights), and multiple prescribed medications—including the medications used to treat sleeplessness (National Sleep Foundation, 2015). Additionally, the daily rhythm of sleep and wakefulness may change with age to an earlier to bed and earlier to rise pattern. Thus, older adults may feel less satisfied with their sleep pattern and nap during the day, further disturbing nighttime sleeping.

Problems that are caused by nighttime sleeplessness in long-term care affect the quality of life of residents and the work environment of staff. Medication issues that can affect sleep patterns are partially addressed through the monthly medication reviews and the Omnibus Budget Reconciliation Act (OBRA) regulations placing limits on the use of psychotropic medications in regulated long-term care settings. Administrators and medical and nursing directors should also evaluate current research and anecdotal information on non-pharmacological interventions to promote residents' sleep. These may include exposing residents to bright, natural, and/or artificial light during the day; planned daytime activities; decreased nighttime noise and light by limiting staff induced wake periods throughout the night; and a structured and predictable bedtime routine that corresponds to the resident's usual habits or establishes new ones (Martin & Ancoli-Isreal, 2008).

Illness Presentations in Older Adults

Changes with aging and disease may affect how illness symptoms present in the LTC resident. Symptoms of acute illness may be as expected. For example, a **heart attack** may present with severe chest pressure, pain in jaw and left arm, sweating, and nausea. This will alert the healthcare staff to seek immediate help. Conversely, traditional symptoms may be absent, and a heart attack may be silent and discovered only when more serious complications occur, such as symptoms of **congestive heart failure** or **cardiac arrhythmia**.

Symptoms in older adults may also be atypical. The presentation of a respiratory or urinary tract infection in an older adult may be only mild confusion, **lethargy**, or loss of appetite rather than the expected cough and fever in respiratory infection, or pain with urination in bladder infection. This requires that staff be vigilant in looking for subtle changes in behavior that may signal an acute illness. Early recognition of infection may prevent unnecessary hospitalizations.

Identification of symptoms becomes more challenging when the resident has dementia and may not be able to identify or express symptoms verbally. Residents' cultural beliefs may also influence their willingness to discuss symptoms with staff, family, or someone of the opposite sex. In such instances the staff must look for subtle nonverbal clues, such as changes in activity level, and respond to family/friend caregivers' observations and concerns, in order to recognize illness signs and symptoms. This requires diligence in the training and awareness of staff to such subtle changes.

Responses to Medications in Older Adults

Until recently drug trials did not include women or those over the age of 65. No distinctions were made in drug types or dosages appropriate for the older adult. We now know because of normal changes with aging, effects of acute and chronic conditions on drug actions, and the potential interactions of drugs with each other, that **adverse drug reactions** (ADRs) can cause unnecessary hospitalizations and even death for this older adult population (White & Truax, 2007). Major causes of adverse drug reactions in older adults result from (a) changes in the way drugs are processed by the aging body, (b) prescription of inappropriate drugs for this population, and (c) **polypharmacy**.

Changes in Absorption, Distribution, Metabolism, Elimination, and Action

Due to changes with age and illness, oral drugs may absorb more slowly through the gastrointestinal (GI) tract. This may be due to altered gastric motility or regularly scheduled antacid use that alters gastric secretions and absorptive functions. Topical drugs may absorb more slowly through skin due to poor blood circulation.

Once a drug is absorbed into the body, it must be distributed. Most drugs are distributed bound to the protein **albumin**, which is limited in frail older adults. Unbound drugs circulate immediately in an active state, leading to higher than expected concentrations in the blood stream at a more rapid than predicted rate. Drugs are also distributed in body water, which may be limited in residents who are dehydrated. Other drugs are distributed in body fat. Altered amounts of body water or fat affect the concentration of a given dose of a drug, causing an unexpected response and speed of action. **Therapeutic levels** of a drug may be reached more rapidly or more slowly than predicted.

Most drugs are **metabolized** (broken down) in the liver. Liver disease, shock, or **congestive heart failure** can alter this process and cause drugs to remain in circulation longer than expected. This can result in **drug toxicity** and an adverse drug reaction.

Most drugs are eliminated through the kidneys. With aging there is an expected decrease in blood flow and filtration of blood through the kidneys that may slow drug elimination. Elimination is further compromised with any condition that alters kidney function, such as congestive heart failure, diabetes, and dehydration. Repeated doses of a drug without the expected distribution, metabolism, and elimination put the resident at risk for **toxic** (adverse) side effects.

Inappropriate Drug Prescribing

In response to these considerations, a consensus panel has periodically reviewed drugs and drug classes that they consider to be inappropriate for older adults, as well as certain conditions that should not be treated with certain drug classes. These are known as the Beers Criteria for Potentially Inappropriate Medication Use for Older Adults (American Geriatrics Society, 2012). These criteria should be prominently displayed and referred to in long-term care settings.

Polypharmacy

The use of nine or more drugs or the inappropriate prescribing of drugs in the long-term care setting has been defined as polypharmacy (Tamura et al., 2011). This includes not only prescription medications but also vitamin and mineral supplements. Despite 30- to 60-day treatment plan reviews by primary care physicians and nurse practitioners/physicians assistants, monthly pharmacy reviews, periodic minimum data set assessments, and strict rules about the use of chemical restraints (psychotropic medications) to control behavior—often for staff convenience—it has been reported that one-third of long-term care residents are subjected to polypharmacy (Doshi, Shaffer, & Briesacher, 2005). Long-term care community staff must be trained to follow the federal and state regulations that restrict the use of certain medications for the elderly population and in the regulations for the use of psychotropic drugs to control behavior.

Additionally, the opportunity for error in dispensing/administering this volume of medications by the licensed nursing staff creates an added risk to the residents and liability for the staff. In this situation, the risk of adverse drug reactions is high and is reportedly the most clinically significant and costly medication-related unfavorable event in U.S. nursing homes (Handler, 2010; Handler, Wright, Ruby, & Hanlon, 2006). Long-term care administrators and staff continue to be challenged by this situation.

Changes in Older Adult and Family Relations in Long-Term Care

The move to a long-term care community is a life-altering event for both the older adult and any family or friend caregivers involved in the decision. Long-term care staff play an integral role in the outcome of this process.

Why Move to Long-Term Care Placement

For most older adults and families, the move to a long-term care setting is not a "destination" but a necessity, potentiated by increasing frailty of the older adult and compromised safety in remaining at home. A move to long-term care may be initiated by the older adult's family, a healthcare provider, or a legal guardian. Ideally, the decision is made collaboratively. At times, however, the proposed move may bring long-standing family issues to the surface, making a decision difficult for all parties, particularly if the move must be made quickly in a moment of crisis. Ideally over time, the move to a long-term care community will enhance the individual's and family's relationship and quality of life.

There are a number of reasons for a move to assisted living or to a nursing home. These include the older adult's recognized difficulties with **basic self-care activities of daily living (BADLs)**, such as bathing, eating, dressing/grooming, toileting, and ambulation; or **instrumental activities of daily living (IADLs)**, such as housekeeping, finances, shopping, meal preparation, medication and transportation management, and telephone use. Losses in **advanced activities of daily living (AADLs)**, such as social engagement in the community, may also suggest the need to consider a move to a more communal setting that will provide and support continued interaction with others. The level of loss of functional daily living activities will determine the level of long-term care required. The need for minimal or occasional support suggests a move to assisted living, including monitoring and coordination of care. If 24-hour healthcare monitoring and services are required, a nursing home setting may be the most appropriate choice. A move to long-term care is indicated with the following:

- Deterioration of physical functions, such as changes in weight associated with poor dietary management, inattention to or inability to perform bathing and grooming activities, difficulty with ambulation.

- Difficulty managing home maintenance.

- Problems managing finances.

- Worsening of a chronic health condition, requiring regular medical supervision.

- Incontinence.

- Medication mismanagement.

- Frequent falls or other issues of safety.

- Behavioral or mental problems: worsening memory problems, confusion, or wandering, not associated with a correctable condition.

- Withdrawal from usual activities and interests.

Caregiver Burden

Caregiver burden is often the impetus for the decision to admit a family member to a long-term care facility. Family may be attempting caregiving at a distance or be burdened by the number of hours a week required to provide supportive care in a home setting. Expanded need for care may also disrupt the caregiver's employment and family obligations. The cost of in-home help can place an additional burden on older adult and family resources. These situations may trigger consideration of long-term care as a viable solution.

Admission to a long-term care community may also be triggered by a family's intentional neglect of a frail older adult, or by the older adult's self-neglect and inability to care for himself. As the number of activities of daily living that require assistance increases, likelihood of placement increases. While the older adult has the right to **self-determination**, in serious cases of neglect or endangerment, legal interventions may be warranted.

A qualitative study by Bern-Klug (2008) articulated normal changes in family dynamics precipitated by admission to long-term care, and what caregivers need from the facility administrator, healthcare professionals, and ancillary staff in order to smooth the transition for both parties. In addition to providing clear information about the facility and the care provided, the following issues related to caregiver stress should be addressed:

- Competing concerns for their family member and other life obligations.

- Distress at witnessing decline in their family member.

- Feelings of guilt about the decision for placement in long-term care coupled with uncomfortable feelings of relief with the decision.

- Assistance with decisions that need to be made within the setting, including those related to end-of-life care.

These issues are especially stressful when the family member is resistant to the move.

Suicide

An additional burden associated with the decision for a move to long-term care is **suicide**. A recent study in the State of Virginia analyzed suicide rates among residents of assisted living and nursing home facilities in Virginia over a 9-year period. Among the findings were that those who committed suicide had a history of treatment for depression, one or more prior suicide attempts while in LTC, and complaints of chronic pain. Others committed suicide when anticipating entry into a long-term care community with resistance to the move, a poor family support system, and despondence at the loss of home, family, friends, and mobility. Finally, caregivers of relatives entered into long-term care were also vulnerable to suicide. Risk factors included despondence over the relative's move, personal failing health, and a history of depression (Jancin, 2014).

Acquired Conditions as Consequences of Long-Term Care Placement

While many physical and mental conditions can be improved with a move to long-term care, some of the changes with aging and certain disease states can be exacerbated in this setting. Physical conditions can worsen in a long-term care setting without vigilant evaluation by staff. Skin breakdown, dehydration, incontinence, **nosocomial infections** (acquired from the long-term care setting), elder abuse, and adverse drug reactions are among the conditions that require careful assessment and intervention for each resident.

Problems may also surface when a resident is transferred to an acute care facility only to return to another room and roommate upon discharge. This may require a new orientation and reintegration of the resident into the setting. This can be avoided if prior arrangements are made with the facility to reserve the original room for the resident's return.

Interventions to Maintain Quality of Life After a Move to Long-Term Care

The goal of any long-term care community should be to provide its residents with an environment that not only is safe but also provides dignity, autonomy, and a good quality of life. To accomplish this requires a culture change in long-term care—a shift in focus from an environment designed for staff convenience to one that is resident-focused and consumer-oriented. Several strategies, in addition to those discussed earlier, can be considered.

Initial Orientation/Transition

The most vulnerable time for a long-term care resident is the first week in a long-term care community. The new resident may experience a battery of emotions that can affect family dynamics and successful integration into the setting. Individuals who functioned well in familiar surroundings may become confused in the new, unfamiliar environment. This may last until the resident is sufficiently oriented to the facility, staff, and other residents. Other normal emotions for a new resident may include, anger, anxiety, depression, and feelings of abandonment that may lead to withdrawal. These feelings may be short-lived if the new resident participates in the setting.

Longer-lasting behavioral problems may need family and professional interventions. Family outings that reinforce the resident's place in the family structure as well as family participation in facility orientation and events may assist in the adjustment.

Conversely, it is possible that the new resident finds relief in being in a setting where his needs will be met, and where family caregivers are no longer burdened with the responsibility for day-to-day care. In this instance the new resident may cooperate fully in the activities at the new location. This may also provide an opportunity to rekindle family relationships strained by the moving process.

Organizations that have successfully transformed their cultures have implemented resident and family mentor programs to assist in the transition. **Resident mentors** welcome and support the new resident to socialize him into the community. Examples of this support include attending activities together, touring the community, introducing staff, and joining the new resident for meals. **Family mentors** function in a similar manner. Family mentors are individuals who can empathically assist the new family member with the transition; they are individuals who know the emotion and the pain that the new family member may be feeling. Family mentors assist new families in identifying key staff to contact, explain community norms, and assist with questions that may arise through the transition process.

Personal Possessions

Upon admission to long-term care, many personal possessions need to be left behind. Familiar objects should be encouraged, including photographs, special objects, familiar clothing, and where possible, familiar furniture and bedding. Creating an environment where residents feel they belong and where they can identify with their surroundings may support them during this transition.

A homelike atmosphere within the long-term care community enhances a feeling of belonging. The Eden Alternative is one example of a redesign of a facility that supports the elder in an environment of safety, belonging, and inclusion rather than in a hospital-like atmosphere (see Chapter 3).

Staffing

Staffing levels vary according to state regulations and level of care (see Chapter 1). Within a long-term care community's staffing parameters, introducing **consistent care models** is a beneficial approach for the resident, staff, and family members. Having the same caregivers on a routine basis usually allows for relationship development between caregivers and residents, and enables staff identification of subtle changes in their physical and psychosocial needs. Additionally, residents experiencing consistent caregivers feel as if their care is more personalized.

Language barriers can also present a difficulty for the resident and staff. Either a staff or resident may have primary language differences. At the least this can cause mutual frustration in trying to be understood; at the most, a misinterpretation in communication can lead to serious consequences. This may be overcome with a respectful approach to the resident by staff, attention to some of the hearing and eyesight problems of residents that may further potentiate ineffective communication, and a staff/resident clarification of needs with a native speaker, where possible.

Feelings of Self-Worth, Independence, and Choice

Research indicates that residents need to have some control over themselves and their environment. It is, therefore, important to give residents opportunities to make choices in their activities of daily living (Doty, Koren, & Sturla, 2008; Kranz, 2011). Research also indicates that residents have a better quality of life when they can take responsibility for something or someone in their long-term care community. This allows the residents to feel that they are contributing to their environment. The culture change associated with the resident-centered care philosophy supports resident preferences for liberalized diets, waking, sleep, activities, and bathing times (Koren, 2010). Among its many benefits are decreased needs for certain medications, especially those that control behavior (psychotropic drugs). Consistent with this philosophy, aging is not viewed as a time of decline, loneliness, helplessness, and boredom, but a time of continued growth and contribution.

Assessment and Care Planning

Because health conditions can change rapidly in an older adult, professional staff, in consultation with ancillary and support staff, should routinely evaluate residents for physical and mental changes. Working with older adults with multiple chronic conditions, in settings with few professional staff available on a daily basis, presents challenges not experienced in acute care settings. It is essential that the healthcare team remains as stable as possible, knows the federal and state regulations required of the long-term care community, and receives regular in-service education on topics related to care of the aging adult. Because long-term care communities increasingly care for residents in **hospice** and **palliative care** programs, it is important for staff to learn about end-of-life care for the resident and family. This should also include support for staff who must deal with resident deaths (Brenner, 2014). Staff should frequently consult with each other about individual patients, both informally and during structured care planning conferences. Staff should also listen to and consult with family caregivers about changes in a resident's condition or behaviors. To these ends it is important for the long-term care community to invest in staff retention and empowerment in their jobs. Research indicates that a **staff peer mentoring program** can be effective in maintaining and growing staff, and preventing staff turnover.

Because of the suicide risk among residents and their family caregivers, concurrent with and following a move to a long-term care community, staff must be vigilant in recognizing signs and symptoms of depression. Section D (Mood) of the Resident Assessment Instrument 3.0 provides staff a formal opportunity to assess for depression and suicide ideation, using the Patient Health Questionnaire (PHQ) screening tool. Both licensed and non-licensed staff should receive training in appropriate interventions when a resident or family member expresses suicidal thoughts, including **passive suicide ideation** (life is no longer worth living; I wish I were dead) and **active suicide ideation** (I want to find a way to kill myself; I am going to kill myself). Protocols should be in place to immediately address suicide ideation, including referral to a trained professional and protection of the resident from immediate harm.

Geriatric psychiatry is a growing specialty in medicine, nursing, psychology, and family therapy. Every long-term care community should have one or more of these professionals on call to address acute incidents and to provide longer-term therapy and medication management to manage depression and suicide risk.

Summary

Because the majority of residents in long-term care are older adults, these settings present incredible challenges to administrators, healthcare staff, and ancillary personnel to provide safety, dignity, choice, and quality of life for their residents, each of whom has a life history that is deserving of respect. An understanding of the bio-psycho-social changes with normal aging can suggest simple, cost-effective interventions that can contribute to disease prevention, enhance quality of life, and prevent unnecessary hospitalizations. Understanding basic principles of gerontology and geriatric care can also prevent misdiagnosis of certain behaviors as pathological conditions when they may be the result of expected changes with aging that can be solved with simple, non-drug interventions.

Healthcare personnel and ancillary staff are on the front lines of this care continuum and should be educated and supported to provide nurturing care to both residents and their families. Attention by administrators to new and innovative designs in the delivery of long-term care services can also enhance life for residents of these facilities. These innovations can address some of the quality of life issues experienced by aging individuals.

Key Terms

Active suicide ideation: Desire to commit suicide, including a plan to accomplish it.

Acute illness: One with a rapid onset and short course, such as a common cold.

Advanced activities of daily living (AADLs): Telephoning, shopping, food preparation, housekeeping, laundry, transportation, medication management, managing finances.

Adverse drug reaction (ADR): Reactions to a drug or the interaction of drugs with each other or with foods that produces illness, hospitalizations, and even death.

Albumin: Protein in the blood stream that helps move drugs to their site of action.

Alzheimer's disease: Most common form of dementia that progressively affects memory, thinking, and the ability to perform simple tasks.

Anergic: Unable to react to an antigen.

Antibodies: Proteins produced by the body to neutralize harmful substances.

Anticoagulation: Prevention of blood clots with the use of medications.

Antigens: Foreign substances, such as a chemical, bacteria or its toxin, virus, or pollen, that enter the body and stimulate the production of an antibody to fight it.

Anxiety: Feelings of stress, fear, and nervousness.

Aseptic technique: Procedures designed to prevent contamination by pathogens.

Aspiration: Breathing contents of the mouth/throat or stomach into the lungs.

Autonomic nervous system: Part of the peripheral nervous system that regulates involuntary activities, such as heart rate and digestion.

Basic activities of daily living (BADLs): Bathing, dressing, eating, toileting, transferring, and continence.

Benign prostatic hyperplasia (BPH): Enlargement of the prostate gland at the base of the bladder in a male.

Blanch: Pressure applied to skin, causing it to lose its pink color. Dark skin will usually not blanch.

Capillaries: The smallest blood vessels.

Cardiac arrhythmia: Irregular heart rate or rhythm that interrupts efficient blood flow to the body.

Cataract: Yellowing, cloudiness, and eventually opacity of the lens of the eye that distorts colors and blurs vision.

Cerumen: Ear wax.

Chemical restraints: Medications used to control behavior.

Chronic illness: One with a long course and continuing process, such as diabetes mellitus.

Circulatory system: Body system including the heart and blood and lymph systems that transports oxygen, nutrients, and waste products to support life.

Congestive heart failure: Condition in which the heart is unable to pump effectively to supply blood to the body, resulting in congestion of blood and fluid in the lungs, abdomen, and extremities.

Consistent care models: Staffing models that provide a team approach and predictable patient care assignments that allow a staff and a patient to get to know one another.

Constipation: Difficulty in having a bowel movement.

Crystallized intelligence: Knowledge from past learning and experience that may become better with age.

Dehydration: A condition in which water loss exceeds water intake.

Delirium: An acute and usually reversible state of confusion that may be caused by drugs, chemical imbalances, or infection.

Dementia: An irreversible decline in mental ability that interferes with daily functioning.

Depression: Disorder of mood characterized by a persistent feeling of sadness and disinterest in life.

Dermis: Middle layer of the skin.

Diarrhea: Stools that are watery.

Diverticulitis: Infection of the colon caused by trapping of undigested food particles in diverticula, allowing bacteria to grow. This requires medical treatment.

Diverticulosis: Weakened musculature in the colon (large intestine), causing pockets to form that can collect undigested food particles. This can produce pain in the lower left abdomen.

Drug toxicity: Adverse drug reaction caused by too much drug in the blood stream.

Dysmotility of the esophagus: A condition in which the esophagus does not transit food efficiently from the mouth to the stomach.

Epidermis: Outer layer of the skin.

Eschar: Thick, leathery, dark-colored dead tissue usually found in Stage IV pressure ulcers.

Esophageal sphincter: Circular ring of muscles that prevents backflow of stomach contents into the esophagus.

Estrogen: A female hormone that influences sexual development and regulates the release of eggs from the ovaries during reproductive years. Following menopause it diminishes and increases the risk of heart disease and osteoporosis.

Family mentor: Selected long-term care resident families who assist new families to socialize into the long-term care setting.

Fluid intelligence: Problem-solving ability that declines with aging.

Gait: The pattern of walking.

Gastrointestinal system: Organs responsible for ingestion of food, digestion, and elimination of food waste.

Gastroparesis: Slowed emptying of contents of the stomach into the intestines.

Genitourinary system: Anatomical system that includes both reproductive and urinary organs.

Geriatrics: Diagnosis and treatment of illnesses common in the older adult, usually by a geriatrician or nurse practitioner/physician's assistant trained and certified in this specialty.

Gerontology: The study of aging.

Heart attack: Damage to the heart caused by a blockage in a blood vessel that supplies the heart muscle. Also called a myocardial infarction.

Hemorrhage: Profuse bleeding.

Hiatial hernia: The stomach pushing upward into the chest, above the diaphragm and causing symptoms of indigestion.

Hospice: An interdisciplinary program designed to provide comfort care for a person and their family diagnosed with a terminal illness, with expected death within an estimated time.

Hyperthermia: Elevated body temperature that occurs when the body produces more heat than it eliminates.

Hypertrophy: Thickening and discoloration of a tissue, such as a toenail.

Hypotension: Low blood pressure that may cause dizziness and fainting.

Hypothermia: A medical emergency when a body loses more heat than it produces and temperature falls below 95° Fahrenheit (37° Centigrade).

Immune system: A network of cells, tissues, and organs that defends the body against disease.

Immuno-senescence: Age-related dysfunction of the immune system that is intended to provide protection against disease-producing organisms.

Instrumental activities of daily living (IADLs): Engagement in social activities.

Lethargy: A lack of energy.

Lewy body dementia: Second most prevalent form of dementia, characterized by protein deposits, called Lewy Bodies, in the area of the brain that affects thinking memory and movement.

Liberalized diet: Diet with few or no restrictions in kinds of food or fluids allowed.

Macular degeneration: Eye disease of aging that limits central vision and may cause blindness.

Malignancy: Cancer.

Menopause: Cessation of menstruation and the ability of a woman to produce an egg and bear a child.

Metabolic processes: The chemical processes in cells and organisms that are necessary for life.

Metabolize: To change the form of a drug or food so that it can be used by the body.

Morbidity: The number of cases of a disease.

Mortality: The number of deaths in a population.

Musculoskeletal system: Body system that includes muscles, tendons, bones, and ligaments that give the body structure and movement.

Necrotic: Tissue that is dead, and usually black in color.

Nervous system: Body system, including the brain, spinal cord peripheral nerves, and sensory organs, that coordinates voluntary and involuntary activities.

Nosocomial infection: Infection acquired in a hospital or long-term care community, usually due to carelessness of staff in maintaining aseptic or sterile technique.

Obesity: Excessive body fat.

Onychomycoses: A fungal infection of the nail, usually of the toes.

Osteopenia: A mild decrease in bone mineral density that can lead to osteoporosis.

Osteoporosis: A major decrease in bone mineral density that increases the risk of bone fracture, especially of the hips and spine.

Palliative care: An interdisciplinary program designed to provide comfort care/pain management for a person at any stage of an acute or chronic illness.

Parkinson's disease: Progressive disorder of the nervous system that is characterized by shaking of the hands, stiffness of the body, and possibly dementia.

Paronychia: Inflammation and infection of the skin around the nail.

Passive suicide ideation: Desire to commit suicide with no plan to accomplish it.

Pathogens: Disease-producing organisms, such as a bacteria, fungus, or virus.

Peripheral nervous system: Nerves outside the brain and spinal cord that provide communication with the central nervous system from internal and external organs.

Peripheral vascular disease: Disorder that affects blood vessels in the arms and legs.

Peripheral vision: Side vision.

Physical changes with aging: Expected changes in body systems that accompany the aging process.

Podiatrist: Physician specializing in care of foot structures.

Polypharmacy: Use of multiple medications that may cause adverse drug reactions.

Presbycusis: A normal change with aging characterized by difficulty hearing high-frequency sounds.

Psychological changes with aging: Changes in mood or behavior that may accompany the aging process.

Psychotropic drugs: Drugs that control mood and behavior.

Refractive error: Vision problem caused by changes in the shape of the eye that do not allow the eye to focus clearly.

Resident mentors: Long-term care residents who help to socialize new residents.

Respiratory system: System that supports breathing and the delivery of oxygen to the blood stream, and removal of carbon dioxide from the body.

Sarcopenia: Loss of muscle mass and strength with aging.

Sebaceous glands: Oil glands in the skin that secrete sebum to lubricate and protect the skin.

Seborrheic keratoses: Raised, wart-like lesions that appear greasy and stuck on aging skin in sun-exposed areas.

Self-determination: Process in which the person controls his own life.

Senile lentigo: Flat, pigmented, freckle-like lesions that appear on sun-exposed areas of aging skin.

Senile purpura: Purple discoloration of aging skin due to leakage of blood from fragile capillaries with minor injury.

Sibilant sounds: High-frequency sounds in words that include *s, f, sh, th, z,* and *ch* that are difficult to understand for someone with presbycusis.

Sleep apnea: Condition in which the individual stops breathing for intervals of time while sleeping. Usually recognized by periods of loud snoring.

Slough: Light-colored, soft, moist tissue remnants in the process of separating from healthier tissue in a pressure ulcer.

Social changes with aging: Changes in interactions with others that may accompany the aging process.

Somatic nervous system: Part of the peripheral nervous system that controls voluntary movement.

Staff peer mentoring: Selected staff who welcome, socialize, and support staff into the long-term care setting.

Subcutaneous: Inner layer of the skin composed mostly of fat cells.

Sudoriferous glands: Sweat glands that provide cooling of the body in hot environments.

Therapeutic level: Level of a drug in the blood stream that causes the desired effect but does not cause an adverse drug reaction.

Thymus gland: A gland located in the chest that assists in providing immunity from diseases.

Tinnitus: Ringing in the ears.

Toxic: Poisonous.

Tuberculosis: Lung infection caused by a bacteria and spread by coughing, sneezing, or other methods of transmitting fluids from the lungs.

Urinary catheter: Sterile tube inserted in the bladder to allow it to drain urine by gravity.

Urinary incontinence: Inability to retain urine in the bladder.

Urinary retention: Inability to completely empty the bladder.

Urinary tract: Body system responsible for eliminating urine from the body.

Urinary tract infection: Infection of the kidneys, ureters, bladder, or urethra.

White blood cells: Blood cells that protect the body from infections and foreign bodies (antigens).

Xerosis: Abnormal dryness of the skin.

Review Questions

1. Describe the normal/expected physical changes with aging that you consider to be the most important for staff to know.

2. Describe the normal/expected **psychological changes with aging** that you consider to be the most important for staff to know.

3. Describe the normal/expected **social changes with aging** that you consider to be the most important for staff to know.

4. Identify three common ways illness can be presented in the older adult.

5. List three reasons for possible adverse reactions to medications in the older adult and interventions to prevent them.

6. Describe the impact of a move into long-term care on family caregivers and on the new resident.

7. Design staff and management interventions to provide resident centered care to the older/disabled adult in long-term care.

Case Study

Mrs. Smith, a widow with an attentive family, has lived in your long-term care facility for 10 months. The staff notices that she has been confused for the last 2 days and needs to be reminded where the dining room is located.

1. What are the possible causes for this confusion?

2. What interventions would you recommend?

References

Alzheimer's Association. (2013). Alzheimer's disease facts and figures. *Alzheimer's & Dementia, 9*(2). Retrieved from http://www.alz.org/downloads/facts_figures_2013.pdf

The American Geriatrics Society. (2012). Beers Criteria update expert panel: American Geriatrics Society updated Beers Criteria for potentially inappropriate medication use in older adults. *Journal of the American Geriatrics Society, 60,* 616–631. doi:10.1111/j.1532-5415.2012.03923.x

American Psychological Association. (2006, June 11). *Memory changes in older adults. Research in Action.* Retrieved from https://www.apa.org/research/action/memory-changes.aspx

Bern-Klug, M. (2008). The emotional context facing nursing home residents' families: A call for role reinforcement strategies from nursing homes and the community. *Journal of the American Medical Directors Association, 9,* 36–44.

Brenner, J. (2014). *An educational curriculum on death and dying for caregivers in California assisted living* (Unpublished master's thesis). California State University, Long Beach.

Centers for Disease Control and Prevention. (2015). *Falls in nursing homes. Home and Recreational Safety.* Retrieved from http://www.cdc.gov/homeandrecreationalsafety/falls/nursing.html

Centers for Disease Control and Prevention National Healthcare Safety Network. (n.d.). *Tracking infections in long-term care facilities.* Retrieved from http://www.cdc.gov/nhsn/LTC/index.html

Danon, G. (2007). Podiatry. In B. White & D. Truax (Eds.), *The nurse practitioner in long term care: Guidelines for clinical practice* (pp. 495–513). Sudbury, MA: Jones & Bartlett.

Doshi, J. A., Shaffer, T., & Briesacher, B. A. (2005). National estimates of medication use in nursing homes: Findings from the 1997 Medicare Current Beneficiary Survey and the 1996 Medical Expenditure Survey. *Journal of the American Geriatrics Society, 53,* 438–443. doi:10.1111/j.1532-5415.2005.53161.x

Doty, M. M., Koren, M. J., & Sturla, E. L. (2008). *Culture change in nursing homes: How far have we come?* (Commonwealth Fund Pub. No. 1131). Retrieved from http://www.commonwealthfund.org/%7E/media/Files/Publications/Fund%20Report/2008/May/Culture%20Change%20in%20Nursing%20Homes%20%20How%20Far%20Have%20We%20Come%20%20Findings%20From%20The%20Commonwealth%20Fund%202007%20Nati/Doty_culturechangenursinghomes_1131%20pdf.pdf

Gellis, Z. D., & McCracken, S. G. (2008). Depressive disorders in older adults. *Mental Health and Older Adults.* CSWE Gero-Ed Center. Retrieved from www.gero-edcenter.org

Geriatric Mental Health Foundation. (n.d.) Overcoming worry and fear. *Anxiety and Older Adults.* Retrieved from http://www.gmhfonline.org

Handler, S. M. & Hanlon, J. T. (2010). Detecting adverse drug reactions in the nursing home setting using a nursing home specific trigger tool. *Annals of Long Term Care, 18*(5), 17–22.

Handler, S. M., Wright, R. M., Ruby, C. M., & Hanlon, J. T. (2006). Epidemiology of medication related adverse events in nursing homes. *American Journal of Geriatric Pharmacotherapy, 4,* 264–272.

Harris-Kojetin, L., Sengupta, M., Park-Lee, E., & Valverde, R. (2013). *Long-term care services in the United States: 2013 overview.* Hyattsville, MD: National Center for Health Statistics.

Hefland, A. E. (2003). Podiatric assessment of the geriatric patient. *Clinics in Podiatry Medicine and Surgery, 20,* 407–429.

High, K. P., Bradley, S. F., Gravenstein, S., Mehr, D. R., Quagliarello, V. J., Richards, C., & Yoshikawa, T. T. (2009). Clinical practice guideline for the evaluation of fever and infection in older adult residents of long-term care facilities. *Clinical Infectious Diseases, 48,* 149–171.

Jancin, B. (2014). Elderly suicide prevention: Focus on change in living location. *Caring for the Ages, 15*(8), 7.

Koren, M. J. (2010). Person-centered care for nursing home residents: The culture change movement. *Health Affairs, 29*(2), 1–6. doi:10.1377/hlthaff.2009.0966

Kranz, K. (2011). The relationship between empowerment care and quality of life among members of assisted living facilities. *Journal of Undergraduate Research, 14*, 1–5.

Martin, J. L., & Ancoli-Israel, S. (2008). Sleep disturbances in long-term care. *Clinics in Geriatric Medicine, 24*, 39–50. Retrieved from http://www.ncbi.nlm.nih.gov/pmc/articles/PMC2215778/pdf/nihms36700.pdf

National Eye Institute. (n.d.). *Fact sheet: Refractive errors.* Retrieved from https://nei.nih.gov/sites/default/files/health-pdfs/HVM09_Fact_Sheet_Final_tagged.pdf

National Pressure Ulcer Advisory Panel. (2007). NPUAP pressure ulcer stages/categories. Retrieved from http://www.npuap.org/resources/educational-and-clinical-resources/npuap-pressure-ulcer-stagescategories/

National Pressure Ulcer Advisory Panel. (2014, March). *The NPUAP selected "Quality of Care Regulations" made easy.* Retrieved from http://www.npuap.org/resources/educational-and-clinical-resources/npuap-selected-quality-of-care-regulations-made-easy/

National Sleep Foundation. (2015). *Aging and sleep.* Retrieved from http://sleepfoundation.org/sleep-topics/aging-and-sleep

Tamura, B. K., Bell, C. L., Lubimir, K., Iwasaki, W. N, Ziegler, L. A., & Masaki, K. H. (2011). Physician intervention for medication reduction in a nursing home: The polypharmacy outcomes project. *Journal of the American Medical Directors Association, 12*, 326–330. doi:10.1016/j.jamda.2010.08.013

White, B., & Truax, D. (2007). *The nurse practitioner in long-term care: Guidelines for clinical practice.* Sudbury, MA: Jones & Bartlett.

Xue, Q. (2011). The frailty syndrome: Definition and natural history. *Clinics in Geriatric Medicine, 27*, 1–15. doi:10.1016/j.cger.2010.08.009

Zimmerman S., Anderson, W., Brode, S., Jonas, D., Lux, L., Beeber, A., . . . Sloane, P. (2012, October). *Comparison of characteristics of nursing homes and other residential long-term care settings for people with dementia: Comparative effectiveness review* (Prepared by the RTI International–University of North Carolina Evidence-Based Practice Center under Contract No. 290-2007-10056-I; AHRQ Publication No. 12(13)-EHC127-EF). Rockville, MD: Agency for Healthcare Research and Quality. Retrieved from www.effectivehealthcare.ahrq.gov/reports/final/cfm

Acknowledgment

I would like to thank Jim Kinsey, Director of Member Experience at Planetree, an organization that fosters creation of patient-centered care, for his thoughtful review and contributions to this chapter.

CHAPTER 12

RESIDENT-CENTERED CLINICAL OPERATIONS

Paige Hector

The nursing facility is a dynamic environment with staff committed to caring for the residents who live there. As in many healthcare environments, the interprofessional team is paramount and together these individuals share the responsibility of caring for some of the most vulnerable adults in our society. As the leader of this dynamic team, the administrator must understand every aspect of the clinical operations and demonstrate proficiency in critical thinking processes.

Clinical Operations

Clinical operations encompass the tasks that ensure resident care not only meets regulatory standards, facility policies and procedures, and standards of practice but also ensures the highest practicable functioning of each resident. From medication administration to advance care planning, clinical operations management is integral to a successful facility and requires strong leadership.

Role of the Administrator

As the leader of a nursing facility, the administrator must be closely involved in the clinical operations, even if she does not have medical training. While medical training can certainly make it easier to understand the clinical complexity of resident care, it is not a requisite. The role of the administrator is to teach and support critical thinking, which results in good clinical judgment. The administrator is ultimately responsible for ensuring that the hundreds

LEARNING OBJECTIVES

- Explain why critical thinking is the foundation of good clinical judgment.

- Understand the importance of policies and procedures and how the administrator ensures they are accurate.

- Identify the components that make up a comprehensive care plan.

- Describe the elements of a medical record audit and why this process is important.

- Explain the difference between subjective and objective documentation and when staff should use each type.

- Detail the steps to facilitate a safe leave of absence for a resident and the facility.

of details that make up daily life in the facility are put into operation and documented appropriately.

Critical Thinking and Clinical Judgment

Alfaro-LeFevre (2009) describes **critical thinking** as reasoning, and **clinical judgment** as a result of that reasoning. Critical thinking is more than common sense; it is learned from experience. Critical thinking is an ability to evaluate a situation objectively and decide the next steps. Clinical judgment is a conclusion based on observation, reflection, and analysis of available information. In the clinical setting like a nursing facility, the steps taken are the evidence of that clinical judgment. Let's look at some examples.

A nurse documents that a resident eloped from the building and that the **wander guard** (electronic safety device) did not trigger the alarm at the front entrance. Security and maintenance were notified of the problem with the system after it happened. So, what is missing? The outcome of ensuring the resident's continued safety. The documentation should also include a resident assessment to determine if injury was sustained, repair of the faulty device, and notification of the administrator, physician, and responsible party.

In another example, a nurse documents, "Foley is draining dark brown urine with a malodor" without documenting the follow-up of physician notification and outcome. This entry demonstrates lack of critical thinking and is a red flag for a potentially poor outcome. Consider this revised entry in comparison with the original. "Foley is draining dark brown urine with a malodor. Spoke with Dr. Smith, gave history, vital signs and described acute symptom of bladder spasms. Requested orders for urinalysis and culture and sensitivity if indicated. Dr. Smith agreed and orders written."

In a third example, a social worker meets with a resident who stated she was not feeling well, which the social worker documents in the medical record. Again, what is missing? The documentation of what the social worker did about the resident's complaint. Here's an improved entry: "Met with resident to discuss advance directives, and she stated she was not feeling well with complaints of right hip pain. Notified charge nurse, who went to assess the resident."

Critical thinking applies to all staff, not just clinical staff. If a house-keeper is cleaning a resident's room and notices a bottle of medication on the nightstand, he must immediately notify the charge nurse. If the business office manager discovers that a resident was incorrectly billed for another resident's supplies, it needs to be determined if this is a one-time error or if there is a problem with the tracking and billing of supplies in general.

Critical thinking is a skill that takes practice and coaching to develop. The administrator and director of nurses must model this skill daily and be alert to coaching opportunities for all staff.

Federal and State Regulations

The nursing home industry is heavily regulated by federal and state governments. Appendix PP of the State Operations Manual (SOM) outlines thousands of federal regulations that each facility must meet. Some states mandate additional regulatory standards.

From a clinical operations perspective, the administrator must demonstrate thorough knowledge of the regulations and ensure they are followed daily. Periodically there are updates or revisions to the regulations, so it is important to stay abreast of any changes through the Centers for Medicare and Medicaid Survey and Certification transmittals (Centers for Medicare and Medicaid Services [CMS], 2012).

Maintain a current set of the regulations, and provide staff with the appropriate sections to help ensure a successfully run department. For example, the dietary manager must have copies of regulations, such as Standard Menus and Nutritional Adequacy (CMS, 2014, F363) and Nutrition (CMS, 2014, F325). The social worker should have copies of Quality of Life (CMS, 2014, F309), Medically Related Social Services (CMS, 2014, F250), and Mental and Psychosocial Functioning (CMS, 2014, F319), to name just a few.

Policies and Procedures

Policies and procedures (P&P) are essential components of each facility and address the processes in every department, such as infection control, fire safety, psychosocial assessment, resident bathing, and change of diet. Unfortunately, facilities are frequently cited for not following their own policies and procedures. Similar to the regulations, the role of the administrator is to empower staff by providing them with current P&P and ensuring they are operationalized.

P&P should be reviewed on a yearly basis in conjunction with the Quality Assurance and Performance Improvement (QAPI) program. Be alert for instances when the P&P do not match what staff are actually doing or where they might have developed work-arounds. Sometimes a P&P is cumbersome or it causes unintended risk with complex steps or ambiguous language. For the facility that is part of a larger corporation, the P&P are usually developed and modified at a corporate level so changes by the individual facility may require approval. It is important to note, however, that P&P must be individualized for each facility. A one-size-fits-all approach is not a good approach to developing or updating P&P. There may be cultural, regional, or even resource differences that make adopting one set of P&P throughout an entire corporation unrealistic.

Let's look at an example of when a P&P actually generates more work for staff. Included in the Minimum Data Set (MDS) is the **Patient Health Questionnaire** (PHQ-9), which screens for depression. It is an excellent tool and contributes valuable information for the resident's mood assessment. The facility also requires a **Geriatric Depression Scale** (GDS) to be completed upon admission. While the GDS is also an excellent tool and widely used, there is no practical reason to require the completion of an additional tool when staff is already screening for depression using the mandated PHQ-9. This P&P creates more work for staff that is already pressured for time.

P&P for tasks such as vital signs and **alert charting** (documentation for a **change of condition**) are good examples of P&P that typically have requisite time frames. For a new patient, vital signs may be taken each shift for the first week unless otherwise directed by the medical provider. Alert charting usually occurs throughout the duration of the clinical change, such as an infection and then a few days following the completion of the antibiotic treatment. Staff must know what is expected, and leadership needs to conduct regular audits to determine that the P&P are being followed.

When a P&P is updated, the change should be reflected in the minutes for the QAPI meeting. Include the rationale for the change, the effective date, and the plan for staff training. Changes to some P&P necessitate residents being informed, which may include written notification. For record-keeping purposes, have the resident, responsible party, and the staff member explaining the change sign a copy of the relevant P&P.

In an informational toolkit titled, "The Younger Adult in the Long-Term Care Setting" (American Medical Directors Association, 2013), the authors advise meeting individually with residents regarding policy changes for issues that are particularly emotionally charged, such as electric wheelchairs, smoking, and storage of belongings.

Admission to Facility

Admitting a new resident or patient to the facility is time-intensive and requires input from different staff to ensure an appropriate and successful admission. This chapter will focus on the clinical operations once the person has already been admitted to the facility.

Care Plan

A resident's care plan or plan of care is one of the most important, and scrutinized, documents in the medical record. Regulations provide guidance for general care plan components and the overall expectation that care and services help the resident achieve the highest practicable well-being. Unfortunately, staff often receive little or no training on how to properly write and update a care plan.

Care plan development depends upon comprehensive assessments by all disciplines. It is illogical to write a care plan for an issue or problem that has not been properly assessed. Consider this example: A resident demonstrates "calling out behavior." While that behavior can be problematic, not only for the resident but also for other residents and staff, without a thorough assessment to determine why the resident is calling out, a reduction in the behavior may actually be undesirable, especially if it is how the resident is communicating pain or other distress.

Care planning a medical issue, such as **edema** (swelling caused by fluid retention), is expected but unless the reason for the edema is identified, an accurate care plan cannot be written. If the edema is due to a **deep vein thrombosis** (DVT) (blood clot in the vein), the goal and interventions will be very different than if the edema is due to congestive heart failure (CHF). The significance of critical thinking must be evident throughout the assessment and care plan process.

Repeatedly, the regulations state that the facility must help residents achieve the highest practicable well-being. The care plan demonstrates how staff intends to achieve this for each resident. Each problem or need, once resolved or even improved, must somehow improve the resident's quality of life. Continuing with the edema example, to resolve or reduce the edema provides relief for the resident, which may result in more independence with ambulation or perhaps an easier time breathing.

Each care plan must be individualized, which means that the plan is unique to the resident and based on the information learned from the resident, responsible party, and staff during the assessment process and general interactions. Depression is a common problem, yet the way that each person manifests depression is different or unique to his personality, history, circumstances, cognitive abilities, and more. These areas must be assessed before an individualized care plan can be developed.

Initial care plan. The **initial care plan** is a document started immediately upon admission. A common initial care plan includes several potential problems on one page. The problem statements are generic, with simple goals and a limited number of interventions. The initial care plan statement may differ from what is eventually developed for the comprehensive care plan, but it is a starting point upon admission. For example, a resident may have a care plan for "Cardiac Problem" due to "Congestive Heart Failure" and "Mood Disorder" related to "Schizophrenia." As staff get to know the resident, a comprehensive plan (with greater detail) is formulated that accurately reflects the individual resident.

Comprehensive plan. After a few weeks, staff has gotten to know the resident much better, including his specific needs and desires. A comprehensive care plan is now developed with input from all disciplines, the resident, and responsible party. Do not be mistaken, however, that once the comprehensive care plan is developed that it is done. A true care plan is a working tool—that is, it changes. Staff must be adept at modifying the care plan as needed, which requires the support of clinical leadership to help stay abreast of this ever-changing document.

Temporary plan. The **temporary care plan** is a very useful tool. Sometimes a resident has a time-limited issue to be addressed, such as an infection, that does not require a comprehensive care plan. A temporary care plan (sometimes referred to as a temporary problem list) is an abbreviated care plan in which the issue or problem is expected to resolve within a short time frame, such as 14 days. It still contains a problem statement, a goal, and a few interventions. Common temporary care plans address issues such as a urinary tract infection, a skin tear, or a rash.

Care plan components. A care plan consists of specific components: a date of initiation, the problem or needs statement, goal(s) or objective(s), **target date** (review date for the care plan), interventions or approaches, responsible discipline(s), and the initials of the person initiating the plan.

Each care plan entry must be dated to indicate the onset of the issue and initialed by the person writing the plan. The timeliness of identifying issues and prompt care plan development is important and demonstrates good clinical judgment.

The problem or needs statement should be sufficiently detailed to explain how the issue is problematic for the resident. Determine specifics, such as the etiology of the problem or diagnosis, the impact of the problem on the resident, the time of day when it might be more problematic, and contributing factors. This information helps make the care plan individualized.

The goal must be measurable, realistic, and time-specific. It is helpful to think of goals as things that can be observed, actually hearing or seeing the resident accomplishing the goal. For the resident with edema in the lower legs, the edema resolves and her legs are no longer filled with fluid. A resident who yells at staff now uses a calm voice at least some of the time. The resident who is depressed makes a statement about enjoying a new hobby.

What does it mean that a goal should be realistic? It means that accomplishing the goal is within the capacity of the resident. For a resident with bladder spasms who is also cognitively impaired, it is not realistic that she is a candidate for maintaining a toileting schedule by herself. Goals must also be reviewed, typically each quarter at the resident's care conference, unless indicated sooner, such as with the completion of an antibiotic treatment or monitoring of a new medication.

"All goals, no matter what problem or need they address, are the resident's" (Davis, Greenwald, & Pareti, 2011, p. B.12). Once a goal is accomplished (or even improved), the resident's quality of life will improve. The goals are all about the resident, not the staff!

The **approaches or interventions** are what the *staff will do* to help the resident meet the goal, like in this example: "The resident will be encouraged to choose activities of interest." Encouraging the resident to choose activities of interest is an approach because the staff will do it, not the resident. Goals are what the resident will do, and approaches are what staff will do. See Exhibit 12.1.

Exhibit 12.1 Sample Care Plan for Depression

Comprehensive Care Plan

Date	Physical & Psychosocial Needs	Goals/Objectives	Approaches/Interventions	Responsible Discipline
	The resident demonstrates significant mood distress related to: ☑ A diagnosis and/or history of depressive illness. ☑ A difficult time adjusting to losses, placement and changes in roles/status. ☐ Feeling angry, guilty and/or out of control (e.g., powerless, hopeless, incomplete, incompetent). ☐ A previous diagnosis of dementia or psychopathology (e.g., schizophrenia, bipolar disorder, personality disorder). ☐ Other: ____ Problems/needs are manifested by: ☐ An inability to mobilize strengths and inner resources towards treatment and recovery. ☑ Remaining secluded in his/her room for the majority of the day. ☐ Seemingly unable to experience pleasure. ☑ Decreased interest in various activities and the environment (profound sense of indifference). ☐ Apathy; the resident does not appear to care about very much. ☐ Angry, abusive outbursts in which the resident "projects" own feelings of misery and distress onto other persons. ☐ Consuming approximately 25% of meals and is at risk for weight loss. ☐ The resident is seen regularly by the psychiatrist. ☐ Presently receives anti-depressant medication. ☐ Other: ____ Strengths and Abilities: Decision-making capacity, engages in conversation easily	☑ The resident will engage in a counseling/supportive relationship by the next review... ☑ The resident will verbalize the thoughts and feelings that contribute to remaining depressed, by ~~mldly...~~ next review ☐ The resident will identify inner resources and strengths in order to take a step towards recovery and self-improvement, during a counseling session, by... ☐ The resident will ____ by...	☑ Counseling/support sessions, [one] times per week. Specify group, individual, prn treatment. ☑ Use open-ended questions during counseling sessions such as, "How can you take advantage of your strengths?" "How can you take control over life and improve your day-to-day functioning?" ☐ If the resident is having trouble discussing/identifying several means of mobilizing his strengths or is not doing this, staff should list several ways he/she can improve the quality of his/her life, including: ✓ Admitting/recognizing that depression is a serious problem, however it is a problem that responds to treatment (i.e., many people with Depression are able to live a fulfilling, meaningful life). ✓ Speaking about feelings/emotions instead of withdrawing and allowing feelings to become repressed and "bottled up." ✓ Planning and attempting to accomplish one small change at a time, focusing on a one-day-at-a-time attitude. This will help minimize the fear of failure and keep expectations reasonable. ✓ Focus on strengths and accomplishments. Help the resident avoid or minimizing lamenting on failures/challenges. Re-frame failures as components of learning and development. ☐ Discuss the resident's situation with the psychiatrist and the IDT. ☐ Consider utilizing a variety approaches to "reach" and "connect" with the resident. This includes the staff member changing from a supportive role to a more confrontative role or a "cognitive behavioral" approach (insight oriented). ☑ Try alternative theCAAies such as music, art, inter-generational, animal interventions, horticulture, empowerment activities (e.g., volunteer jobs, assisting staff, newsletter, music/singing, resident council) ☐ ____	soc work ▼ ▼ soc work nursing MD-psych act ▼ ▼ soc work act
SwCG, Inc. ©	Resident Doe, Jane	Signs and Symptoms of Depression	Mood State CAA's 7,8	Care Plan No. 34 May 16, 2015

Source: Adapted from *Revolutionary OBRA & JCAHO Formatted Care Plans* (2015).

Each entry in the care plan must indicate which staff are responsible for the intervention. Sometimes only one discipline is responsible for the intervention, such as nursing administering medication or a social worker meeting weekly with the resident to discuss grief related to placement. Other times, multiple disciplines are responsible for the intervention, such as reminding the resident to use a quiet voice when making requests rather than screaming at staff.

There are care plan pitfalls that staff need to avoid. A common mistake is when staff care plan the administration of a medication or the potential for side effects as the problem statement itself—for example, "Resident takes Ativan for anxiety." The problem is not that the resident takes the medication but rather the diagnosis (anxiety) for which the medication is prescribed and how the symptoms manifest for this resident. Care plan the anxiety specific to the resident, and list medication administration as an *approach*.

Another pitfall is redundant care plans. Combine similar problems into one comprehensive care plan rather than write separate plans. For example, a resident has pain associated with recent hip surgery, pain related to chronic back problems, pain from migraines, and arthritic pain. Combine all the types of pain into one comprehensive pain problem statement with a limited number of goals and a reasonable number of interventions.

A third pitfall and one that is very important from a risk management perspective is a seemingly harmless term: *prevent*. While staff certainly do everything possible to prevent harm from befalling residents, there are certain situations in which it is not preventable. A good example of when to avoid the term "prevent" is with a fall risk care plan. For a resident who is at risk of falls, unless a facility offers one-on-one care 24 hours a day, the likelihood of preventing a fall is not realistic. What is realistic is that we *minimize* injury from a fall.

A fourth pitfall is when staff state the name of the medication on the care plan itself instead of the category, such as diuretic, antipsychotic, or pain. Do not state the actual medication and certainly not the dose. In the event the medication or dose changes, the care plan would need to be revised to reflect the new name and dose. The class of medication suffices by itself.

Yet a fifth pitfall is a care plan that places the facility under unnecessary scrutiny. Take this care plan statement, for example: "Resident is experiencing severe weight loss related to poor food intake." A chart review revealed that this resident is on hospice with diagnoses of advanced dementia and failure to thrive. The weight loss is *expected*. Unfortunately, the way it reads in the care plan attributes fault to the facility. An appropriate problem statement would be, "Resident is on hospice for diagnoses of advanced dementia and failure to thrive. Appetite is poor and weight loss is expected."

A sixth pitfall is a care plan with conflicting information regarding the resident's status or abilities. Consider this example of an actual resident's care plan that demonstrates the problems associated with conflicting information. The activities care plan states that the resident is dependent on staff for mobility; however, the impaired mobility plan states the resident propels her own wheelchair. Yet in the interventions of the mobility plan, the word "wheelchair" is crossed through and "walker" is indicated instead. So, what is this resident's mobility status? How do staff know what to do and how is the correct information communicated to all staff on all shifts?

Strengths-based plans. Utilizing a **strengths-based assessment** whereby staff identify resident strengths and use them in the care plan helps ensure a positive, individualized approach to care. Strengths can be identified in many categories, like personality traits, intellectual abilities, physical condition, lifestyles and roles, support systems, and ability to draw upon supportive relationships (Davis et al., 2011). Learning a resident's strengths can be as simple as just asking, "What do you consider your strengths?" If the person has endured a hardship in the past or a medical challenge, how did he get though it? What helped? Questions like these also help remind people that they have coping abilities no matter the age or debility. Even for a resident with advanced dementia, the ability to smile or respond to gentle touch is a wonderful strength that can be used throughout the care plan.

Care plan for mood disorders. **Mood disorders** (a psychological disorder characterized by the elevation or lowering of a person's mood) are perhaps the most difficult area for staff to write a care plan.

Mood disorders require a unique approach, and it is not completely intuitive. Take the diagnosis of depression. Unfortunately, a typical care plan may just list "depression" as a problem statement and then a generic goal, such as "reduce crying episodes." Staff may reason that crying episodes are measurable, and are therefore an appropriate goal.

The problem statement for a mood disorder should be sufficiently detailed so the problem is very clear in terms of severity, time of day, symptoms, effect on the resident, and any other information that conveys important details. Based on a comprehensive assessment, the depression problem statement might look like this: "Resident has a diagnosis of depression with symptoms of tearfulness, self-isolation, lack of interest in usual activities. The symptoms are more evident in the evening around bedtime. Resident has stated she feels depressed but 'doesn't care.'" Wow! That is a comprehensive statement that paints a picture of the resident.

Goals for mood disorders should not focus on reducing symptoms, such as the number of crying episodes. "Mood distress expressions, such as tearfulness, negative statements, frequent complaints, unrealistic fears, and apathy for example, are a means of communication. It is not acceptable to develop care plans that inhibit or restrict expression of these feelings" (Greenwald, 2002, p. 6.7). Staff must assess and understand why the resident is displaying the symptoms and then develop a comprehensive care plan, including goals to resolve or relieve the underlying issue. The emphasis is on improving the resident's quality of life, not just reducing symptoms. So, a depression goal might read, "Resident will discuss thoughts and feelings related to placement." This goal is simple, measurable, and within the resident's capability to achieve.

Another complication in care planning mood disorders occurs when staff care plans a medication, such as an antidepressant, anxiolytic, or an antipsychotic *as the problem itself*. The problem statement should be the diagnosis for which the medication is ordered and how it manifests specifically for that resident. The medication, monitoring for side effects, and any related dose reductions are *interventions*, not problems and not goals.

CMS established a national goal that unnecessary antipsychotic medications be reduced in nursing homes. While many facilities have made great strides in reducing these mediations, there is still much room for improvement in assessing and utilizing nonpharmacological interventions in relation to mood and behavior challenges. This is where the interdisciplinary approach to assessment and care planning should be evident.

Nurses, social services, nursing assistants, and activity and dietary staff can all contribute to mood and behavior care plans. In other words, everyone has responsibility to identify nonpharmacological interventions that might be successful for each resident. For one resident, music might help provide a calming effect, or perhaps petting an animal. For another resident, a stroll outside might prove calming. The care plan must reflect an individualized, person-centered assessment.

Updating the care plan. The care plan is a working document. As the resident's needs evolve, changes of condition occur, and staff learn more about the resident, the care plan needs to be revised. Staff should be accustomed to hearing the administrator and DON ask, "Is a care plan in place?" or "Does the care plan need to be updated?"

Let's look at an example. A resident is diagnosed with a lower respiratory tract infection. A care plan is initiated on January 16 and includes the intervention of antibiotic treatment for 7 days. After the completion of the antibiotic treatment, the provider determines that the infection is resolved. The nurse then discontinues the care plan by indicating the date of the resolution and initials the updated information.

What about updating a care plan for a behavioral problem? A resident who chooses to yell at staff when she needs something has a goal to use a respectful volume and tone of voice when making a request. She has been doing very well and consistently achieves the goal at least once a day. She is ready to progress to a more challenging goal! Staff revise the care plan with a goal to achieve success twice a day.

One of the challenges when updating the care plan occurs when information is written in multiple areas. Consider the resident with declining health who is approved for hospice. Many medications and treatments are discontinued, including weekly weights. Unfortunately, "obtain weekly weights" was written in several places in the care plan and not all entries were revised or discontinued. The facility was then cited for weight loss as the resident continued to lose weight (although everyone agreed that weight loss was expected) as the care plan was not updated properly.

The stand-up meeting is a comprehensive process to stay abreast of care plan development and ensure accuracy. Refer to Chapter 13 for in-depth discussion on stand-up.

Medical Record Audit

Regular medical records audits are intrinsic to successful clinical operations and performance improvement. Auditing the record for a newly admitted resident is one of the best strategies for identifying incomplete areas, missing documents, and general issues or liability concerns. The key is to be proactive and identify areas sooner rather than later. Although the timing of an audit may differ between facilities, doing an audit in the first 24 hours of the stay is recommended. The admission audit is an integral part of the stand-up meeting and will be discussed in Chapter 13.

This section of the text will discuss how to perform an admission audit. Each facility should have policies and procedures that address each of the following sections of the medical record, and it is imperative that the administrator and director of nurses be familiar with these policies and ensure they are followed.

Face sheet. The face sheet orients the reader to important information, like the resident's name, date of birth, payer source, and responsible party. This information must be accurate. One facility was cited when the power of attorney information was inaccurate and the appropriate individual could not be notified when the resident had a sudden change of condition (any symptom, sign, or apparent discomfort that is sudden in onset, is a marked change, and is unrelieved by measures already prescribed) (American Medical Directors Association, 2003).

Advance directives. **Advance directives** are documents that convey a person's healthcare wishes. Documents may include a **healthcare power of attorney** (document that allows a person to designate a spokesperson to make healthcare decisions), **living will** (document that provides guidelines for resident's wishes regarding life-sustaining treatment), and **code status** (decision regarding wishes for resuscitation measures in the event of cardiac or respiratory arrest). Refer to Chapter 8 for information on the individual documents.

Upon admission, it is the nurse's responsibility to determine code status—that is, whether the resident wishes to undergo resuscitation measures in the event of cardiac or respiratory failure. Some facilities make the mistake of assigning code status responsibility to the social worker; while this individual should be adept at having this conversation with a resident or responsible party, the conversation should occur upon admission with the nurse, not a day later.

If someone is listed as a power of attorney in the medical records, there must be a copy of the appropriate document in the advance directives section. While obtaining code status is the responsibility of the nurse upon admission, the social worker is responsible for assisting the resident to complete other advance directives documents if desired.

Provider orders. A medical provider (typically a hospital provider or the person's primary care physician) must write admission orders to admit a person to the skilled nursing facility. Admission orders must include specific information, such as diagnoses, medications, treatments, equipment, and any other special instructions, such as follow-up appointments. The admitting nurse must sign, date, note, and verify each page of the orders. If the provider has already signed these orders, the process of **verifying the orders** means the nurse reviewed them with the provider who will be caring for the resident and any changes were made such as discontinuing a medication or adding a physical therapy consult or wound care orders. **Noting the orders** includes tasks such as transferring medications to the **medication administration record** (MAR) (legal record of drugs administered) and treatments to the **treatment administration record** (TAR) (record that lists procedural orders, separate from the MAR), faxing medication orders to the pharmacy, and obtaining equipment.

Throughout the resident's stay in the facility, either medical providers give orders verbally, which the nurse (or another clinical staff member, like a therapist or dietitian) writes in the chart, or the provider writes the order herself. These instructions are simply referred to as "orders."

Catheters. Sometimes a person is admitted with a Foley catheter, a tube inserted into the bladder to assist with voiding urine. There must be a diagnosis that justifies the use of the catheter. Typically, it is a good idea whenever possible to discontinue the use of the catheter to minimize the potential for infection. For the resident who needs to continue its use, in addition to the diagnosis, there must be a size for the tube, often written as a number with an "F," which indicates French (e.g., a common size is 16F). There must also be a balloon size designated with cubic centimeters, such as 10cc. The last component that must be part of the order and checked during the audit is instruction to change the catheter, typically on a monthly basis. All of this information must also be reflected on the care plan.

Medications. Each medication, including over-the-counter medications, herbal supplements, and creams, must have a corresponding diagnosis—that is, rationale for the administration of the medication. For example, atrial fibrillation is one diagnosis to justify taking Coumadin. Prednisone may be ordered for rheumatoid arthritis and hydrocortisone cream for a rash. Each medication should be accompanied by a diagnosis.

The laws that govern medication administration in the nursing facility are stringent. For example, narcotics can be ordered only with an actual hard copy prescription rather than just ordering the medication over the phone or fax to the pharmacy. The orders must include exact parameters that guide the nurse when to administer specific doses. For example, one tablet for moderate pain between 4 and 7 out of 10 on the pain scale and two tablets for severe pain between 8 and 10 out of 10 on the pain scale.

Psychotropic medications. **Psychotropic medications** are those classes of medications such as antidepressants, anxiolytics, and antipsychotics that alter an individual's mood or thought processes. In the nursing facility, these medications are highly scrutinized and require additional documentation to justify their use. On the order, include the **target behaviors** (behavior identified for change), such as yelling out or anxiety as evidenced by rapid speech. That way, the target behaviors are entered into the electronic record and will then be included on the monthly **recapitulation** (orders printed at the start of the month and signed by the provider).

Psychotropic medications also require that the resident or responsible party give consent for the medication to be administered. That is, they must be made aware of the potential risks and side effects and sign a form to acknowledge such understanding before the medication is given. If a resident receives psychotropic medication without consent, it is a medication error and an **incident report** (record of an unusual event) must be completed.

Consent forms must be completed accurately. Only one medication should be listed per consent form. If multiple medications are ordered that require consent, staff should complete one consent form for each medication. And it is not recommended to include the dose on the consent (only the name of the medication) so in the event the dose changes, the consent remains valid.

For purposes of the chart audit, determine if any medications require consent and then determine if the consent form is completed properly.

History and physical. The history and physical (H&P) is a detailed document that outlines important information about the resident. It includes a history of the present illness (e.g., why the person was in the hospital), past medical and surgical history, allergies, medications, physical examination, social issues, lab and imaging studies, and the overall assessment and recommendations or plan. Typically, the H&P is obtained from the transferring facility before the person actually arrives in the facility, which provides valuable information to the receiving provider and staff. Regulations stipulate that the H&P can be done within 30 days of the admission date, but many companies have a policy that the H&P must be done within a much shorter time frame, such as 24 to 72 hours from admission. The audit ensures that the H&P is on the chart and within the specified time frame.

Restraints. Many nursing facilities have committed to a restraint-free environment, while others permit their use. Restraints can be physical devices, such as **lap buddies** (cushion that snugs into the frame of the wheelchair to serve as a reminder to not get up without assistance; **wedges** (seat cushion to promote proper positioning) in a wheelchair and seatbelts in a wheelchair and side rails on a bed; even a bed pushed against a wall can be considered a restraint in certain circumstances. **Chemical restraints** are medications used with the intention of altering an undesirable behavior, such as aggression or sexual inhibition. There are extensive regulations that govern residents' rights and restraints, which will not be discussed in this chapter; instead, this chapter will focus on the clinical operation elements of restraints.

Staff must realize that a device for one resident may meet the definition of a physical restraint but for another resident it may not. A restraint requires consent, either by the resident or the responsible party, *prior to its use*. A device meets the criteria of a physical restraint if the resident is unable to remove the device so freedom of movement is restricted and the resident does not have normal access to his body.

An example of a physical restraint is bed side rails. For some residents, side rails actually facilitate independence with bed mobility and are beneficial. For other residents, the side rails prevent the resident from exiting the bed (a restraint) and may actually endanger the resident should he attempt to climb over or become stuck between the rails. Therefore, it is incumbent on leadership to provide ongoing coaching in this area as well as clinical oversight to ensure that restraints, when used, are done so properly with corresponding assessments, documentation, and care plans.

For purposes of the chart audit, identify either from the admitting orders, orders since admission, or interdisciplinary assessments and progress notes if the resident is using a device that may be considered a restraint. Determine if a prerestraint assessment was completed, whether a consent form was signed, and if the restraint is on the care plan. If the device in question is being used to facilitate independence with mobility or another function, there must be clear documentation of this assessment as well as documentation on the care plan. For the example with the side rails, if the rails are not a restraint, indicate their function on the care plan, such as "side rails are for mobility purposes." Do not be surprised if a surveyor asks this resident to demonstrate the use of the rails to enable independence with mobility.

Record of current immunization. There are extensive regulations governing pneumococcal and influenza immunizations and the responsibility of the facility to offer these vaccines as well as to provide education regarding the benefits and potential side effects. For purposes of the chart audit, determine if the resident was queried about his immunizations and offered the missing immunizations and the outcome is documented.

Evidence of being free of tuberculosis (TB). It is a federal requirement that a person admitted to the nursing facility be free of TB. There are two ways this can be determined: (1) by a chest x-ray or (2) with a purified protein derivative (PPD) skin test. Documentation from one of these tests must state that the resident is negative for (or free from) TB.

Nursing admission note. The nursing admission note sets the stage for the admission. This entry contains critical assessment information as well as paints a clear picture of the resident upon arrival at the facility. Typically the nursing admission note includes: date and time of admission; location admitted from and mode of transportation; who accompanied the resident; age, sex, race, and a general description; condition of skin, hygiene, breaks or bruises, or contractures; mobility status, prosthetic devices, skin dressings, bandages and sutures, in-dwelling tubes, ostomy, hearing aid, eye glasses, and any other devices; cognitive status and ability to communicate; known allergies; attending physician; resident's response or reaction to admission; and vital signs (Beicher, 2003a).

For admission audit purposes, read the nurse's admission note to determine if it contains the necessary information.

Height and weight. Upon admission, the resident's height and weight must be recorded. The facility should have a policy on how weights are obtained to best ensure accurate and consistent readings. Do not use the hospital weight, but reweigh the resident upon admission to your facility.

Medicare certification. In order for a person to qualify for skilled care under the Medicare benefit, the medical provider must certify that the service is necessary. The **Medicare certification** form is signed upon admission and at specific time intervals throughout the stay. It is illegal to predate or presign this document. For admission chart audit purposes, make sure the provider has signed the first section of the form for certification upon admission.

Preadmission Screening and Resident Review (PASRR). The purpose of the **PASRR** is to ensure that the nursing facility is an appropriate setting for individuals who have a serious mental illness (SMI) or mental retardation (MR) as a primary diagnosis. The PASRR should be completed before the person is transferred to the facility, such as by the discharge planner in the hospital—hence the first word, *preadmission.* While the general function of the PASRR is the same, some states have laws governing its completion. For the purpose of the chart audit, ensure that the document is present and completed accurately.

Rehabilitation

Most skilled nursing facilities offer rehabilitation services, such as physical, occupational, and speech therapy. Orders for these services may be present upon admission or they may be written at another point during the resident's stay, depending on the individual's condition and goals.

Evaluations

All payer sources require justification in order for therapy services to be covered. Before a patient receives therapy services, an evaluation must be completed to assess areas such as prior and current level of functioning, short and long-term goals, resident goals, muscle strength, range of motion, and balance. Some facilities require the medical provider to sign this evaluation, which acknowledges agreement with and need for therapy service.

In order for a person to receive physical, occupational, or speech therapy, the therapist must write a clarification order that specifies the reason for the therapy, the frequency (how many times per week), and the duration (how many weeks) of the therapy service.

Treatment Plans

When therapy is asked to screen a resident to determine rehabilitation potential, it is important from a clinical operations standpoint that the assessment information be shared with the team. Let's look at an example of recommendations written by a speech therapist. The resident was evaluated for difficulty swallowing and risk of aspiration (choking). The therapist determined that the resident would benefit from sitting at a supervised table in the dining room and from staff providing reminders to take small bites. The facility must have a process in place to ensure that recommendations like these are reflected in the care plan and that staff is made aware of the changes in care or treatment.

Supportive Devices

Supportive devices include items such as braces, slings, casts, and prosthetic limbs. Devices or interventions that help prevent contractures or skin damage due to contractures, such as a rolled washcloth placed in the palm of a hand, require care plan interventions. For audit purposes, make sure the order for these devices must also include instructions for time frames that the resident should wear the device—for example, "during waking hours." Anytime a resident has such a device, leadership must determine if staff require training on the proper way to **don** (put on) and **doff** (remove) the device according to manufacturer's recommendations.

Skin monitoring. Any time a supportive device is used on the resident's body, staff must pay close attention to the resident's skin condition beneath the device. Sometimes the friction between the device and the body can result in skin tears, rashes, or even pressure sores. A care plan is written for the actual device and to monitor the skin.

Documentation

Documentation in the medical record can be challenging and even intimidating at times, especially in circumstances when a resident, family member, or provider is upset, or when there is an incident or a crisis. Documentation must demonstrate the critical thinking by staff, accurately record the resident's condition and response to intervention, and be written in such a way that it is defensible. Many individuals outside the facility may read the medical record, including the **ombudsman** (resident advocate), an insurance case manager, providers, surveyors, and sometimes attorneys.

Staff must be taught how to document in the medical record, and leadership must remain diligent in conducting regular audits of the documentation to identify opportunities for coaching and improvement. This section will provide a brief overview of some of the complexities of documentation as well as guidance to help make it easier.

Interdisciplinary Focus

What does interdisciplinary mean? Staff in the nursing facility have different areas of expertise, in social work, activities, dietary, therapy, nursing, mental health, and more. Each person has training and experience unique to his role. Sometimes there is overlap, such as with a nurse who assesses aspects of psychosocial functioning or the social worker who contributes to a pain care plan.

Rather than each person functioning in his own "silo," he is expected to communicate and contribute to a comprehensive assessment and care plan. Each person's contribution is important, and together these contributions create an interdisciplinary approach to care. Documentation in the medical record should reflect an interdisciplinary focus, meet standard guidelines that demonstrate the care provided, and create a defensible record.

Dos and Don'ts

Critical thinking skills and good clinical judgment must be reflected in each person's documentation. Another way to think of this is to avoid red flags—that is, documentation that describes a problem (or even a potential problem) but lacks an assessment, intervention, and outcome.

If it is documented that the resident's glasses are broken, there should be information that includes what is being done about the problem, by whom and when. If the resident depends on the glasses to read the newspaper each morning, what is staff doing in the meantime while the glasses are repaired to facilitate the resident's activity?

An area of documentation that is easily overlooked is the use of forms. Forms are valuable and necessary, but when used inappropriately or unnecessarily, they can lead to a host of problems. For example, when information is documented in multiple places in the medical record, one area or another is likely to be missed (Beicher, 2003a). Missing information or blank sections on a form make it easy for surveyors or attorneys to argue that the care was not provided. Every form and every assessment should have a clear and functional purpose.

Another area that is problematic with documentation is the use of certain phrases or words. Some words undermine the credibility of the writer, such as apparently, accident, mistake, confusing, abuse, grievance, and assumed. These words should not be used in the medical record.

There is an interesting caveat with the word "incident." When a resident has an incident or accident, staff completes an incident report. Since incident reports are typically part of the facility quality assurance process, these reports do not have to be made available for review by the surveyors. "Records of the committee meetings identifying quality deficiencies, by statute, may not be reviewed by surveyors unless the facility chooses to provide them" (CMS, 2014, F520). However, if staff documents "incident report completed" or otherwise references an incident report, that document is now **discoverable**—that is, it would have to be provided to the surveyor if requested. The same is true if staff documents "grievance report." Sometimes during a survey, it might be in the facility's best interest to share selected incident and grievance reports, but this decision is made by the administrator, not inadvertently by unknowing staff. Do not document "incident report" or "grievance report" in the medical record.

A phrase seen quite frequently in documentation is "will continue to monitor" or any related variation, such as "close supervision continues." These phrases are red flags since it is unclear what is being monitored, how frequently, and for what purpose. Rather than writing "will continue to monitor," be more precise with a statement such as "nursing will monitor the edema and the effect of the diuretic." "Implied monitoring should be followed up with intervention, and the interventions should be documented until the event can be brought to closure" (Beicher, 2003a).

Subjective Versus Objective

Documentation must be primarily objective—that is, what can be seen, heard, smelled, counted, touched, or otherwise collected using the senses. **Objective documentation** does not include staff opinion about an event or resident. Opinion or information not based in fact is called subjective. "The resident appeared sad today" is subjective as it is based on the writer's opinion. To make this entry objective, the writer could state, "The resident did not engage easily in conversation today and cried after her daughter left at 11 A.M." Another clue that an entry is subjective is use of the term "appears."

Anger (and other feelings including positive ones) is subjective and can be defined differently by different people. One person may define anger as a loud voice, whereas another person may define it by a penetrating glare. Rather than use a subjective term like anger, simply describe the mood. What does the staff member see or hear? What is the resident doing—striking out, yelling, spitting, or not interacting with staff?

Subjective documentation has a place in the medical record when the writer records what the resident or family member actually states. Consider these examples: "Resident stated she is so angry," or resident said, "I would rather go on the outing than to dialysis." Both statements offer valuable information about the resident's state of mind and originate directly from the resident.

When a resident uses profanity or says something offensive, staff may be hesitant to document it. While it may be uncomfortable to record profanity, it is appropriate to capture this in the medical record. If it is easier, use symbols to convey profane terms, like "s**t." The use of profanity conveys the resident's state of mind at the time, and it is okay to write it in the medical record.

Late Entry

Sometimes, despite staff's best intentions, timely documentation may not be possible. In these instances, a **late entry** must be indicated when documenting in the medical record. The current date and time of the entry are recorded, but right at the beginning of the note, the writer indicates the date that the entry references:

> 4/7/15 1100 Late Entry for 4/6/15 (Begin narrative entry)

Ideally, staff documents in a timely manner. The more time that passes between an event and the recording of the event, the easier it is to challenge the credibility of the writer and the documentation. The role of the administrator is to help ensure that staff have sufficient time to document during a shift. Not only does timely and accurate documentation demonstrate competent resident care, but also it can protect the facility in the event of a lawsuit or inquiry during a survey.

Summarizing Event Entry

When a situation is unfolding very quickly (resuscitation efforts for a resident found not breathing, a resident-to-resident altercation, or a resident with out-of-control behavior), it is not possible to document each interaction or phone call in the moment. But it is important that these events are captured in the correct time order to demonstrate appropriate staff intervention and the resident's response. The documentation technique used in these situations is called a **summarizing event entry** (Peterson, 2004). Staff jot down notes on a piece of paper and pay close attention to the times, what is being said, who is being notified, their response, and other important information, which will then be used later to compose a summary of the event. Here is an example of this technique by a social worker.

> 04/1/14 1135 Summary Entry-------------
>
> 0830 Notified by charge nurse that patient's son was on the unit, yelling at his mom and demanding she give him her wallet.
>
> 0835 Arrived on unit to talk with son. His appearance was disheveled and the smell of alcohol was on his person. Several attempts were made to talk with son, but he continued yelling and interrupting this writer. His speech was rapid, and he was pacing the room.
>
> 0840 Call placed to administrator from patient's room. Charge nurse also present, and both she and this writer were positioned between the son and patient as he was increasingly agitated, pointing his finger at his mom, cursing and threatening to not take her home.
>
> 0843 Administrator and maintenance director arrived and persuaded son to leave facility.
>
> 0845 Met with patient. She cried and shared that her son has addiction problems. He has stolen things from her on many occasions, and she has had to call the police from home.

Take note of the clear writing that paints a picture of the events in specific and, very importantly, time-sequenced order.

Complaints

Documenting complaints, and staff response, is necessary not only to demonstrate provision of quality care and service but also to identify opportunities for improvement. Documenting complaints can be tricky, but with a little guidance staff can do this successfully. First, keep in mind that a complaint is a form of feedback, which in essence is a perception. Think of it this way: feedback (a complaint in this example) is a perception being shared, not a truth being declared. "The food here is terrible!" or "That physician doesn't know what he's doing!" These statements represent a person's opinion or perception; however, do not make the mistake of assuming the complaint is not valid. Staff at all levels should receive training on how to handle complaints effectively and to defuse escalating situations.

After the complaint has been investigated, it must be documented. Document the person's perception of the situation, and then document the reality (Beicher, 2003b). Objectivity is key. Sometimes the perception is the reality, and sometimes the perception is very different from the reality. Let's look at an example.

The charge nurse observed a resident yelling at the medication nurse, "You're an idiot! I haven't gotten my pain medicine all day!" That is the complaint or the perception. Upon investigation, the nurse determined that the resident received pain medication at 0800 and 1600. Additionally, a **rescue dose** (medication administered between routinely scheduled doses) was administered at 1330. While the perception and reality are quite different, it would be a mistake to stop the investigation here. There is an opportunity to talk with the resident to see if the pain medication is not working adequately. Perhaps the dose needs to be changed or maybe social services and activities need to help identify additional **non-drug interventions** to help the resident. Maybe something else has happened in the resident's life that is the source of her anger and it has nothing to do with pain medication. But, again, the assessment is how staff uncover the underlying issues that need to be addressed.

Contributory Negligence

The term **contributory negligence** describes the situation when a person makes a choice that may cause or worsen a potentially negative outcome. For example, a resident who has diabetes chooses to eat snacks from the vending machine or a resident with a sacral pressure ulcer prefers to stay up in the wheelchair for long stretches at a time. Residents have the right to make choices regarding their care, and this fact is not in dispute. But when these choices cause or contribute to a negative outcome, or have the potential to do so, the facility has responsibility to ensure that the resident and sometimes the responsible party clearly understand the impact of the choices, to offer alternatives, and to document all discussions.

Resident, Patient, and Family Education

Education constitutes a large part of effective clinical operations. Residents, family, and staff need education in different areas. Whether it is to notify and get permission to administer a new medication or start a different treatment, staff are constantly providing information and education. From a clinical operations perspective, capturing all attempts at education in the medical record is of utmost importance.

Documentation

Often, education is documented with a simple entry, such as, "Informed daughter, Sue, of the side effects of the antidepressant and answered her questions. No concerns expressed. She is in agreement with trying the medication for her mom and signed the consent."

At other times, the education provided to the resident or family is more extensive or repetitive, and in these instances, it is helpful to consolidate the interactions into one location in the record. There are various forms that accomplish this, but the components of any form must include the date of the interaction, who it was with, the type of information provided (dietary, medication, equipment, discharge planning, etc.), what information was shared, how it was shared (written, verbal, video, etc.), the response, and the signature of the person providing the education.

Staff from different disciplines take responsibility for providing education, sometimes on the same topic. For example, a resident has diabetes with uncontrolled blood sugars and chooses to eat snacks from the vending machine or the sweet treats provided in activities (even if sugar-free options are available). The nurse counsels the resident on the health impact of his choices and how they may affect him. The activities director educates the resident that sugar-free treats are available. The social worker discusses the complications of uncontrolled blood sugars in terms of his goal to discharge home with his wife. Each discipline provides important education, and consolidating it on one form makes it is easy to locate, especially during a survey or a care conference.

Care Conference

Sometimes it is necessary to schedule an interim care conference so the whole team, including the resident and family, can discuss the issues, risks, and benefits and everyone hears the same information simultaneously. A care conference allows staff to present information and seek understanding from the resident or family regarding their choices.

Leave of Absence (LOA)

Residents in nursing facilities enjoy going on outings, just like an individual living in his own home. Attending an outing with a group of residents and staff from the facility can be a wonderful way for residents to stay connected and participate in events outside the nursing facility.

Sometimes a resident wants to go on a LOA by himself or with a family member or friend, perhaps for a few hours or even overnight. Facilitating an LOA takes planning and preparation on behalf of staff and sometimes the resident and family. It must be done correctly to ensure the greatest chance success of the LOA as well as resident safety. Depending on whether the resident is able to go on an LOA independently or requires assistance, there are certain tasks that must be accomplished and documented in the medical record.

Community Survival Skills Assessment

If the resident plans on an independent LOA, perhaps to a neighborhood store or restaurant, it is recommended that staff complete a **community survival skills assessment**. There are many areas that must be assessed in order to identify potential risks with the outing and to help make it safe for the resident. A member of the therapy team may assess the resident's ability to maneuver the electric wheelchair around obstacles and to safely cross a street, and what to do if the wheelchair wheel gets stuck. The nurse may assess his ability to transfer from the wheelchair to a toilet and provide education on what symptoms signify dehydration. The social worker may assess the resident's problem-solving ability in the event the wheelchair battery dies, whether he can manage a monetary transaction, or what to do if he needs help when away from the facility.

If a family member is taking the resident on an LOA, perhaps there is medication that must be administered during this time, so the nurse teaches the family how to do this. There may need to be instruction on how to safely transfer the resident from the wheelchair to the car or what to do if the resident becomes agitated on the LOA.

What about the resident who enjoys taking a stroll on the facility campus? Again, critical thinking skills must be evident and staff must plan for contingencies. Does the resident wear sunscreen or proper clothing to be protected from the elements? Does she need to carry a water bottle? Does she walk in the parking lot or does she stay on the sidewalk? How long does she stay out at a time? Does she sign out each time? Do staff check on her if she is gone too long? How long is too long? While this line of questioning may seem exhausting, this is the level of critical thinking necessary in order to provide care and services to vulnerable adults.

Provider Order

In order for a resident to go on an LOA, the medical provider must give an order that acknowledges an LOA is permissible. The provider may also indicate that staff must provide caregiver or resident training in the order. For people unfamiliar with the long-term care setting, it may seem paternalistic that the medical provider must give an order, somewhat akin to permission, to allow the resident to leave the building. The reality is that most everything, from over-the-counter medications to an LOA, requires an order.

Role of Payer Source

An LOA can be for a few hours or overnight. Before going on an LOA, be sure to check the policy of the payer source. Most Medicaid plans allow a certain number of overnight LOAs, but beyond that the payer source may not cover additional bed holds during an absence. Medicare is much more lenient today than years ago with allowing patients to go on short-term day passes or LOAs as long as the patient is back in the facility by midnight. An LOA during a patient's rehabilitative stay can help identify areas of success as well as barriers that the patient or caregiver still needs to work on, such as car transfers or medication management.

Tending to a resident's psychosocial well-being by facilitating an outside visit to a family gathering or an event or to go shopping is applauded, and staff should make reasonable efforts to arrange an LOA.

Summary

Clinical operations in the nursing facility are complex, but with strong leadership they can be managed successfully. As a leader, the administrator incorporates policies, procedures, and regulations into daily operations and coaches all staff to employ critical thinking skills. The administrator helps ensure that care plans and documentation not only meet the needs of the residents but also demonstrate good clinical judgment.

Key Terms

Advance directives: Documents that convey a person's healthcare wishes.

Alert charting: Documentation of a change of condition for a specified time period.

Approaches or interventions: Tasks that staff will do to help the resident achieve a care plan goal.

Change of condition: Any symptom, sign, or apparent discomfort that is sudden in onset, is a marked change, and is unrelieved by measures already prescribed.

Chemical restraints: Medications used to modify a patient's undesirable behavior.

Clinical judgment: Result of critical thinking that yields a decision.

Clinical operations: Tasks to ensure resident care meets regulatory standards, facility policies and procedures, and standards of practice and ensure the highest practicable functioning of each resident.

Code status: Outcome of decision of whether resident wants resuscitation measures in the event of cardiac or respiratory arrest.

Community Survival Skills Assessment: Assessment tool to identify potential risks for the resident who wants to go on an outing.

Contributory negligence: Situation when a person makes a choice that may impact a poor outcome.

Critical thinking: The process of reasoning based on experience.

Deep vein thrombosis: Blood clot in a vein.

Discoverable: Document that would not usually be available for review by a surveyor but if mentioned in the medical record would have to be provided.

Doff: Remove something from the body.

Don: Put something on the body.

Edema: Swelling caused by fluid retention.

Facility survival skills assessment: Tool to determine if a resident has the necessary skills to safely manage a leave of absence independently.

Geriatric Depression Scale: Depression screening tool.

Healthcare power of attorney: Document that allows a person to designate a spokesperson to make healthcare decisions.

Incident report: Record of an unusual event, such as a fall.

Initial care plan: Document started upon admission to address immediate care needs.

Lap buddy: Cushion that snugs into the frame of the wheelchair to serve as a reminder to not get up without assistance.

Late entry: Technique for documenting information in the medical record a period of time after the event occurrence.

Leave of absence: When a resident leaves the facility for a period of a time.

Living will: Document that provides guidelines for resident wishes regarding life-sustaining treatment.

Medicare certification: Verification by the medical provider that skilled services are necessary.

Medication administration record: Legal record of drugs administered.

Mood disorder: A psychological disorder characterized by the elevation or lowering of a person's mood.

Non-drug interventions: Interventions that should be tried before administering psychotropic medication.

Noting orders: Process of following through with the admission orders.

Objective documentation: Information based on what is seen, heard, smelled, counted, touched, or otherwise collected using the senses.

Ombudsman: Resident advocate.

Patient health questionnaire: Depression screening tool.

Preadmission Screening and Resident Review (PASRR): Process to ensure that the nursing facility is an appropriate setting for an individual with a serious mental illness or mental retardation.

Psychotropic medications: Medications that alter a person's mood or behavior.

Recapitulation: Orders printed at the start of the month and signed by the provider.

Rescue dose: Medication administered between routinely scheduled doses.

Strengths-based assessment: Process to identify a resident's strengths to cope with a problem.

Subjective documentation: Based on an opinion or can also be a statement by a resident or family member.

Summarizing event entry: Technique for documenting a series of events in the medical record.

Target behaviors: Behaviors identified for change.

Target date: The date when a care plan will be reviewed.

Temporary care plan: Process to address a problem that is of a short duration, such as an infection.

Treatment administration record: Record that lists procedural orders, separate from the MAR.

Verifying orders: Process of reviewing orders with the medical provider.

Wander guard: Safety device for an individual at risk of elopement.

Wedge: Seat cushion to promote proper positioning.

Review Questions

1. Why are critical thinking skills so important?
   a. Demonstrate mental discipline to evaluate a situation objectively.
   b. Combine analysis of available information with a person's experience.
   c. Both a and b.
   d. None of the above.

2. When can a policy become problematic?
   a. When it creates more work for staff.
   b. When it does not reflect actual practice.
   c. When it is not individualized to the facility.
   d. All of the above.

3. Which is an appropriate care plan goal?
   a. Resident will demonstrate the ability to speak calmly to staff daily.
   b. Yelling out episodes will decrease to two times a day.
   c. Encourage resident to speak calmly to staff daily.
   d. None of the above.

4. What is not an important reason for auditing a medical record?
   a. To identify missing components.
   b. To determine if assessments correlate to the care plan.
   c. To identify staff who did not follow a facility policy.
   d. To identify performance improvement projects.

5. Which one is the reason that justifies documentation in the medical record?
   a. To demonstrate critical thinking skills and good clinical judgment.
   b. To establish timely response to resident needs.
   c. To communicate with staff about resident care.
   d. All of the above.

Case Study

As a newly hired administrator to a 90-bed facility, you have reviewed several resident records and identified that the care plans do not reflect the care being provided to some residents and that the goals for mood and behavior issues are inappropriate. You also identified that the documentation across all disciplines is sparse and there are specific instances where staff has written information that is not defensible. What are some ideas of how to correct these problems? How can you as the administrator be involved in the solutions?

References

Alfaro-LeFevre, R. (2009). *Critical thinking and clinical judgment: A practical approach to outcome-focused thinking. St.* Louis, MO: Saunders Elsevier.

American Medical Directors Association. (2003). *Clinical practice guideline: Acute change of condition.* Retrieved from http://www.amda.com/tools/guidelines.cfm#acoc

American Medical Directors Association. (2013). *The younger adult in the long-term care setting.* Columbia, MD: AMDA.

Beicher, T. (2003a). *Defensive documentation for long-term care: Strategies for creating a more lawsuit-proof resident record.* Marblehead, MA: hcPro.

Beicher, T. (2003b). *A facility-based risk management program: A practical guide for LTC providers.* Washington, DC: American Health Care Association.

Centers for Medicare and Medicaid Services. (2012). *SNF program transmittals.* Retrieved from http://www.cms.gov/Medicare/Medicare-Fee-for-Service-Payment/SNFPPS/SNF-Program-Transmittals.html

Centers for Medicare and Medicaid Services (CMS). (2014). *State operation manual: Appendix PP—guidance to surveyors for long-term care facilities.* Retrieved from http://www.cms.gov/Regulations-and-Guidance/Guidance/Manuals/downloads/som107ap_pp_guidelines_ltcf.pdf

Davis, E. J., Greenwald, S. C., & Pareti, T. (2011). *The new care plan answer book for activity, psychosocial and social work programs MDS 3.0 Edition: A partner in definitive OBRA care plan compliance.* Glenview, IL: Social Work Consultation Group.

Greenwald, S. C. (2002). *Social work policies, procedures and guidelines for long-term care.* Glenview, IL: Social Work Consultation Group.

Peterson, E. (2004). *Long-term care pocket guide to nursing documentation.* Marblehead, MA: hcPro.

Revolutionary OBRA & JCAHO Formatted Care Plans. (2015). Glenview, IL: Social-Work Consultation Group. Available at http://swcginc.com/store/manuals-c-1/revolutionary-obra-and-jcaho-formatted-care-plans-p-6

Acknowledgment

With deepest gratitude to my husband and best friend, Dr. Mel Hector, for his insights and edits as well as his patience for the hours I spent on this project. To my dear friend and colleague, Barbara Viggiano, RN, for her honest critique and suggestions. And, to both of you for all the laughs along the way!

CHAPTER 13

FACILITY-CENTERED CLINICAL OPERATIONS

Paige Hector

Managing clinical operations requires a broad base of knowledge across many disciplines and the expertise to synthesize that knowledge into good resident care and a defensible medical record. Dividing tasks into daily, weekly, and monthly responsibilities helps organize the huge volume of information. This chapter demonstrates some of the key components of clinical operations, using examples of medical record audits. The second part of the chapter teaches how to use the **stand-up meeting** as an integral part of managing the complexities of clinical operations.

Weekly Operations

The enormity of clinical operations management necessitates tasks be divided into manageable components. Some tasks require daily attention, as will be discussed extensively in the stand-up section of this chapter, while others only require weekly discussion. Each week, clinical leadership should discuss residents who are "at risk"—that is, residents who already display a risk factor or who are at risk of developing one, such as poor nutrition, skin or pressure issues, behaviors, and falls. Consider including staff from social work, activities, and dietary in these meetings.

Wound Rounds

As a person loses functionality, the risk of pressure ulcers increases, especially in prominent areas of the body that bear weight, such as the coccyx, heels, and spine. For some

LEARNING OBJECTIVES

- Describe the tasks completed in weekly and monthly clinical operations.

- Explain the process to audit a medical record and why it is valuable in managing risk.

- Understand the process to utilize the stand-up meeting as an integral part of clinical operations.

- Discuss the Critical Elements of Care and how to operationalize the first three in the stand-up meeting.

- Explain the importance of the 24-hour report and how to use it successfully in the stand-up meeting.

people, even pressure from oxygen tubing resting atop the ear can result in a pressure ulcer. Staff require training and ongoing supervision to manage skin issues and to ensure that pressure ulcers that are preventable are indeed prevented. When skin breakdown is expected, such as with someone whose disease process is progressing, the medical provider and staff must be diligent to document this expected decline and ensure the care plan also reflects this anticipated outcome.

Many facilities engage in weekly wound rounds led by the medical director or another qualified physician to examine every resident who has a wound. The purpose is to determine if changes to the treatment plan are necessary and to evaluate the overall plan for the resident, including pain management.

Nutrition at Risk

Another area that must be closely monitored is nutrition. For various reasons, such as disease progression and depression, a resident's appetite may diminish and eventually result in significant weight loss or other nutritional imbalances that affect other aspects of care, like wound healing. Food carries a high symbolic attachment in many cultures, and when a person loses weight, it can cause alarm in family members and warrant attention from surveyors if not communicated and documented properly.

Many facilities hold weekly meetings to discuss residents who are losing weight, calculated as a percentage of weight loss over a period of time, and residents whose appetite is poor. Since nutrition and wound healing are closely associated, often residents who are followed by the wound team are also discussed in the nutrition-at-risk meeting.

Falls

Falls are an area closely scrutinized by oversight agencies as well as the general public. While all residents have some risk of falls, for various reasons, including certain medical diagnoses and cognitive and functional impairments, some residents are at higher risk of falling. Each resident's fall risk must be assessed upon admission and then regularly throughout the stay. Just as wounds are followed on a weekly basis, falls should be as well.

When a resident falls, an incident report is completed that describes the fall, including where it occurred, if equipment was involved, and a number of other factors, such as use of the call light, lighting, floor hazards, and if there were any interventions in place at the time. Also included in the assessment is the resident's cognitive and functional status, any recent changes, such as with medications, diagnoses, and vital signs. For each fall, the care plan must be reviewed to determine if there are new interventions to try.

Restorative Nursing

Restorative nursing includes services to help residents achieve or maintain their highest practicable level of functioning. Services can involve activities of daily living, such as ambulation, transfers, and bathing, or range of motion and eating. Restorative nursing is different from the daily care provided by the nursing assistants, and while it is supervised by the director of nurses, the physical or occupational therapist is also involved. Residents receiving restorative nursing services must demonstrate the ability to regain or relearn a task—hence the term "restorative."

In many facilities, the restorative nursing aides, the nursing supervisor, and sometimes a therapist meet weekly to discuss the treatment plan for each resident on caseload, as well as identify other residents who would benefit from the service.

Monthly Operations

The regulation for Quality Assessment and Assurance (Centers for Medicare and Medicaid Services [CMS], 2014, F520) stipulates that the facility maintain a committee and that it meet at least quarterly. Yet, many facilities choose to meet on a monthly basis. Data in key areas are gathered and analyzed, such as infections, falls, wounds, weight loss, admissions and discharges, grievances, and incident reports. Performance improvement and data analysis are discussed in Chapter 14.

Another monthly task is a comprehensive assessment for each resident (completed by the nurse), which includes information such as a review of systems, ADLs, mood, and behavior as well as a narrative summary. Typically, every month residents are weighed and vital signs are taken. This information is used by interdisciplinary team members, including the medical providers.

The director of nurses or a designee should maintain an accurate list of residents who have a device in place either as a restraint or that might become a restraint. Such devices include bed side rails, wedge cushions, Geri chairs, a bed placed against the wall, and seat belts. From an operations perspective it is advisable to monitor residents who have other interventions in place, such as floor mats, specialized call buttons (e.g., the pad variety instead of the push button), specialized footwear, heel protectors, and braces. At least once a month, do visual checks of the residents and their rooms to ensure that each resident has what is ordered, the items are in good working condition, the care plan is correct, and the list is accurate.

Medical Record Audit

A very effective strategy to mitigate risk factors and improve clinical operations is to audit the medical record. This process is similar to the admission audit but is much more in-depth. Auditing a record is not completely intuitive, and it takes practice and coaching to uncover the inconsistencies that can lead to a poor resident outcome, inadequate documentation, or deficient practice.

Auditing an entire medical record is time-intensive but will yield valuable information to guide clinical operations as well as identify performance improvement opportunities. Sometimes a modified audit is needed to address a single area, like monthly nursing summaries, or a specific section, such as advance directives or the behavior management program.

A significant part of the audit will center on the care plan. Determine if assessments, progress notes, and providers' orders are consistent with the care plan. Here is an example of when these elements are not consistent: A constipation care plan states the resident is on a routine narcotic medication (for which a common side effect is constipation), yet the orders reflect only a PRN narcotic medication. The discrepant information indicates a process breakdown with communication that must be corrected.

In a different example, the nutrition care plan says that the resident's intake and output (I&O) will be monitored. Yet, the I&O flow sheet is blank. For this same resident, the cardiac care plan includes interventions for a diet restriction, fluid limit, oxygen, and to elevate legs, yet none of these interventions are reflected in the monthly orders. Upon viewing the resident in her room, there is no oxygen concentrator in the room, she has a pitcher of water at bedside, and there are no wedge cushions or extra pillows in her bed to elevate her legs. These inconsistencies can lead to resident harm and deficient practice citations.

In this audit example, the hospital H&P indicates the resident was interested in smoking cessation, yet there is no documentation that such education or resources were offered. Staff at the nursing facility documented they saw the resident smoking between the cars in the parking lot. The social work note states that the resident was smoking with his oxygen on, yet the smoking evaluation indicates he is a safe smoker. The risks associated with this situation affect the safety of the resident and the nursing facility.

When auditing a record, be sure to read progress notes from the medical provider as well as consulting providers. The provider wrote that the resident wanders and "has gone outside in the midsummer heat." For this same resident, the situation becomes more complicated with the elopement assessment on which staff indicates that the resident is not an elopement risk (yet the provider wrote the resident wanders and went outside in the heat).

The provider also wrote in the progress notes that the antipsychotic medication, BuSpar, was started to control the wandering (which is not an appropriate reason to prescribe that medication). The orders, however, indicate the rationale for the medication is anxiety with depression. A third discrepancy occurs on the medication consent, which states the medication is for inability to relax, repetitive questions, and pacing.

There are numerous problems with this medical record. It seems that communication between the medical provider and staff is lacking as well as consensus regarding the level of elopement risk.

In another example a nurse on the evening shift wrote "Resident refused eye drops tonight. He says they make his eyes 'hurt' in the morning. Charge nurse aware." Yet, there is no documentation that the pain was assessed, the provider notified, or the care plan updated. Subsequent entries in the medical record state that the resident declined eye drops for the next two days, but there was no assessment or notification to the provider.

In this next example, the activity director documents, "The resident is very involved with **resident council** (group of residents who meet regularly to discuss concerns and develop suggestions). He has very high expectations for his care. He has had issues with staff on difference of opinions on what has and has not occurred." Missing from this entry is how staff is addressing the concerns. The phrase "high expectations" is subjective (an opinion), and more information is needed regarding what the resident expects. Furthermore, the care plan does not address the resident's expectations or how the differences are being resolved.

Reading all staff progress notes is important to identify documentation that is incomplete or unclear or documentation that might indicate resident care concerns or be problematic from a survey perspective. For example, a resident was admitted for an incomplete healing of the distal humerus (elbow) and was non-weight-bearing (NWB) on the right side. Unfortunately, one nurse repeatedly documented that the resident was weight-bearing as tolerated (WBAT).

Be sure to audit discharged charts as well. The health information manager or medical records department manager should have an extensive checklist of items to audit upon discharge. When the administrator or designee reviews a discharged chart, one of the most important documents to review is the **discharge summary**. The discharge summary is a review of the resident's stay in the facility, which should be written for the resident and responsible party in "a language and manner they understand" (CMS, 2014, F203). There should be no medical jargon or abbreviations. Let's look at some examples from actual discharge summaries.

In this example, there are two red flags with the discharge summary: (1) numerous blanks on the form, and (2) staff do not provide clear instructions for the caregivers at home. Rather than leave a section on any document or assessment form blank, indicate the area is not applicable or "n/a" so the resident and caregiver do not have to guess the meaning of missing information.

The discharge summary should reflect any care and services that will be provided or that will continue in the home setting. A resident who had regular labs drawn each month in the facility is discharged home, but the summary does not address the labs. Should the labs continue? If so, that should be explained on the summary, including where the resident should get the labs drawn. If the labs are no longer necessary, that should also be indicated so the resident and caregiver have no questions about what they need to do post-discharge.

If the resident must follow up with specialists after discharge, that information should be clear and include the name of the physician, the phone number, and time frame in which the appointment should be made. If home health will be provided, the name of the agency, phone number, and start date should be written on the summary. For the resident who requires medical equipment, indicate which company will provide the equipment, when, and where will it be delivered.

Staff must be diligent about writing all information on the summary in layperson terms, not medical jargon or legalese. The list of discharge medications must be easy to understand and to follow. In the facility a nurse would write, "i tab BID," but on a discharge summary it should be written as, "one tablet twice a day."

Pharmacy

The regulations that govern pharmacy services are extensive and are summarized in this statement in Pharmacy Services (CMS, 2014, F425): "The overall goal of the pharmaceutical services system within a facility is to ensure the safe and effective use of medications." The processes associated with the safe administration of medication depend upon staff members who are properly trained and knowledgeable about the medications, contraindications, and side effects.

Each month the pharmacist (either through direct employment or a contractual arrangement) must review each resident's medications in what is known as a **medication regime review** (MRR). The pharmacist reviews the medications to determine if some can be discontinued, whether the doses need to be titrated (increased or decreased), side effects, drug-drug interactions, drug food interactions, expiration dates, contraindications, and overall efficacy of the regime. The pharmacist then writes recommendations for the medical provider to review. If the provider is in agreement with the recommendation, an order is written per the suggestion. If the provider is not in agreement, this needs to be reflected on the recommendation from the pharmacist and explained in some detail in the provider's progress note.

Medication Error Rate

Every facility strives to have a 0% medication errors rate, but the reality is that errors will occur. The medication error rate is defined as the percentage of errors calculated by dividing the number of errors by the number of medication opportunities and multiplied by 100. The administrator should monitor the facility error rate to make the facility a safe environment, to identify opportunities for coaching and improvement and because medication administration is a significant part of the survey process. The facility must have a viable reporting process to capture all errors. Medication errors range from outcomes in which the resident suffers no harm all the way to significant harm, even including death. Managing medication errors is beyond the scope of this book but when an error occurs, it is important that the administrator and director of nurses approach the situation, the resident, and the nurse with compassion. One must understand that the nurse already feels bad about the error and may worry about possible repercussions. Errors are inevitable. How they are managed to prevent further recurrences is instructive and critical.

Recapitulation (Recap)

At the beginning of each month, a new set of orders is printed for each resident, which are called recaps. Any changes made over the previous month, such as new medications, dose changes, and new treatments, should be reflected on the current set of orders or recaps. The nurse checks the previous month's orders to ensure the current month's information is accurate.

When the medical provider reviews the recaps, she looks for unnecessary or redundant medications that can be discontinued and signs each page, indicating the information is accurate and acceptable.

Nursing Assistant Flow Sheets

Nursing assistants document the care they provide and the resident's activities of daily living on flow sheets. Information such as bathing, bowel movements, mobility, behaviors, and percentage of meals consumed is recorded in these records. Often, nursing aides document information that provides insightful information regarding a resident's mood, behavior, and general daily life issues. A nursing supervisor should review the flow sheets monthly. Information may be documented that requires intervention from the clinical team, but unless there is a consistent plan to review these records, these opportunities will be missed.

For example, the nursing assistant documented how a resident with moderate dementia continues to pack her belongings as she is convinced that she is going home. The resident wanders into other people's rooms and takes their items. Upon investigation, it is discovered that the elopement risk assessment indicates this resident is *not at risk*. And the care plan does not indicate any of the behaviors—the packing of bags, the potential elopement risk, the wandering into other residents' rooms and taking their belongings. The administrator and director of nurses need to evaluate the communication process and institute a new process, such as a more robust 24-hour report and stand-up meeting that will bring these issues to light, ensure they are handled in a timely manner, ensure the resident's well-being and safety, and protect the facility from liability.

Quarterly Operations

It is a standard of practice that each quarter, interdisciplinary staff complete updated assessments to identify changes in the resident's status. Most of these assessments are similar to those done upon admission.

Individual Discipline Summaries

The nursing assessments done quarterly include fall risk, skin integrity, bowel and bladder issues, elopement risk, pain management, smoking safety, restraints, and any other assessments mandated by the facility P&P. Typically, the assessments are divided and assigned to individual nurses or shifts who know the resident best. Each set of assessments should be compared to previous assessments to identify changes and establish a time perspective.

For example, a resident who was not a fall risk in the previous quarter has slowly declined over the past 3 months and with the current assessment scored in the high fall risk range. With this assessment information, staff need to determine if any of these fall risk factors can be mitigated or even reversed. Would the resident benefit from physical therapy or restorative nursing? How is her pain? Are there changes in her room or environment in general that would make it safer for her? Answering these questions demonstrates critical thinking skills that result in good clinical judgment.

The dietary manager summarizes the past quarter for food preferences, dietary compliance, and weight gain or loss. The care plan is then examined and updated as needed.

The activities manager reviews the past quarter to determine what events the resident participated in, and if there are new interests or a need to adapt or modify activities to facilitate participation. Again, the care plan is examined and updated as needed.

The social worker completes a quarterly assessment, with focus on areas such as mood, behavior, adjustment to life in the facility, family, and relationships (Greenwald, 1999), and updates the care plan.

For purposes of clinical operations, a quarterly audit should be completed to ensure that assessments are in place and inform the plan of care. Teach staff to view the assessments as one part of the bigger picture for each resident. Make sure the assessments directly correlate with the care plan. Consider what each staff member can contribute to the plan of care to ensure the resident's highest practicable well-being.

Changes of Condition

A **change of condition** is any symptom, sign, or apparent discomfort that is (a) sudden in onset, (b) a marked change that is more severe in relation to usual symptoms and signs, and (c) unrelieved by measures already prescribed (American Medical Director's Association, 2003). Prompt notification to the medical provider of a change of condition is expected.

Changes of condition are exhibited in a variety of ways by clinical and behavioral manifestations, such as shortness of breath, confusion, delusions, pain, lethargy, and anxiety. Nurses are trained to identify and respond to changes of condition. So, too, must staff members from other disciplines, like social work, dietary, and activities.

Consider this activity note that states, "Resident displays a change in cognitive impairment, gets very anxious and upset at times, cannot stay on task, and her attention span is very short, she gets lost and can't remember what she is doing." This valuable information should be shared with the interdisciplinary team to ensure that a comprehensive assessment is done and the medical provider and family are notified of the change.

Keep in mind that a change of condition can also be an improvement, which may necessitate notification to the resident, responsible party, and physician as well as updating the care plan. An example of an improvement is when a resident who was relying on artificial food supplementation is eating sufficiently to discontinue the tube feedings or the resident who was unable to get out of bed without assistance can do so independently now.

Notifications

When a resident's condition changes, such as a life-threatening event or clinical complication, staff are required to notify the resident, the responsible party when appropriate, and the physician (CMS, 2014, F157). Notification can be done in person or via the phone.

If a phone call is placed to the provider or responsible party and they are not available, a message on voice mail or with an answering service does not meet the definition of notification (Beicher, 2003). Staff must speak with the person to constitute notification. Be sure to document all attempts, times, and method of communication. This time line helps build a defensible medical record and demonstrate staff response to changes. When the individual is reached, document the content of the conversation, including the response and next steps, if any.

Alert Charting

Alert charting is the process of tracking changes of condition for a period of time and documenting the resident's status. Each facility should have a P&P for alert charting. Typically, it stipulates that for a change of condition the nurse will document information related to the change, such as vital signs, reaction to a medication, reaction to a behavioral intervention, labs/diagnostics, and signs and symptoms of the condition. The P&P should also provide guidance on how long the alert charting will continue. If a resident is being treated for an infection and is taking an antibiotic, the period of alert charting lasts for the duration of the treatment and then a couple days beyond the stop date to determine if any symptoms return. For incidents such as elopement attempts and falls, a standard duration of documentation is each shift for 72 hours following the event.

24-Hour Report

The **24-hour report** is a communication tool that facilitates the flow of information (e.g., a change of condition) from the nursing units to the department managers, director of nurses, and administrator. The 24-hour report is a vital component of successful clinical operations, and the role of the administrator and DON is to establish this tool and its use as a priority for staff.

There are a number of different types of 24-hour report forms; leadership needs to choose one that works well for their facility. Typically, the form will include areas for information, such as new admissions, discharges, antibiotics, labs, skin issues, and other changes of condition. Refer to Exhibit 13.1.

Nursing staff must be trained to utilize this document as a communication tool and understand how important such communication is to the well-being of the facility and positive resident outcomes. Even if an issue is resolved during a shift, it is still important to write it on the 24-hour report. The administrator must be aware that some staff might feel it unnecessary to include things that are resolved or perhaps even become defensive if questioned. This perception must not be ignored but addressed openly and honestly.

Exhibit 13.1   Sample 24-Hour Report

24 Hour Report

Day Nurse: *John Kline*   Eve Nurse: *Sue Martinez*   Noc Nurse: *Mary Bell*

Date:	Unit: 200		
Admissions: Jones, Mary - 208B	Discharges, Room Changes: Cleaver, Susan (212A) to home Brown, Cleo to Room 216B	Labs, xrays, tests: Chest x-ray, Mr. Preston Smith, F. u/A Shirley, J. CBC - BMP	PT/INRs: N/A
	Plant/facility issues: Ran out of towels for evening showers Med cart wheel broken	Lab Results: Frank, G. Hgb 7.2 - Dr. S notified	ABT Therapy: 208B - IV abt q6°

Include: Falls, new skin issues, new infections/ABTs, changes in condition, mood/behaviour issues, resident/family concerns.

	Alert Charting
207A - fall c̄ hematoma and skin tear @ forearm, Tx Order, family notified	Ⓨ N N/A
	Y N N/A
201A - diarrhea x2, fluids encouraged	Ⓨ N N/A
213B - wandering into other peoples' rooms, tried talking to activities and offering snack - need social worker to review	Y Ⓝ N/A
	Y N N/A
	Y N N/A
	Y N N/A

A 24-hour report is not a regurgitation of every progress note or order given during the previous 24 hours. Instead, it provides key information to be shared from shift to shift and with leadership. Here are some examples of issues that should be captured on the report.

- Green family requested consult with hospice.

- Jones rolled out of bed three times tonight, bed arranged on the floor.

- Goss upset that call light wasn't answered quickly, requires much attention.

- Shields refused a shower this evening.

- Gomez with intractable pain, medicated without effect, physician notified.

- McNab declined medications after three attempts with different staff and times.

- Johnson pacing up and down the halls at 2 A.M., difficult to redirect.

- O'Keefe and Nunez heard arguing in dining room, nurse intervened before escalation.

- Marks was short of breath, attempted to reach physician 3x but no answer.

- Proust went to an ortho appt and was gone for 6 hours, skin check negative upon return.

Each of these entries requires discussion and possibly additional follow-up, even if staff resolved the issue in the moment. The follow-up for each entry will be explained in the stand-up section later in this chapter.

Process

Each unit should complete its own 24-hour report. This information is then discussed daily in the stand-up meeting. Staff is apprised of changes of condition, and issues are tracked through resolution. It is a communication tool that when used properly can help facilitate wonderful discussion that improves resident care and guides effective risk management. Historically, the 24-hour report is used by nursing staff, but consider encouraging other departments to use this tool as well, which helps facilitate interdisciplinary communication.

Shift Change

Shift change (sometimes referred to as "huddles") can be a hectic time in the facility as one group of staff is leaving and another group is arriving.

Shift change is a critical time as staff must report important information, such as changes of condition and the status of unfinished tasks. Information shared during shift change should also be recorded on the 24-hour report.

The administrator and director of nurses must establish shift change communication as a high priority. It may also be necessary for the administrator to help minimize or even eliminate interruptions so staff can focus on sharing important details from the previous shift.

Stand-Up Meeting

Long-term care is a complex industry with thousands of rules and regulations, policies, and procedures. Daily existence and success depend upon the successful interaction and choreographing of residents, patients, medical providers, service providers, staff, and family members. The volume and complexity of information exchanged each day in the nursing facility are enormous. From new admissions to changes of condition and chronic disease management, staff are responsible for each aspect of the resident's well-being. No one staff member is solely responsible for the success or failure of a facility. Each staff member is an integral part of the interdisciplinary team and is interdependent with the others.

Staff must have a venue in which to communicate information with the interdisciplinary team. Given the complexity of this business and the constant demand to reprioritize and demonstrate incredible flexibility, there must be a system in place, a check-and-balance system, to manage the details that make up the everyday reality of life in long-term care.

Purpose

That system is the **stand-up meeting**. Stand-up is the forum in which staff can discuss issues, decide how to approach problems, and be held accountable for the policies, procedures, and regulations that govern the facility. The hundreds of details, like proper assessments, documentation, care plans, and notification, are discussed.

Unfortunately, few facilities maximize the potential of the stand-up meeting. Staff filter into the meeting as their schedule allows, and only the barest of information is shared, often without follow-up discussion over consecutive days.

Efficiency and strong leadership are keys to running an effective stand-up meeting. Discussions should be brief and outcome-driven, with clear task assignments and responsibility. Stand-up is not the time for lengthy discussion or debate. The administrator is the primary facilitator of this meeting. As needed, the director of nurses will step in as facilitator, but, again, it is important that the administrator take primary responsibility for this role.

Color-Coding System

Keeping track of details necessitates a system that makes it easy for the administrator to categorize the volume of information. There are two categories of information discussed in stand-up: (1) tasks/issues that are resolved and (2) tasks/issues that are unresolved or pending. The goal of stand-up is complete resolution of all issues.

Implementing a color-coding system provides a simple method to track information. The facilitator uses two highlighter colors; one color indicates resolution and the other color indicates resolution pending. An issue is never "dropped" from stand-up until necessary resolution is verbalized by the department manager. If an action is still pending, such as writing a care plan or documenting an outcome, indicate as such by writing a brief note and highlight it as "resolution pending." It is the responsibility of the assigned staff member to work toward resolution and give a status report in stand-up the next day. If an item is resolved (no further action is necessary), use another color highlighter to indicate it as "resolved."

Part I—General Issues

There are two parts to the stand-up meeting. Part I includes all department managers and other key staff, like a charge nurse or a nursing assistant. During Part I, general facility business is discussed and staff provide brief updates on their departments. The majority of clinical discussion takes place in Part II, but there are some issues that warrant discussion during Part I, especially when they impact nonclinical staff. For example, if a resident had an elopement attempt, all staff need to be aware of this event. Or if a resident has an infectious process and staff must use special precautions, housekeeping and maintenance also need to be apprised.

Each staff member takes a moment to report specific information, which includes updates from the previous day's pending issues. For example, when discussing room changes, the social worker may need to report that documentation is complete for a room change from 2 days ago. If the maintenance director is working on an air conditioner, a progress report is given each day until the unit is fixed. If a resident grievance was discussed 3 days ago and resolution is still pending, it should be discussed each day until resolved.

Sometimes, issues are "brought forward" or "carried" for many days. Again, nothing is dropped from stand-up until resolution is achieved. The administrator may fret that staff will think she is micromanaging. While this process may be new to staff, they will eventually come to appreciate the check-and-balance function it serves. And by encouraging staff to come prepared with care plans already written or revised, notification and documentation already done, staff will trust that it is not micromanagement but supporting each other in this most complex business. The process will be streamlined in no time at all. It also helps when the administrator regularly acknowledges a job well done! An administrator who regularly and sincerely praises staff is a good role model and appreciated by employees.

In this next section, we will discuss each staff member's responsibility during stand-up. The areas identified correlate with significant resident care areas as well as areas frequently cited for deficient practice. While the staff member responsible is indicated for each section, this assignment may vary from facility to facility. The most important point is that the information is discussed.

Census. The day just cannot start properly if the **census** is inaccurate. The census is basically a head count, the number of residents in the facility as of the immediate midnight past. An inaccurate census wreaks havoc for the business office from a billing perspective, for the admission director as it is unclear what beds are available for new admissions, for the staffing coordinator, who needs to determine how many nursing assistants to staff on each unit, and for nursing staff in the event of an emergency, when residents need to be accounted for.

Besides the total number of residents, the census is divided into categories, such as payer sources. Medicare, Medicaid, hospice, managed care, and private pay are common payers. Administrators are very conscious of the number of residents with each payer source as these numbers directly impact the budget.

New admissions. Reported by the health information manager (medical records), the new admissions are the residents who arrived on the previous day by midnight. Information reported includes the person's name, room number, payer source, diagnosis, and the status of the admissions paperwork. Refer to Chapter 14 to learn about the admission process and required paperwork. From a clinical operations perspective, this packet of information is important as it includes acknowledgment of resident's rights and a wealth of other information to help orient the new resident and family. If this packet of information is not complete, the administrator must ask when it will be completed and by whom (either the resident or responsible party). In some facilities the consent to treat form might be completed by the admissions director or by the admitting nurse, but no matter who is responsible, it must be done in a timely manner.

Actual discharges. Reported by medical records or the health information manager, the actual discharges are the residents who have physically left the facility, regardless of whether they are expected to return, such as following a hospitalization. Information reported includes the resident's name, room number, payer source, destination, whether the discharge order is written, if the nursing discharge note is complete, if the discharge paperwork is signed, whether a bed hold was needed and signed, and whether the room is deep-cleaned (ready for a new admission).

Similar to the nursing admission note, a thorough nursing discharge note must include specific details. The writer must paint a picture of the resident's status at discharge so that no questions are left unanswered. Such details include the provider's order to discharge; date and time of discharge; physical and mental condition, including skin condition; method of transportation; if accompanied, name of person; destination; post-discharge plan that has been developed with the resident and family; disposition of remaining medications; and disposition of personal belongings (Beicher, 2003).

Room changes made. Room changes are inevitable in the life of the facility. Finding compatible roommates can prove challenging, and when changes need to be made, staff must be diligent in meeting the regulation called Accommodation of Needs (CMS, 2014, F247). In stand-up, the social worker reports who moved rooms, the status of notification, documentation of the move, and social work documentation 2 to 3 days following the room change, addressing resident adjustment following the move. Documentation of notification is the responsibility of the staff member who actually talked with the resident or responsible party. It is important to also notify the family of the change so they are not startled when they come for a visit and cannot find their loved one.

There is an important caveat to the notification requirement. Not only must staff obtain agreement from the resident who is actually moving rooms but also they must notify the resident who will be receiving a new roommate (just to be clear, the expectation is notification, not permission).

Room changes pending. The social worker also reports any pending room changes, the anticipated room number, reason for the move, and expected date of the move, notification, and documentation. Room change information is essential to the admissions director so there is no confusion about bed availability and room numbers. It is important to the housekeeping staff so they can plan extra time to deep-clean (more extensive cleaning and sanitization) a room after a move. For the central supply manager, room changes are important so the correct resident is billed for supplies.

Pending admissions. The admissions director reports any referrals, including the potential resident's name, referral source, pending admission date, payer source, diagnoses and skilled need if for rehabilitation, **Class II prescriptions** (a prescription for a medication that is a controlled substance, such as a narcotic), anticipated discharge plan following the skilled stay, whether it is necessary to start the Medicaid process, behavioral health concerns, whether restraints or a sitter were required while hospitalized, special needs (bariatric equipment, oxygen, colostomy supplies, breathing treatments), any unusual medications or nursing needs, the PASRR, and whether the family or responsible party is involved. That is a lot of information!

When the administrator fails to ask these questions and allow the interdisciplinary team to discuss the potential admission, problems that would have been identified prior to arrival go undiscovered until the resident is in the facility. Administrators are under enormous pressure to maintain census and meet budget, which means the beds need to be filled. But beds filled with patients whose needs cannot be met, whose behaviors take so much staff time that other responsibilities go undone and liability skyrockets, are problems no administrator needs or facility wants.

Pending discharges. Pending discharges are reported by the social worker and include the resident's name, room number, payer source, anticipated date of discharge, destination, date of issuance for the **notice of noncoverage** (NONC) (letter specifying the last covered day of payment), and the status of the discharge.

If the patient plans to remain in the facility as a long-term care resident, the provider should write an order to reflect the date for the payer source change—that is, the date when the resident transitions to long-term care and another payer source. Sometimes this order is written as "last covered day of [name of payer source] is [date]."

Financial issues. The business office manager reports financial issues, such as payer source changes and effective dates, outstanding balances, problems with obtaining authorization for continued stay, and any patients getting close to exhausting their benefit period. These issues affect other departments, and the purpose of discussing them in stand-up is so everyone is apprised of the same information and a plan is developed. It is very important for therapy staff to know when a payer source changes as there may be different requirements for documentation or a different therapy benefit to track. Although the social worker should never be asked to collect payment, he can ensure that all other resources for payment have been explored. He is also closely involved in the discharge planning process should a 30-day notice of discharge for nonpayment be issued. (Refer to Chapter 6 for more information on payer sources.)

Maintenance/housekeeping/central supply. Although these three departments are not considered "clinical," they are integral to clinical operations. In the stand-up meeting, each department manager reports any facility or equipment issues and supply issues. Clinical staff may have requests for equipment repairs, so the maintenance director needs to be involved. The night shift may have run out of towels, so housekeeping needs to be involved in the discussion and resolution. A provider may have ordered an unusual wound care product, so central supply needs to discuss this with the director of nurses. While these discussions may have taken place prior to or outside of stand-up, it is imperative that they are also addressed in the meeting itself so the administrator is always kept apprised and can ensure that appropriate resolutions occur.

Nursing. Clinical discussion in Part I of stand-up is limited to those issues that involve nonclinical staff. From a nursing perspective, there might have been an incident involving a faulty piece of equipment or a slippery floor and maintenance or housekeeping needs to be involved in the discussion and resolution. Otherwise, all incident reports and clinical issues are held for discussion in Part II of the meeting.

Dietary. The dietary manager addresses any issues, problems, and special requests. Perhaps a family asked the night nurse if they could join Mom for dinner the next evening, so an extra meal needs to be ordered and charged to the resident's account. Or there was a problem with lunch trays yesterday, and several residents expressed dissatisfaction that needs to be addressed.

Activities. The activities director shares the agenda for the day. If there is a special event, department managers are expected to assist in transporting residents. Managers may need to finalize coordination of snacks for an event or logistics of having residents ready for an outing.

Therapy. The therapy director informs the group if there are any resident issues, problems, or concerns. Perhaps there needs to be a brief discussion regarding a therapy schedule for a new resident who goes to dialysis three times a week. Maybe a patient had a difficult time participating in therapy yesterday due to pain and needs to be premedicated.

MDS assessments. The MDS coordinator shares what assessments are due today and which ones are past due. Take care that this is not the time or place to reprimand a staff member whose assessments are past due. The purpose of the discussion in stand-up is to help everyone orient their day and keep the administrator apprised of the status of assessments due.

Scheduled days off and staffing. Staffing issues are discussed only as they impact the facility and resident care, not to share private staff information with the whole group. If there are holidays coming up, the administrator needs to know who plans to take the day off and how job responsibilities will be covered.

General events. This is a good time to remind staff of any special events or meetings for the day, such as an in-service. Are there visitors scheduled for the day, like a consultant or corporate staff? Are there any concerns or complaints from residents, family, or staff? And do not forget to ask for compliments! Take time to acknowledge and praise staff. These are tough jobs, and compliments help maintain morale.

Part II—Clinical Review

After Part I is complete, the administrator excuses nonclinical staff from the meeting. The concept of which department managers are defined as clinical staff needs clarification. Nursing and therapy staff are easily defined as clinical, as might be the dietary manager. Social services and activities are the other two department managers who must also be included in the clinical part of this meeting. Changes of condition, new medications, nonparticipation with therapy, falls, and accidents impact many departments. Remember, the purpose of stand-up is to achieve interdisciplinary communication.

Consider the social worker who is making arrangements for Mr. Smith's discharge plan. If Mr. Smith fell overnight when his spouse tried to transfer him from the bed to the wheelchair and an x-ray of the hip is pending, clearly this situation impacts the discharge plan. Even if the x-ray is negative for a fracture, additional caregiver training may be necessary to facilitate a safe discharge, which could mean an extended stay in the facility.

Here is an example that impacts the activity department. A resident has a change of condition and is now on a mechanically altered diet (food is chopped instead of served whole) due to aspiration risk. This resident loves to attend activities, and today is one of his favorites, but there will be snacks served. Activity staff must be notified of the new diet orders so they can ensure his participation and safety in the event.

In Part II of stand-up, there are specific components of clinical operations that are discussed, which include chart audits for new admissions, incident reports, 24-hour reports, new orders, lab tests, and resident appointments. Serving as the foundation of resident care are the Critical Elements of Care.

Critical Elements of Care. In 2010 when Centers for Medicare and Medicaid (CMS) began using the Quality Indicator Survey (QIS) process, facilities were introduced to the **Critical Elements of Care**, a group of regulations deemed to be at the center of the resident care process. While these regulations are certainly not new, the difference is how they are organized and the added emphasis placed on each element.

The Critical Elements of Care are as follows:

1. Comprehensive Assessment (CMS, Centers for Medicare and Medicaid Services, 2014, F272)

2. Comprehensive Care Plan (CMS, Centers for Medicare and Medicaid Services, 2014, F279)

3. Care Plan Implementation by Qualified Persons (CMS, Centers for Medicare and Medicaid Services, 2014, F282)

4. Care Plan Revisions (CMS, Centers for Medicare and Medicaid Services, 2014, F280)

5. Care Plan Provision (varies but usually includes Quality of Care) (CMS, Centers for Medicare and Medicaid Services, 2014, F309)

Basing the clinical operations and the stand-up meeting on the Critical Elements of Care is an excellent way to organize the hundreds of details that must be managed each day and to ensure robust discussion among the interdisciplinary team.

The Critical Elements of Care are arranged in a logical numerical order. Until a comprehensive assessment is completed, a care plan cannot be implemented. That makes sense! Staff should become accustomed to being asked, "What is your assessment of that?" Depending on the situation, the answer might include the score or outcome of a specific assessment tool. It might include a set of vital signs or a conversation with the resident, family, or other staff. The point is that staff must learn to thoroughly assess a situation as part of the critical thinking process and before proceeding to the care plan step. The role of the administrator is to help guide staff through this process and identify areas that might need additional investigation and follow-up.

Chart audit for new admission. In Chapter 12, the chart audit for a new admission was explained in detail. Now is the time in stand-up where each audit (one for each new resident) is reviewed. The administrator quickly scans the document to identify incomplete areas. Perhaps a DNR order is missing, a fall risk care plan needs to be done, or not all medications have diagnoses. Whatever the issue, resolution is assigned to the appropriate person and recorded on the administrator's copy of the audit, which is then discussed the next day.

To make the stand-up meeting more efficient, some facilities bring the medical charts for all new admissions to stand-up or have a computer with access to the electronic medical record available. Many issues can be resolved immediately and eliminate the need for follow-up the next day.

Incident reports. The administrator asks if there were any incident reports from yesterday. If so, they are briefly discussed to ensure all components were addressed, including necessary assessments, care plans, notifications, and documentation. Based on the assessment information, any follow-up is assigned, which is then discussed in stand-up the next day. Here are examples of issues, followed by a brief discussion.

24-hour reports. The 24-hour report is one of the most critical components in managing clinical operations, and it gets center stage in stand-up. Earlier we looked at examples of information that should be recorded on the 24-hour report. Now, let's take the next step and discuss why each of those issues is important, what questions need to be asked, and what follow-up is necessary.

- Green family requested consult with hospice.

- Jones rolled out of bed three times tonight, bed arranged on the floor.

- Goss upset that call light wasn't answered quickly, requires much attention.

- Gomez with intractable pain, medicated without effect, physician notified.

- McNab declined medications after three attempts with different staff and times.

- Johnson pacing up and down the halls at 2 A.M., difficult to redirect. Ativan ordered.

- O'Keefe and Nunez heard arguing in dining room, nurse intervened before escalation.

- Marks was short of breath, attempted to reach physician 3x but no answer.

  - "Green Family Requested Consult With Hospice"

Has Mr. Green had a sudden change of condition or is a hospice (a program for intense palliative care) consult request expected? Is the resident cognizant and if so, in agreement with the consult? Do staff and the medical provider agree that hospice is an appropriate transition? Does the resident or family have a preference for a hospice agency? If not, what is the facility protocol for making a referral? Is the resident's decline documented by a member of the interdisciplinary team and does the care plan reflect the decline? Is a change of condition MDS necessary?

- "Jones Rolled Out of Bed Three Times Tonight, Bed Arranged on the Floor"

The assessment in this scenario is important. Why was he rolling out of bed? What was he trying to do? What did he need? Were incident reports completed each time? Did he sustain injury? Is he experiencing a change of condition? Is he able to get up from the bed on the floor? If not, the bed is considered a restraint and there should be a prerestraint assessment. How did the resident react to the bed on the floor? Were the provider and family notified and is it documented? Is the care plan completed? Are there other interventions that might work better? Are there dignity issues?

- "Goss Upset That Call Light Wasn't Answered Quickly, Requires Much Attention"

What did Ms. Goss need when she used the call light? How did staff react? Were her requests reasonable? What does "require much attention" mean? Is there another underlying issue, such as fear of being alone or pain, that is driving the repetitive requests? Is this behavior typical for her? Should a grievance report be completed? Is documentation done? If this is more of an attention-seeking type behavior, it should also be care planned.

- "Gomez With Intractable Pain, Medicated Without Effect, Physician Notified"

Is this a change of condition for Mr. Gomez? What is the assessment of the pain? What was the outcome of the conversation with the physician? Are there new orders? Is a pain care plan in place? Is he on alert charting? How is he feeling this morning?

- "McNab Declined Medications After Three Attempts With Different Staff and Times"

Unfortunately, many facilities read that entry on the report and simply move on to the next item. Further discussion is necessary to determine what medications she did not receive. Is it of concern that she did not take those medications? Was the family and physician notified? What is the assessment of her choice? Is this the first time or a regular occurrence? If a regular occurrence, what interventions do staff try to encourage her to take the medications? Is the issue care planned? Is a review of the medications by the physician and pharmacist necessary to determine if the medications are vital to her well-being or can some be discontinued, thereby simplifying the medication pass?

- "Johnson Pacing Up and Down the Halls at 2 A.M., Difficult to Redirect. Ativan Ordered"

Is it unusual for Mr. Johnson to pace the halls? Or pace the halls at 2 A.M.? What interventions did staff try for redirection? What exactly was the outcome? What is the assessment of the pacing? Was he looking for something or someone? Was pain or fear an issue? Was he trying to get somewhere? Why? Is he a fall risk? If so, is it care planned? Was a consent in place before the Ativan was administered? What other interventions can staff try? What are his strengths that staff can use to help reduce the pacing? Is the care plan accurate?

- "O'Keefe and Nunez Heard Arguing in Dining Room, Nurse Intervened Before Escalation"

Do these two residents have a history of altercations? What was the issue that resulted in an argument? In other words, the assessment? How did staff intervene? What was the outcome? Do these two residents need to be separated when dining or during activities? How close are their rooms? Do all staff know what to do in case of an altercation? Are the issues care planned on both charts?

- "Marks Was Short of Breath, Attempted to Reach Physician 3x but No Answer"

What did the nurse do when the physician could not be reached? What was the assessment of the patient's shortness of breath? Are all three attempts documented (including the times of the calls)? Staff need to know that anytime a physician cannot be reached, the medical director should be contacted to provide orders. No matter the time of day or night, the administrator should be notified of problems such as this one. The administrator and DON will need to investigate why the physician did not respond and what to do next.

Now, for one last example, recall the documentation example from the activity director about the resident with a cognitive change of condition (restless, inability to focus, forgetful, gets lost) earlier in this chapter. Let's examine this situation in light of the Critical Elements of Care.

What do the different disciplines (nursing, social work, therapy, and dietary) think may be contributing to the change? Ask questions that yield clues about the assessment. Did something happen recently in her life to cause a grief-like response? Might she have an infection? Has the provider been notified? Would talking with the family to see if they've noticed a change be helpful? Should the elopement risk assessment be redone, given her increased agitation that may result in exit-seeking behavior? Does the care plan need to be updated? This is an excellent example of the benefit of stand-up and staff from different disciplines communicating about residents and patients.

New orders. Whether the facility is entirely paperless or still uses hard-copy providers' orders, reviewing orders is another main part of stand-up. Each morning prior to the meeting, the DON or designee gathers the orders from each unit (or runs a report with all the orders) and quickly reviews them. The goal is to investigate and resolve as much as possible before the meeting starts, which improves efficiency and reduces the amount of follow-up the next day.

Refer to the order written by a physician in Exhibit 13.2. An order to start antibiotics is multilayered, and while this order may appear complete at first glance, it is not. There is a diagnosis (UTI) and duration (10 days) for the medication. But there are two components that need to be clarified: (1) the route to administer the medication, which in this case is likely to be oral or "by mouth" (PO), and (2) "DS" should be written out as double strength or a milligram equivalent.

Once the nurse writes a clarification order, there are three more areas to check: (1) nursing documentation summarizing the change of condition and notification of the resident and responsible party if necessary; (2) alert charting per P&P to make sure nursing staff continue to document the medication administration and response to the antibiotic; and (3) care plan to ensure the change of condition and treatment are documented.

Let's look at one more example that demonstrates the importance of an interdisciplinary response to a provider's order. Refer to Exhibit 13.3.

A novice administrator might simply assume the unit clerk would make an appointment with a dentist to get new dentures, when, in fact, this "simple" order is infinitely more complex. Consider the first Critical Element of Care, comprehensive assessment. In this case, *why* are the resident's dentures not fitting properly? Has he lost weight? If so, is it

Exhibit 13.2 Provider Order for Antibiotic Medication

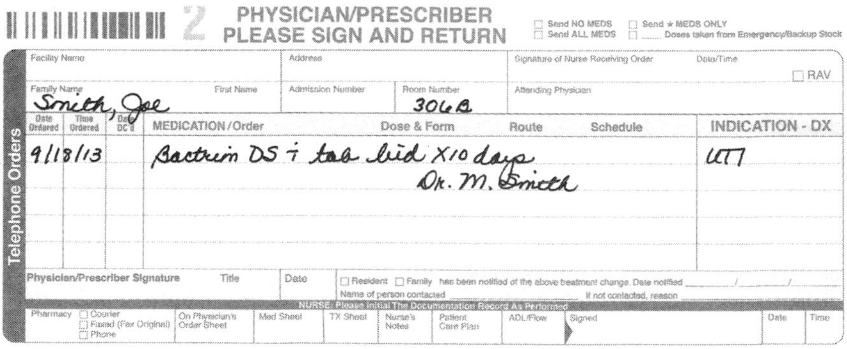
2 PHYSICIAN/PRESCRIBER PLEASE SIGN AND RETURN

☐ Send NO MEDS ☐ Send ALL MEDS ☐ Send ★ MEDS ONLY ☐ ____ Doses taken from Emergency/Backup Stock

ORIGINAL) COPY — Telephone Orders

Facility Name | Address | Signature of Nurse Receiving Order | Date/Time | ☐ RAV

Family Name: Smith, Joe | First Name | Admission Number | Room Number: 306B | Attending Physician

Date Ordered	Time Ordered	Date DC'd	MEDICATION/Order Dose & Form Route Schedule	INDICATION - DX
9/18/13			Bactrim DS i tab bid X10 days Dr. M. Smith	UTI

Physician/Prescriber Signature | Title | Date | ☐ Resident ☐ Family has been notified of the above treatment change. Date notified ___/___/___ Name of person contacted ______ If not contacted, reason ______

NURSE: Please Initial The Documentation Record As Performed

Pharmacy ☐ Courier ☐ Faxed (Fax Original) ☐ Phone | On Physician's Order Sheet | Med Sheet | TX Sheet | Nurse's Notes | Patient Care Plan | ADL/Flow | Signed | Date | Time

Exhibit 13.3 Provider Order for Dental Consultation

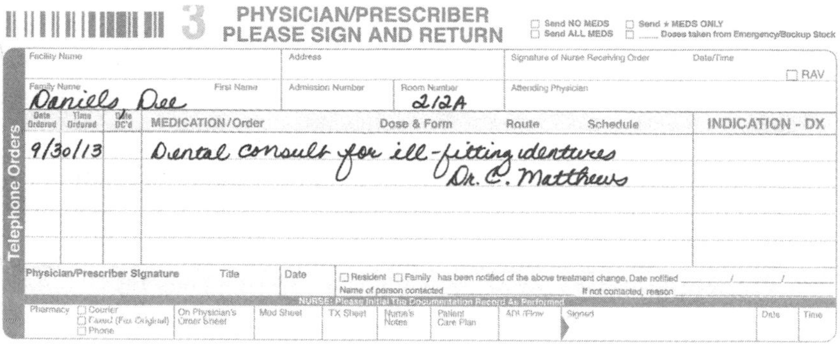
3 PHYSICIAN/PRESCRIBER PLEASE SIGN AND RETURN

☐ Send NO MEDS ☐ Send ALL MEDS ☐ Send * MEDS ONLY ☐ ___ Doses taken from Emergency/Backup Stock

ORIGINAL COPY — Telephone Orders

Facility Name | Address | Signature of Nurse Receiving Order | Date/Time | ☐ RAV

Family Name: Daniels | First Name: Dee | Admission Number | Room Number: 212A | Attending Physician

Date Ordered	Time Ordered	Date DC'd	MEDICATION/Order	Dose & Form	Route	Schedule	INDICATION - DX
9/30/13			Dental consult for ill-fitting dentures Dr. C. Matthews				

Physician/Prescriber Signature | Title | Date | ☐ Resident ☐ Family has been notified of the above treatment change. Date notified ___/___/___ Name of person contacted ___ If not contacted, reason ___

NURSE: Please Initial The Documentation Record As Performed

Pharmacy ☐ Courier ☐ Faxed (Fax Original) ☐ Phone | On Physician's Order Sheet | Med Sheet | TX Sheet | Nurse's Notes | Patient Care Plan | ADL/Flow | Signed | Date | Time

a desired weight loss or is there another etiology to consider? Are his dentures broken or damaged? If so, why? Did the nurse do an assessment to determine if there are oral problems, such as ulcers or a possible infection? Is it due to pain?

During the stand-up meeting other department managers will need to be involved in the assessment process. The dietitian will need to investigate the resident's intake. Is a diet consistency change necessary (e.g., chopped food) or is the resident able to eat regular-texture food without the dentures? Should the speech therapist evaluate the resident?

The social worker will need to investigate the financial aspects of obtaining new dentures. What is the payer source? It is also important to ask the resident if he even wants new dentures. Does the family need to be involved? Investigation of these questions will yield valuable information, which is then discussed in the stand-up meeting and agreement for a plan is established. Each manager needs to document his findings in the medical record and contribute to a comprehensive care plan.

As demonstrated with just one order, there are numerous issues to be considered, and the administrator is responsible for asking the questions and guiding staff to engage in the critical thinking processes that ultimately result in good clinical judgment, thorough and defensible documentation, and robust care plans.

Lab tests. In some facilities with a caseload of high-acuity patients on a skilled stay, there might be dozens of lab tests ordered each day, while in other facilities, labs are infrequent. Regardless, there must be a system to ensure the timeliness of lab draws, reporting, and follow-up. When labs are ordered and when results are received, they are typically written in the 24-hour report or perhaps in a lab log book.

The DON or designee brings the lab book and the labs to stand-up. It is not necessary to report on each lab result in the meeting. Instead, the nurse determines if all the labs ordered were drawn and which results were received. The nurse reports labs that were outside normal limits, either high or low. For example, a white blood count (WBC) of 19,000 is high and would necessitate follow-up from the provider. A potassium level of 2.9 is low and would need follow-up from the provider. In both cases, there must be documentation in the resident's medical record that the provider was notified and what, if any, follow-up is needed.

Resident appointments and consultations. Each facility needs a process to manage the residents' appointments and consultations. Residents see a variety of specialists and have tests or procedures outside the facility, such as CTs, MRIs, blood transfusions, and dialysis. Getting a resident to an appointment outside the facility can be time-consuming and requires detailed coordination. Sometimes the appointments or consultations occur in the facility, such as with a podiatrist or mental health professional.

For purposes of clinical operations, we will focus on the steps once a resident has had a consultation or appointment. Before stand-up, the DON or designee checks the scheduling book to see what appointments were scheduled on the previous day. For each resident who had an appointment, there are several things that must be investigated. Is there a progress note from the specialist that reports what was done in the appointment, recommendations, and whether follow-up is necessary? The provider in the nursing facility needs to be notified of the outcome, which is then documented. The outcome and recommendations may need to be discussed with the resident or responsible party. The resident's provider may need to give orders in response to the specialist's recommendations, and depending on the orders, staff may need to notify and obtain consent from the resident or responsible party. Members of the interdisciplinary team may need to document in the record, and the care plan may need to be updated.

Let's look at an example. Mr. Jones sees an ophthalmologist and on the report it states, "Cataract surgery may not be that beneficial since macular problem would need further evaluation." The facility nurse and the provider need to acknowledge the outcome of the visit with a signature. Given his moderate dementia, Mr. Jones may not be a candidate for further work-up, but that needs to be indicated and communicated with everyone, including the resident and family. There is already a vision deficit care plan in place, so the nurse should add the date and outcome of this consultation on the care plan. That way, staff has an up-to-date record of all efforts and interventions. Including the outcome of the consultation on the care plan consolidates this important information in a logical place.

Challenges With Electronic Medical Records

Many facilities have transitioned from paper medical record systems to electronic medical records. While there are benefits to an electronic medical record (EMR), the challenges of selecting the best software are numerous. Some of these challenges impact clinical operations.

While staff usually receives initial training with the implementation of an EMR system, it is also important to schedule interim trainings. The administrator should regularly check with staff to see if they are having any problems with the EMR and work to find resolutions. Perhaps a section is so cumbersome that it takes extraordinary time to complete, or maybe a section does not address all the areas that staff need to assess. Staff get frustrated trying to find areas of the record and instead choose to ignore them.

Another challenge with many EMRs is the care plans. Often, the care plan components are linked to the data inputted on the MDS. Unfortunately, these prepopulated care plans are generic and in some instances may even be incorrect. If the software allows modifications, staff can manually correct each plan, but if the software does not allow modifications, staff can be stuck using what is available. When necessary, print out hard copies of records, such as the care plan, and encourage staff to revise them manually so they accurately reflect the resident, not a preprinted image of a generic person.

For treatments like wound care, which might be ordered a specific number of times per week but not every day, the EMR may not allow "twice a week" as an option but force the nurse to select specific days. If in this facility the wound care nurse is responsible for all wound care and she is absent on a day the dressing should be changed, the facility is not following providers' orders. Issues like these are not insurmountable, but they do require forethought and planning that culminate into a clear process for staff.

Another important issue to consider is a power outage. Of course, the facility will have generators to maintain critical functions, but does this include the EMR? Consider the situation in which staff cannot access the EMR, which is the only record of orders, medications, and treatments. Again, this is not insurmountable but the administrator must plan for all contingencies.

Critical thinking skills must be evident even with documentation in the EMR. We cannot rely so heavily on electronic data systems and software that we forget to use common sense. The administrator should talk with the software vendor, explain the need, and try to identify how it can be met. Then take credit for identifying the problem and solution as a performance improvement project, and submit it in the next QAPI meeting. Refer to Chapter 10 for more information on the EMR.

Summary

Managing clinical operations in the nursing facility is a complex process. Dividing tasks into daily, weekly, and monthly categories helps the administrator and the interdisciplinary team achieve success. Utilizing systems and processes, like the 24-hour report and the stand-up meeting, to facilitate communication will also reduce deficiencies and improve resident outcomes.

Key Terms

24-hour report: Communication tool to record changes of condition and general goings-on for each unit or neighborhood.

Census: Number of resident in the facility at any given time.

Class II prescription: A prescription for a medication that is a controlled substance, such as a narcotic.

Critical Elements of Care: Group of regulations at the center of the resident care process.

Discharge summary: Review of a resident's stay in the nursing facility.

Medication error rate: The percentage of errors calculated by dividing the number of errors by the number of medication opportunities and multiplied by 100.

Medication regime review: Process to review a resident's medications.

Notice of noncoverage: Letter specifying the last covered day of payment.

Resident council: Group of residents who meet regularly to discuss concern and develop suggestions.

Restorative nursing: Specialized nursing services to help resident achieve or maintain their highest level of functioning.

Stand-up meeting: System to manage complex clinical operations.

Review Questions

1. For a change of condition, what is the first step?
   a. Notification of provider
   b. Notification of family
   c. Start alert charting
   d. Assessment

2. What is the driving force of the stand-up meeting?
   a. 24-hour report
   b. Critical Elements of Care
   c. Lab tests
   d. Incident reports

3. What clinical components are reviewed in a medical record audit?
   a. Recaps
   b. Nursing assistant flow sheets
   c. Care plan
   d. All of the above

4. Which one should be recorded on the 24-hour report?
   a. Fall
   b. Resident-to-resident altercation
   c. Upset family
   d. All of the above

5. Which element is not discussed in Part I of stand-up?
   a. 24-hour report
   b. New referrals
   c. Room changes
   d. Staffing issues

Case Study

As a newly hired administrator of a 110-bed facility, you and the director of nurses completed chart audits for several residents and found incomplete orders, missing consents, inadequate documentation, and an overall absence of clinical judgment based in critical thinking skills. The previous administrator held a daily stand-up meeting, but you learned from the department managers that there was very little communication between departments and there was never any follow-through from day-to-day. On the last survey, there were several serious citations for issues, including comprehensive assessment, comprehensive care plan, resident rights, laboratory services, and notification of changes of condition. You want to implement a different stand-up meeting format. What is your plan to address the deficiencies? How will you get started?

References

American Medical Director's Association. (2003). *Clinical practice guideline: Acute change of condition.* Retrieved from http://www.amda.com/tools/guidelines.cfm

Beicher, T. (2003). *Defensive documentation for long-term care: Strategies for creating a more lawsuit-proof resident record.* Marblehead, MA: hcPro, 2003.

Centers for Medicare and Medicaid Services. (2014). *State operation manual: Appendix PP—guidance to surveyors for long-term care facilities.* Retrieved from http://www.cms.gov/Regulations-and-Guidance/Guidance/Manuals/downloads/som107ap_pp_guidelines_ltcf.pdf

Greenwald, S. C. (1999). *Social work policies, procedures and guidelines for long-term care.* Glenview, IL: SocialWork Consultation Group.

Acknowledgment

With deepest gratitude to my husband and best friend, Dr. Mel Hector, for his insights and edits as well as his patience for the hours I spent on this project. To my dear friend and colleague, Barbara Viggiano, RN, for her honest critique and suggestions. And, to both of you for all the laughs along the way!

CHAPTER 14

FACILITY OPERATIONS AND PERFORMANCE IMPROVEMENT

Rebecca Perley
Jim Kinsey
Paige Hector
Jill Harrison

This chapter focuses on facility operations and performance improvement in the skilled nursing facility, a segment of the long-term care continuum that provides the most complex care in the most highly regulated environment. Long-term care facilities strive to provide the best physical and psychosocial care to residents while also meeting operational expenses and revenue goals. Long-term relationships and friendships between residents and staff often develop and are a positive aspect of operating this type of business. When facility operations and performance improvement are exemplary, the facility is a viable and productive organization that provides a home where residents thrive.

Facility Operations

Facility operations include day-to-day activities necessary to provide clinical and nonclinical care for residents. Clinical care is provided by the medical provider (a physician, nurse practitioner, or sometimes a physician assistant), nurses, dietary and social services, pharmacy, and activity staff as well as rehabilitation staff and mental health providers. Nonclinical care includes support services,

LEARNING OBJECTIVES

- Identify the role of the nursing home administrator (NHA) in facility operations and performance improvement.

- Describe the nursing home facility's admission process.

- Incorporate resident's preferences into facility operations.

- Explain how the Quality Assessment and Assurance (QAA) committee implements the Quality Assurance and Performance Improvement (QAPI) program.

- Define the importance of data management.

- Discuss the NHA's role in managing the survey process.

such as plant and equipment maintenance, housekeeping, laundry, business office, front office, and admissions. Ultimately, it is the licensed nursing home administrator (NHA) who must manage both clinical and nonclinical services to ensure that residents receive **quality of care** (medical care that maximizes the physical and mental needs of each resident) and **quality of life** (the enjoyment and happiness a resident experiences from his life), and the facility meets business objectives.

Role of the NHA

The NHA is ultimately responsible for all activities associated with the facility. The education and training of an NHA may be clinical, such as nursing, although many have a business or management background. The primary areas of responsibility for the NHA are to ensure that all staff, resident, family, corporate, and statutory requirements are met. If any of these areas are neglected, the organization may be unable to provide services in a way that would maximize positive outcomes for the residents.

Residents. Taking care of these individuals requires an understanding of their unique status. Residents at the skilled nursing level of care have complex medical requirements resulting from mental and or physical changes, which can cause them to feel frustration, anxiety, and depression. The NHA must be aware that these residents may not be able to articulate their needs and may not have family or friends for advocates. "Stepping into the shoes" of the resident creates a relationship between the resident, NHA, and facility staff that enables a better understanding of the residents' view of the changes in their lifestyle. The NHA needs to form an ongoing relationship that creates feelings of trust within the residents to enable open communication and the discovery of ways to improve their quality of life.

Staff. Critical to success is hiring and training the right people to work in the long-term care environment. The NHA must hire staff who demonstrate empathy and compassion. They must be adept at interacting with residents who may be at a vulnerable time in their lives and are expressing anger, frustration, or grief. Residents may be unhappy about living in a facility or the loss of abilities they once enjoyed. These feelings of sadness or grief can be reduced through the development of positive interactions between staff and residents.

The following are leadership concepts that the NHA can implement. These models move the NHA leadership style away from a hierarchical structure to one that embraces, empowers, and welcomes staff to be integral in decision making.

Leading through collaboration is one leadership concept style promoting interdependence among departments versus independence. Working as a team offers benefits, such as opportunities to collaborate on care, and improves resident outcomes and satisfaction for staff (Frampton et al., 2010).

The NHA's relationship with staff is a relationship-based concept that can establish trust, autonomy, collaboration, and successful outcomes. (Frampton et al., 2010). Mechanisms to support this approach include inviting frontline staff to care plan meetings, **consistent assignment** (when a staff member is assigned to the same resident(s) each shift), flexible work scheduling, and inclusive decision making. If staff do not feel empowered and considered in approaches to care, then they may remain focused on task-based care (Diamond, 1992), which will not maximize outcomes for the resident.

Inclusive decision making is a form of participatory decision making in which no decision is made without staff input when the decision relates to the work they do. This form of decision making ensures that decisions are made with input from the staff who are impacted by the decision. A drawback for this approach is that more time is required to reach a decision due to consideration for all opinions. Achieving consensus, empowering others, and facilitating a team approach will increase staff satisfaction and improve resident outcomes (Kinsey & Manning, 2015).

Family members. Family members play a critical role by easing loneliness and acting as an advocate for the resident. They can offer support by bringing items, such as clothing and personal effects, as well as helping to communicate the resident's needs. They also help by aiding a resident when eating meals and performing other personal tasks, such as brushing hair and getting dressed. Occasionally, tension may arise between family members and facility staff because expectations are perceived as not being met. For example, lost resident laundry or other possessions are a perpetual problem in any facility. Open and ongoing communication is especially important between the NHA and family members because the NHA acts as an advocate for both residents and staff.

Corporate goals. Corporate goals are expressed to the NHA through a variety of documents, including the mission statement, policies and procedures, and budget. The responsibility of the NHA is to manage facility operations to achieve corporate goals, such as low staff turnover and few or no resident medication errors. Consultants may do monthly reviews to assist the NHA in identifying operational areas needing improvement. The NHA is responsible for monitoring all operational and medical outcomes, including census, pharmacy use, budget versus actual results, marketing efforts, inventory, and payroll expenses.

Statutory regulations. The NHA must ensure that the facility complies with state and federal regulations to ensure quality of care and life for residents. Periodic state and federal surveys are performed by the state Department of Public Health to determine if the facility is operating in compliance with statutory regulations established by the state and federal governments. Violations of regulations, called **deficiencies**, can result and must be corrected or the facility may ultimately be at risk of losing its state license and certification from Centers for Medicare and Medicaid Services (CMS). The survey process will be discussed later in this chapter.

Daily NHA Rounds

Daily NHA rounds include physical inspections of the facility and discussions with staff and residents regarding operational performance. These rounds should be completed in rotation by the NHA and members of the management staff. Companies vary in their requirements, but typically a daily inspection schedule is created for all areas frequented by residents, staff, and family members. Such areas include: resident rooms, bathing areas, reception area, courtyard, parking lot, and department areas such as nursing, housekeeping, kitchen, and laundry. Creating a schedule allows for an inspection as frequently as every 4 hours to assess compliance with federal and state regulations, company policies and procedures, and satisfaction levels.

It is necessary for the NHA to orient department managers on how to successfully complete facility rounds. Questions such as the following facilitate conversation and build a team approach: "Who can I thank for helping you today? Do you need anything from me right now? Is there anything I can do to make you feel more comfortable or safe?" The skills for rounding include knowing what to look for and what to listen for.

Rounding for relationship (discussion held during rounds to build trust and communication during this activity) further advances a **resident-centered care** culture (an approach to care that focuses on the resident's preferences and needs) by engaging staff, promoting teamwork, and modeling inclusive decision making. This approach requires a NHA to believe and accept the value of listening to feedback from residents, staff, and family (Frampton et al., 2010).

Preadmission

Prior to admission the prospective resident must be prescreened to determine whether the facility can provide adequate care. The NHA and director of nurses together evaluate the potential resident's health records, which include mental and physical status. Other evaluation methods are in-person visits when possible to assess behavior, and discussions with case managers and family members. This process involves many steps, which are discussed from a clinical perspective in Chapters 12 and 13 and from an operational perspective as follows.

Historically, the preadmission process has been viewed from the perspective of the facility and not the prospective resident. The current emphasis to incorporate resident-centered care requires that resident input is considered along with the needs of the facility.

Preadmission Screening and Resident Review (PASRR)

The PASRR is completed prior to admission for all prospective residents who may be admitted to a Medicaid-certified nursing facility. The purpose of the this screening is to "identify a resident who has a mental illness or is suspected of having a mental illness, an intellectual/developmental disability, or a related condition to determine if specialized services are needed during their stay in a nursing facility" (California Department of Health Care Services, 2015, p. 3). This screening step is important to perform to ensure that for residents with mental or developmental illness, their needs can be met by the nursing facility level of care.

Financial Reimbursement for Treatment

Another important aspect of the admission process is to identify a viable payer source, such as Medicaid or federal Medicare subsidies, private pay, or third-party contracts. A resident and/or the responsible party should receive a detailed cost analysis estimating expenses for the resident's stay at the facility. If the facility is assisting the resident in applying for Medicaid, documents such as bank account balances, Veteran's benefits, and retirement pension may be discussed to make a preliminary determination about Medicaid eligibility.

Facility Tour

The tour is an important step in the preadmission process that helps familiarize prospective residents and family members with the facility environment and provides an opportunity to meet staff and other residents. Engaging in conversation, asking the individual how he feels about the transition, and acknowledging concerns help build trust and rapport. A tour protocol must be established and followed to ensure that all important services of the facility are reviewed with the prospective resident. These services should include an example of a resident's room, shower area, dining room, and activity rooms. The tour is conducted by the admission coordinator or a **manager on duty** (person designated to be in charge in the NHA's absence).

Documentation Required for Admission

The resident may transfer to the facility from a personal residence, hospital, or other setting, such as an assisted living facility. The facility must ensure that the following records accompany the new resident upon transfer.

Physician Order

Per federal regulations (CMS, 2014c, p. 130), "At the time each resident is admitted, the facility must have physician orders for the resident's immediate care." This means that a resident cannot be admitted to a facility without a physician order. Orders should include specifications for diet, medications, treatments, and per State Operations Manual, Appendix PP—Guidance to Surveyors for Long-Term Care Facilities, §483.20(a) (CMS, 2014c, p. 130), "routine care to maintain or improve the resident's functional abilities until staff can conduct a comprehensive assessment and develop an interdisciplinary care plan."

Medication Administration Record (MAR)

The MAR is a record of the medications administered, and with certain medications, the resident's response. The MAR should accurately reflect providers' orders for medications, be updated with any changes, and accompany the resident prior to admission.

Evidence of Being Free of Tuberculosis

Residents should be tested for tuberculosis prior to or upon admission because it is a life-threatening disease that can spread to other residents and staff. This screening is part of the infection prevention and control program that the NHA is responsible for enforcing. Federal regulations, as stated in the State Operations Manual, Appendix PP—Guidance to

Surveyors for Long-Term Care Facilities, Intent: (F441) 42CFR 483.65 Infection Control (CMS, 2014c), require that "Tuberculosis screening on admission and following the discovery of a new case, and managing active cases consistent with State requirements" (p. 630).

History and Physical (H&P)

An H&P is a document reflecting the medical status of a resident at a certain point in time and should be provided to the facility prior to transfer. An H&P outlines the diagnoses, care, and treatment provided in the hospital and recommendations for follow-up. Within a specified time frame, the medical provider in the facility will complete a new H&P upon admission.

Discharge Summary

The **discharge summary** is a document created by a physician or licensed healthcare provider from the transferring setting. This document gives a summary of the resident's prior medical condition and care and can include admission and discharge date, name of physician, initial and final diagnoses, medications, laboratory test results, consultant, physician and nurse's progress notes, x-rays, and discharge instructions. This information is important when creating an initial care plan for the resident.

Admission Packet

Once admitted to the facility, the resident or responsible party completes the **admission packet**. The admission packet contains information that explains the resident's rights and obligations and gives an overview of daily operations in the facility. Items found in the admission packet are as follows.

Identification of Parties

This agreement identifies the names of the facility and the resident or the resident's representative. This is another step that verifies the identity of the resident and prevents such mishaps as billing under the wrong name or administering the wrong care to a resident.

Consent to Treatment

The **consent to treatment** form documents that the resident agrees to undergo routine and emergency nursing care in the facility. This general consent does not supersede the resident's right to decline specific care and treatment once in the facility, however.

Advance healthcare directive is a document that explains the resident's wishes for healthcare treatment in certain circumstances, such as when the resident is unable to make decisions. The directive is not required for admission, but the facility must offer assistance if the resident desires to prepare one. Please refer to Chapters 11 and 12 for additional detail on advance healthcare directives.

Resident Rights

Residents must sign a **resident rights acknowledgment** form that certifies that they have been informed of their individual rights in the facility. These rights should also be posted in an area of the facility visible to public view.

Financial Arrangement

A financial arrangement is a written agreement explaining how the facility will receive reimbursement for services provided to the resident. The facility should monitor the resident's method of payment monthly as it could change.

Transfers and Discharges

This is an explanation of the reasons why a resident can receive a change in room assignment or be transferred or discharged from a facility.

Bed Hold Policy

The facility's bed hold policy requires that the resident or responsible party be informed in writing of the option to reserve his bed prior to hospitalization or going on a therapeutic leave. The number of days a bed is held for a resident and the form of payment varies by state (CMS, 2014c).

Personal Property and Funds

Personal property is tracked on an inventory list, which is divided into two parts, one used upon admission to document resident belongings and the other used to document belongings taken upon discharge. It is important to create and maintain an accurate inventory in the event an item is reported missing. There are no federal regulations mandating a procedure to track resident belongings, but if a policy and procedure is created by the facility then it must be adhered to.

Residents have the option to set up a resident trust account, which is managed by the facility, similar to a bank account in that the resident can withdraw funds during designated times.

Photographs

This is notice that the facility takes the resident's photograph only for identification and healthcare purposes. Photographs taken of the resident cannot be used for any other purpose unless the resident gives prior written consent.

Confidentiality of Medical Information

Medical information must be kept confidential unless the resident gives written consent that the information can be disclosed to a relative, other person, or organization.

Facility Rules and Grievance Procedure

Facility rules, also known as house rules, are a list of expectations for all residents living in the facility. Examples include: no profane or improper language, no smoking inside the facility, and signing out when leaving for an outing.

The grievance procedure details how a resident can report a complaint or concern regarding facility services. A list of agencies is also provided that can be contacted in relation to the complaint.

Admission Agreement

The admission agreement is signed by the resident and representative of the facility, stating that all items in the admission packet have been reviewed and agreed upon.

Resident-Directed Move-In

The NHA directs the facility staff in developing an empathetic move-in process for both the resident and family. It is a good policy for staff to remember that it may be their 100th admission but it is the resident's first and should be treated with respect and dignity. The goal of a successful transition for the resident is aided by trained staff who understand the needs and interventions required by the resident and family. A **resident-directed move-in** is a process in which a resident's preferences are accommodated whenever possible as long as the health and safety of the resident are not at risk. For example, the resident may prefer to wake up later in the morning or go to sleep later in the evening than the other residents. This approach ensures a successful transition for the resident and the start of a trusting relationship between the staff and the resident/family.

Orientation to the Facility

The decision to relocate to a care facility and the subsequent adjustment are complex depending on the health status of the resident, family dynamics, and the circumstances by which the admission occurred. Focus group data indicate that residents and families experience orientation to a care facility as jarring, overwhelming, devastating, guilt-ridden, frightening, anger-provoking, saddening, and relieving all at once (Graneheim, Johansson, & Lindgren, 2013).

Predictors of a resident's successful transition to a facility are having a "buddy" on admission to assist with the adjustment, being involved in decision making, choosing a facility that follows a person-centered care model, and the way in which the orientation process is carried out (Sury, Burns, & Brodaty, 2013). Incorporating family members as care partners and implementing the life story of the resident into daily care can ease the strain of the adjustment period. These lifestyle preferences (e.g., gardening, painting) should then be included into the care plan so that the resident can continue to enjoy these activities (Graneheim et al., 2013; Lepore et al., 2013).

Orientation to the facility includes giving the resident a tour of the facility and introductions to other residents, including a roommate if applicable, and staff members. Orientation may ease the new resident into the facility, helping him feel welcome and more familiar with the surroundings.

Resident's Adjustment, Grief, and Loss

Transitions in life are associated with degrees of anxiety, and staff must be trained to recognize anxiety and the grief that may be present on admission as well as throughout the stay. Some individuals may experience **role exit**, the process of disengaging from central social roles and identities. Some residents will discover new social roles, including friendships, while others may feel helpless and dependent on others for care, which is a documented source of grief and loss for the older adult (Saunders & Heliker, 2008).

Many people express their identity through the display and attachment to material possessions. Adjusting to the physical dimensions of a new room and the regulatory restrictions that limit material possessions can be challenging. Letting go of possessions accumulated over a lifetime and downsizing to those items that will fit into the nursing home room may contribute to feelings of grief and loss.

Resident Assessment Instrument Process

The **Resident Assessment Instrument** (RAI) process includes the Minimum Data Set (MDS), Care Area Assessments (CAA), and the care plan.

The MDS and CAAs are used to assess the medical and psychosocial status of the resident as well as make care plan decisions. Information in the following areas is gathered and evaluated in this process:

1. Identification and demographic information.
2. Customary routine.
3. Cognitive patterns.
4. Communication.
5. Vision.
6. Mood and behavior patterns.
7. Psychological well-being.
8. Physical functioning and structural problems.
9. Continence.
10. Disease diagnosis and health conditions.
11. Dental and nutritional status.
12. Skin conditions.
13. Activity pursuit.
14. Medications.
15. Special treatments and procedures.
16. Discharge potential.
17. Documentation of summary information regarding the additional assessment performed on the care areas triggered by the completion of the Minimum Data Set (MDS).
18. Documentation of participation in assessment.

Observations and discussions with the resident, licensed and non-licensed staff, the resident's physician, family members, outside consultants, and a review of the resident's record can be used to accumulate information needed to address the foregoing areas (CMS, 2014c, p. 131).

Minimum Data Set (MDS)

The MDS is an instrument that contains item sets of information completed during the resident's stay in the facility. Initially, an MDS is done upon admission and then at predetermined intervals based on the payer source. For residents living in the facility (not just a temporary rehabilitative stay), the MDS is completed on a quarterly basis. Anytime a resident has a change in condition, another MDS assessment is completed. This information is entered into a software program chosen by the facility and then transmitted to CMS. For many payer sources, such as Medicare, the MDS drives the rate of reimbursement.

Care Area Assessment (CAA)

CAAs are areas that indicate "conditions, symptoms, and other areas of concern that are common in nursing home residents and are commonly identified or suggested by MDS findings" (CMS, 2013a, p. 2). This information is used in the development of an individualized care plan. Areas assessed include delirium, cognitive loss/dementia, activities of daily living (ADL), functional/rehabilitation potential, urinary incontinence and indwelling catheter, behavioral symptoms, falls, nutritional status, feeding tubes, pressure ulcer, physical restraints, pain, and return to community referral (CMS, 2013a).

Care Plan

The care plan must be developed for "(1) each resident that includes measurable objectives and timetables to meet a resident's medical, nursing, and mental and psychosocial needs that are identified in the comprehensive assessment" (CMS, 2014c, p. 150). The care plan must be developed by the interdisciplinary team and describe the following:

   i. The services that are to be furnished to attain or maintain the resident's highest practicable physical, mental, and psychosocial well-being. . . ; and
   ii. Any services that would otherwise be required .... but are not provided due to the resident's exercise of rights. . . , including the right to refuse treatment. (CMS, 2014c, p. 150)

It is the responsibility of the NHA to ensure that facility staff complete the comprehensive care plan within 7 days after the comprehensive assessment is completed (CMS, 2014c). Care plans are dynamic documents that must be updated if the resident's status changes. Care plans are explained further in Chapters 12 and 13.

Care Plan Conference

Good communication is an essential part of any well-run facility. One way for staff to communicate with residents and families is through individualized care plan conferences that are held quarterly or more often as necessary. Several staff members attend care conferences, including nursing, dietary, social services, activities, and physical therapy. These disciplines, along with the resident and family, attend the meeting to ask questions and provide valuable input that helps individualize the care plan.

Identifying and Honoring the Resident's Voice

Engaging in a resident-centered care model means ensuring that residents' wishes are assessed and incorporated in the plan of care. Residents should be encouraged to make decisions regarding their care to the greatest extent possible. An example of **identifying resident preferences** is when staff inquire about and honor a resident's bathing preferences. Traditional shower and bathing schedules are rarely revisited in care facilities that follow an institutional model. A shift to resident-centered care allows for the revision of shower and bathing schedules to *honor residents' preferences* whenever possible and should be documented in the care plan.

The resident's preferences, such as daily living habits, should be shared with facility staff. These preferences need to be part of a continued dialogue in the facility so adjustments can be made to the care plan as changes occur.

Nursing

Resident respect and dignity should be considered by the nursing staff when completing the physical assessment and delivering care. For example, privacy curtains should be drawn closed when a bed bath or other personal care is given. Residents should not be rushed to respond to questions regarding their medications, pain levels, and cognitive ability but allowed time to carefully consider answers. Remembering events and processing the meaning of past experiences can play an integral role in providing accurate answers to medical questions.

Dietary

As people age or endure the effects of multiple diagnoses, eating preferences and tastes may change (refer to Chapter 11). Medications may impact taste and appetite or cause side effects, like nausea or constipation. A resident's quality of life can be closely associated with food and the overall dining experience. Honoring food preferences and allowing liberalized diets offer residents greater choice. Sometimes, a resident makes a choice contrary to the provider's orders and the facility must demonstrate that the resident has been advised of the risks and benefits of this choice and document the outcome of the conversation. Resident choices should be clearly documented in the comprehensive assessment, care plan, and progress notes and reviewed at least quarterly with the resident, family, and/or responsible party.

Social Services

The social service department is responsible for meeting the psychosocial needs of residents and providing emotional support to residents, families, and staff. Federal regulations mandate that "The facility must provide medically-related social services to attain or maintain the highest practicable physical, mental, and psychosocial well-being of each resident" (CMS, 2014c, p. 119). Social services support residents and families in adjusting to life in the facility, accessing resources, identifying strengths to cope with challenges, and providing emotional support. Social services also support staff through in-service training, and providing grief counseling when residents die.

Activities

The goal of a robust activities department is resident engagement in meaningful activities. Traditional models of long-term care assign staff to choose, plan, and implement the activities and ensure resident attendance. As the traditional model of long-term care evolves to resident-centered care, residents participate in the creation of the activity schedule and decide whether to partake.

Residents in long-term care should be afforded the opportunity to continue to grow and develop through programs and hobbies. The role of the activity professional is to assist in creating an environment in which the residents can embrace lifelong routines and habits, such as hobbies and spiritual practices, as long as they do not interfere with the rights of others. Residents should have time in their day for solitude as well as socializing with friends and family.

Activities should be tailored for residents with dementia and other cognitive impairments that contribute to their quality of life and do not cause frustration. All staff must help each resident find value and have a sense of purpose by engagement in meaningful activities.

Performance Improvement

Quality Assurance (QA)

The QA program is used by the facility to monitor and study the quality of services it delivers, and to make recommendations for improvement (National Association of Long-Term Care Administrator Boards, 2003).

This requirement of the federal regulations for long-term care providers has been in effect since the inception of OBRA in 1987.

Before OBRA, the facility's process to solve quality issues was often a reaction to regulatory deficiencies and other problems. Attempts to resolve these regulatory deficiencies and problems often resulted in blaming staff and additional processes that added complex audits and thresholds that were often unsustainable. QA meetings associated with quality were often data exchanges with little or no discussion or problem solving. Many facilities were successful on the surface, but deep sustainable process change was often not achieved.

Performance Improvement (PI)

PI is also known as quality improvement (QI) and is

a pro-active and continuous study of processes with the intent to prevent or decrease the likelihood of problems by identifying areas of opportunity and testing new approaches to fix underlying causes of persistent/systemic problems. PI in nursing homes aims to improve processes involved in health care delivery and resident quality of life. (CMS, 2014d, p. 1)

Quality Assurance and Performance Improvement (QAPI)

QAPI combines quality assurance and performance improvement to increase the quality of care and services delivered in nursing home facilities. It is accomplished by

a data-driven, proactive approach to improving the quality of life, care, and services in nursing homes. The activities of QAPI involve members at all levels of the organization to: identify opportunities for improvement; address gaps in systems or processes; develop and implement an improvement or corrective plan; and continuously monitor effectiveness of interventions. (CMS, 2014d, p. 1)

The official implementation of QAPI was started on June 7, 2013 (CMS, 2013b).

Five Elements of QAPI

The five elements of QAPI include the following:

1. Design and scope: All services in the facility should be addressed by QAPI. The program goal is to improve management practices and quality of life and enhance resident choices and clinical care.

2. Governance and leadership: Leadership should include staff, residents, and responsible parties or family members. The NHA should maintain responsibility for direction and guidance, but governance should be shared throughout the facility. The environment should welcome and respect all suggestions for improvement projects. Employees should never be subjected to reprisal for identifying areas for improvement or performance concerns.

3. Feedback, data systems, and monitoring: Multiple data sources are used to create performance improvement through evaluating adverse events, addressing performance indicators, and listening to the voice of stakeholders.

4. Performance improvement projects (PIPs): When a problem area is identified, a committee is developed that includes staff affected by the issue, family members, residents, and sometimes even community members. They begin working on a PIP. The project may be concentrated in one area or throughout the facility and involves gathering information to clarify issues and implement solutions.

5. Systematic analysis and systemic action: Highly organized and structured approach to determine whether identified problems and areas needing improvement may be caused or worsened by the way care and services are organized or delivered (CMS, n.d.).

Quality Assessment and Assurance (QAA)

The QAA committee is mandated by federal regulations, and while only required to meet quarterly, many facilities choose to meet monthly. The goal of the committee is to implement the QAPI program by identifying, implementing, and evaluating performance improvement projects. Monitoring the effect of the changes is necessary to ensure enhanced outcomes for residents. If necessary, action plans are revised and implemented. Committee members include the director of nursing, a physician designated by the facility, and at least three other members of the facility's staff (CMS, 2014c).

Quality Measure/Indicator Reports

Quality Measure/Indicator Reports (QM/QIs) contain information such as gender, age, and functional ability and are used by the NHA as indicators of potential problems or concerns in the facility. These reports can be used by the facility as a tool to rate its performance compared to the state and to target areas of care for improvement. Because the data reports can be generated for sequential time frames, they are also useful to track trends. (CMS, 2012, p. 1)

There are three QM/QI reports. The first is the Facility Characteristics Report, which provides demographic information about the resident population, such as gender, age, payment source, and diagnostic characteristics for a selected facility compared to all other facilities in the state. The second is the Facility Quality Measure/Indicator Report, which lists the facility status as a percentile as compared to state and national averages for each of the MDS-based quality measures. Higher percentiles may indicate an area the facility should investigate further using the QAPI process.

The third report is the Resident Level Quality Measure/Indicator Report, which identifies residents (based on MDS data) who may need further assessment of functional abilities (CMS, 2014a).

Program for Evaluating Payment Patterns Electronic Report (PEPPER)

The PEPPER report is used by the NHA to identify potentially incorrect Medicare payments. "Target areas" are identified in the PEPPER data report, which the NHA can use to evaluate payments received for services billed. This task is important because payments received due to inappropriate billing can be construed as an attempt to defraud Medicare. The report also compares the facility to other facilities in the same jurisdiction, state, and nation. These data are important because they aid the NHA in identifying potentially inappropriate billing practices by evaluating the facility's billing practices and comparing them to others. PEPPER is developed and distributed by TMF Health Quality Institute, under contract with the CMS (TMF Health Quality Institute, n.d.).

Data Management

A study done in 2013 found that NHAs may lack basic knowledge of quality improvement tools and overall capability to conform to the new Quality Assurance and Performance Improvement (QAPI) regulations (Smith, Castle, & Hyer, 2013).

This section is going to teach some incredibly powerful, deceptively simple statistical concepts, with very few tools. A mind-set and cultural language of process-oriented thinking will change the focus from "meeting the goal" to creating a culture that is "perfectly designed" to meet any goal.

Regardless of whether people understand statistics, *they are already using statistics.*

Imagine yourself as the facility NHA in a meeting to discuss incident reports. Also in attendance is the director of nurses, the medical director, a few department managers, and key floor staff.

Everyone is looking at the same **data** (a collection of numerical observations) display of incident reports, but what each person might find useful or interesting will differ. You, the NHA, may be most concerned about the number of incidents that resulted in transfer to the hospital and whether it is higher or lower than what you expected. So, you draw a circle around those numbers. The director of nurses may be most concerned about the number of resident-to-resident altercations on the memory care unit, so she circles those numbers and writes notes on her report. She announces that there are "too many" altercations and then asks, "What can we do about it?" The floor nurses are pleased to see that there were fewer falls this month than last month and there go the circles again.

All these different perceptions, opinions, and interpretations describe **human variation**. Conversations are filled with statements like, "There are too many [fill in the blank]" or "What happened that we had so fewer [fill in the blank] than last quarter—what is staff doing differently?" and "Why can't they do that again this month?"

At face value, these may seem like useful statements and questions. They result in well-intentioned people doing the best they can, making decisions about actions that could ultimately cause more disruption and confusion, and adding unnecessary, additional complexity rather than improvement.

Process-Oriented Context

A process is a sequence of tasks that transforms inputs into outputs. For example, transcribing a physician's order, changing a dressing, sending out monthly resident statements, conducting an assessment, and creating the monthly activity calendar or menu are all processes.

Every aspect of every person's job is a process. From housekeeping to dietary, from social work to nursing, every action is part of a process. And guess what? Those processes are perfectly designed to get the results they are already getting. You might be thinking, "You mean to tell me that when a resident falls or when a medication order is not carried out properly, that the system is perfectly designed to do that?" Yes! But do not make the mistake of thinking that the process cannot improve, that the number of falls can't be decreased or the number of medication errors lowered. However, until leadership understands variation in a **process-oriented context** (a framework for considering improvement efforts), they will continue to treat things that "shouldn't" happen as unique events, which, believe it or not, need a totally different approach if the system is perfectly designed to have them (Balestracci, 2015).

By understanding the nature of processes, a deeper question can be asked: Is the *process* that produced the current number different from the *process* that produced the previous numbers? In other words, was there a formal method in place for improvement or was it just exhortation to "get better"? To paraphrase one saying of the late Joseph Juran's (quality giant of the 20th century), "There is no such thing as 'improvement in general'" (Juran, 1995).

Approaching improvement from a process-oriented context means recognizing poor and useless data displays and analyses. In 1995, Dr. Donald Berwick, MD (2002), who may be the leading authority on healthcare improvement in the world, made a profound statement:

> Plotting measurements over time turns out, in my view, to be one of the most powerful devices we have for systemic learning. . . Several important things happen when you plot data over time. First, you have to ask what data to plot. In the exploration of the answer you begin to clarify aims, and also to see the system from a wider viewpoint. Where are the data? What do they mean? To whom? Who should see them? Why? These are questions that integrate and clarify aims and systems all at once. . . When important indicators are continuously monitored, it becomes easier and easier to study the effects of innovation in real time. . . If you follow only one piece of advice from this lecture when you get home, pick a measurement you care about and begin to plot it regularly over time. You won't be sorry. (pp. 82–83)

New results will require new conversations, and this simple technique will create these new conversations.

Here are process-oriented questions that can begin more in-depth discussion on any processes in your facility (Berwick, 1989):

- Do you ever waste time waiting, when you should not have to?

- Do you ever redo your work because something failed the first time?

- Do the procedures you use waste steps, duplicate efforts, or frustrate you through their unpredictability?

- Is information that you need ever lost?

- Does communication ever fail?

What types of things are you observing because of these process breakdowns? How do these events compromise resident care?

Run Charts—Just Plot the Dots!

A **run chart** is the very first step of any analysis. It is a simple yet powerful graph with data plotted in their naturally occurring time order with the **median** (the number at which half of the data fall above the middle data point and half fall below) drawn in as a reference line. For example, the number of pressure ulcers each month, the number of outstanding accounts receivable each week, or the number of antipsychotic medications being administered, to name just a few (see Chapter 15).

The purpose of the run chart is to determine whether process behavior has been consistent over the time period or whether there were shifts in performance. Proper interpretation of the data plotted on the run chart will facilitate a deeper analysis (Balestracci, 2015).

Variation

Think of **variation** as a gap between where a process "is" (the number it is producing) and where it can or should "be." Reducing variation ultimately yields a more predicable process. W. Edwards Deming (another 20th-century statistician) is quoted as saying, "If I had to reduce my message to management to just a few words, I'd say it all has to do with reducing variation" (Snee, 2006). There are two kinds of variation: common cause and special cause. Treating one as the other will generally make things worse (certainly not better), and pretending variation is not there will not make it go away.

Common cause variation. Think of your commute to work. Some days, all the lights are red and you get stuck behind every school bus and encounter three traffic accidents. On other days, you fly to work, zip through green lights, and miss all the buses. You may get to work 10 minutes earlier than "usual." There is nothing special, nothing to explain. It just is. And, especially in the latter case getting all the green lights, it cannot be intentionally reproduced.

Common cause variation refers to the natural range of an output from a stable process. There is an "average," but no one can predict any specific result in advance; however, the naturally encountered range of results is quite predictable.

Further, the ability to explain a change after the fact does not necessarily make it unique or "special": "I was late because I got all the red lights coming to work." You know that will happen a couple of times a year predictably—you just cannot predict exactly when. Another day, you get all green lights coming to work. Super! Can you *make* it happen? Of course not—how absurd. It is still common cause variation (Balestracci, 2015).

Special cause variation. **Special cause variation** means specific issues show up from outside the current process. It can be a one-time event, which would cause a "spike" in the time plot—or a planned intervention, which would cause a shift in the previous process average. It may be unintended or perhaps even desirable and appropriate. These events are outside the norm and can be easily detected by a time plot of data, a run chart (Balestracci, 2015).

Examples of special causes (things acting on the current process) are a new charge nurse, changing a policy or procedure, using a new assessment form, or changing pharmacies. These are events that act on the current process or system that may cause one or more data points to be outside the norm.

Unfortunately, human tendency is to treat *all* variation as special cause (needing a specific explanation). Often, the knee-jerk reaction is to do yet another root cause analysis without examining the system in which the incidents are occurring by asking these questions (Balestracci, 2015): Was this a truly unique event (special cause) or was it waiting to happen (common cause)? If different people had been involved, could it still have happened (common cause)? In fact, is a similar type of incident "waiting" to happen somewhere else (common cause)?

There are two tests to identify special cause variation: (1) statistically defining a **trend** (rarely occurs) and (2) identifying a "**clump of eight**" data points either all *consecutively* above the median or below the median. In either case, some outside force happened to the system and caused it to change and created a new process (Balestracci, 2015).

First, one must understand the deceptiveness of the word "trend" and dispel some common misunderstandings.

Trend. This term is bandied about, masquerading as an "explanation" as people look for reasons why some key indicators went up or down or didn't achieve established targets. And, the problem is that people will find those reasons and treat every assumed "trend" as something special, while more than likely it is not. A widespread misconception of the word "trend" is all, or some, of the data points going up or down. But there is human variation (different perceptions) in how exactly how many data points would make various people conclude a trend existed (Balestracci, 2015).

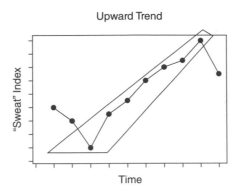

Figure 14.1   Upward Trend

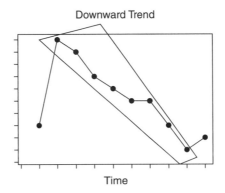

Figure 14.2   Downward Trend

Let's use some simple theory: The statistical definition of a trend is a cluster of seven data points either all going up or all going down (six successive increases or decreases). See Figure 14.1 for an upward trend and Figure 14.2 for a downward trend.

Consider a trend in a process-oriented context as a signal that the process is *in transition*. The process was previously perfectly designed to get the results it was getting, and then an intervention was introduced. The process is transitioning to what it is perfectly designed to get given its new inputs. And here is the key point—the process is transitioning to what it is perfectly designed to get now *and then it will level off again*.

So, for purposes of improvement, trend = transition.

Look at the run chart in Figure 14.3. Notice that time (in this case months) is the horizontal axis. The vertical axis is the indicator being counted, falls. Using the run chart of the falls data, one can see that there are no trends.

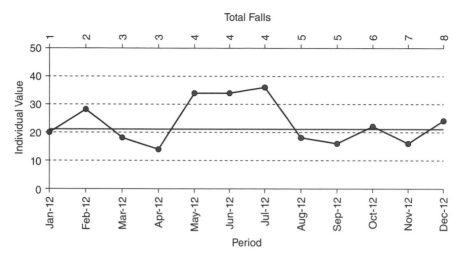

Figure 14.3   Data Shows No Trends

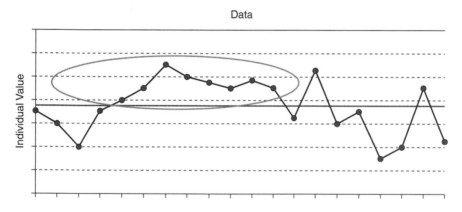

Figure 14.4   Clump of Eight Special Cause

Clump of eight. The second test to determine if there is special cause variation present is the "clump of eight" consecutive data points either all above or all below the median. This indicates the presence of at least one significant shift in the process in the time plotted. "Something" happened! That's all we know at this point. . . that something happened. Figure 14.4 shows a clump of eight special cause (Balestracci, 2015).

Strategies for Improvement: The Fun Stuff!

What happens when staff employs spontaneous reactions and haphazardly implements "improvement" actions? Consider this example of a common problem in nursing facilities, urinary tract infections (UTIs). A facility is experiencing a high number of UTIs. Management immediately jumps to the conclusion that it must be a hand-washing problem and arranges hand-washing in-services for everyone. While hand washing is certainly important, it was not the problem in this case. So, they tried reducing urinary catheters. Yes, another good intervention but still not the problem. So, they tried reviewing the culture and sensitivity (C&S) lab reports, only to find an abundance of a particular bacteria called E. coli. It turns out that the problem was peri-care and that fecal matter was getting into the urinary system—hence the UTIs. Only after wasted time on unnecessary in-services and wasted money paying staff to attend the unnecessary in-services did management "land on the answer."

Wasting time and money is problematic enough, but the biggest negative outcome in this scenario was increased cynicism from staff. Had leadership been trained in how to use a simple run chart and determine what type of variation they were dealing with, the waste would have been detected, acted on appropriately, and eliminated.

Most problems arise from common cause variation. Developing improvement actions for common cause and special cause variation requires distinctly different managerial approaches in order to be effective. The human tendency is to address a "vague" problem with a "vague" solution, guaranteeing a "vague" result, many times a misuse of the currently favored technique of rapid-cycle **Plan-Do-Study-Act** (PDSA) (a process to test an improvement effort; see Balestracci, 2014).

The Pareto principle. Using the key concept of Joseph Juran's beloved **Pareto principle** (Juran, 2002), one can focus improvement efforts by asking—and answering—"What are the 20% of these types of occurrences that cause 80% of the actual occurrences?" The Pareto principle states that 80% of the variation is generally caused by only 20% of the process inputs. Think of it this way (Balestracci, 2015): "What are the 20% of the organizational processes causing 80% of your problems?" Or yet, one more very direct way, "What 20% of the numbers cause 80% of the sweat?"

For example, 80% of the outstanding accounts receivable are from 20% of the payer sources. Or, 80% of the pressure ulcers are associated with 20% use of a particular type of bed. And one more, 80% of the facility's complaints are due to 20% of the potential improvement opportunities. Focusing with laser-like intensity on the data with the most potential yields big payoffs. Now, time, money, and effort are being spent wisely for a good return on investment.

First, always **exhaust in-house data.** That is, use the data you have already collected. This is the initial strategy when considering an improvement action dealing with common cause variation. Begin by look-ing at a sample of raw data from any routine meeting and objectively ask (Balestracci, 2015):

- What could these data tell you?

- What is actually being done with these data?

- What graphical displays are being used?

- What is the reliance on using tables of raw numbers?

- What actions result from these data?

- Does staff consider whether the variation being acted on is common or special cause?

- And the most important question: Does a plot of these data over time exist? If not, how could you construct one? (p. 151)

Answering these questions allows you to do two very important things before involving teams of people or doing cumbersome additional data collections in addition to the routine ones:

1. It allows you to find out what is "wrong" with the data. A very famous statistician once said, "The more you know what is wrong with your data, the more useful it becomes."

2. It allows you to establish a baseline estimate of the extent of the problem, from which to assess the effects of interventions. One of the biggest reasons many projects fail is lack of a good baseline estimate. Teams are working on a "vague" problem with no idea of the extent of the problem, or whether their efforts improved the situation!

Stratification. **Stratification** is a tool that lends focus to a "vague" problem (Balestracci, 2015). What if, instead of looking at only 1 month's falls data, you analyzed 17 months' worth of data for a total of 162 falls? Rather than ask useless questions like, "Why did we have more falls this month/quarter than last month/quarter?" or worse yet, treating every fall as special cause, and doing root cause analysis on each, you looked at the bigger picture and asked meaningful questions. If a run chart of the 17 months showed common cause variation, the result would be a totally more productive set of questions that would then guide the improvement effort.

Now, sort the 162 falls into groups or categories based on different factors:

- Day of the week

- Activity at time of fall

- Type of injury
- Time of day
- Use of assistive device

Encourage staff to get creative! This sorting process is called stratification. The purpose is to look for patterns in the way that the data points cluster or do not cluster, which will lead to yet a more intelligent analysis, as will be demonstrated shortly.

Stratification takes a vague problem, looks at it as a process, and identifies the 20% of the process causing 80% of the problem. It enables specific focus.

Figure 14.5 demonstrates an example of stratification of the falls data. This stratification tool is called a **Pareto matrix** and may very well be one of the most useful diagnostic tools that you can employ as an NHA.

Notice that Unit A has the second highest number of falls but almost 75% come from just two categories, falls while walking and transferring. In fact, all three units had higher numbers of falls while transferring, culminating in almost one-third of the total falls. Take a look at Unit C—this unit had 25 falls from wheelchairs (the other two units combined only had 8), which contributed to the highest number of total falls for the three units, at 44%. How does this focus your improvement plan?

Compare this to more typical, arbitrary interventions like a "falls in-service," or putting every resident on the falls program.

Sometimes, one can further focus on the areas that are causing 80% of the problems. More information may be needed, and getting appropriate staff involved *would not waste their precious time*.

Reducing confusion and complexity through process-oriented thinking will reduce costs and save time. Learn to use data and statistics to simplify

Event	Unit			Total
Type	A	B	C	
Walking	24	2	8	34
Wheelchair	6	2	25	33
Toileting	5	6	2	13
Found on Floor	0	8	11	19
Rolled from Bed	4	0	8	12
Transferring	18	15	18	51
Totals	57	33	72	162

Figure 14.5   Pareto Matrix of the Falls Data

and unify improvement efforts and enjoy the benefits you will ultimately reap. . . as will the residents.

Surveys

Surveys are conducted by state and federal surveyors to determine if the facility is in compliance with CMS participation requirements. Participation requirements set minimum standards of care that the facility must meet to continue receiving reimbursement for its Medicare and Medicaid residents. Facilities strive to exceed these minimum standards since the goal is to continuously improve the quality of care and quality of life for residents.

The survey inspection process is resident-centered, outcome-oriented, and based on information from a sample of residents (CMS, 2014a). Surveys are performed annually within a survey window of 90 days before or after the current facility's licensing expiration date.

The role of the NHA is to ensure that facility policies and procedures are in alignment with state and federal regulations and staff are well trained in their implementation. The NHA must have an in-depth knowledge of the State Operations Manual (SOM), Appendix P—Survey Protocol for Long-Term Care Facilities and State Operations Manual, Appendix PP—Guidance to Surveyors for Long-Term Care Facilities and ensure that department managers have access to those regulations that pertain to their departments.

Survey Management

Once an official survey begins, the NHA or designee becomes the main contact person who communicates with the surveyors and staff. Staff may feel nervous during a survey, and the NHA must maintain an environment that is calm and professional. Residents are also interviewed by surveyors, and the NHA is responsible for ensuring residents do not feel overwhelmed. The NHA should manage the survey process in a manner that creates a non-adversarial relationship with surveyors.

The facility that is always "survey-ready" requires that staff and management have a proficient understanding of the regulations and their implementation. This "always ready" policy is optimum since surveyors can enter the facility unannounced and/or when the NHA is not available.

The NHA must be acutely aware of the performance of each department and monitor facility operations daily. Daily rounds, stand-up meetings with department supervisors, discussions with residents and family members, and periodic checks of equipment and plant maintenance are examples of NHA activities that keep the facility ready for the next survey. Some NHAs and department supervisors perform practice surveys to review clinical and non-clinical operations to identify areas for improvement. Practice surveys offer an opportunity to audit the facility's compliance with federal and state regulations.

Initial Certification Survey

This survey is performed by state and or federal surveyors before a nursing home facility can obtain a license to open and to receive CMS reimbursement for Medicaid- and Medicare-approved services. The surveyors use the Traditional Standard and Extended Survey models, described in the next section, to review the facility for regulatory compliance. Their emphasis during the survey is on the residents, their rights, and the physical environment (CMS, 2014a).

Traditional Survey

The Traditional Survey, used since 1995, refers to the original paper-based survey. The State Operations Manual, Appendix P—Survey Protocol for Long-Term Care Facilities, details the protocol used to identify the number of residents to review and investigate for potentially deficient practices. There are five surveys used in the Traditional Survey model. These surveys gather information and identify nursing, medical, and administrative practices that do not comply with state and federal regulations. The names and purposes of the surveys are as follows:

1. The Traditional Standard Survey is a two-phase process used to complete the survey. Phase I uses data gathered from quality indicator reports routinely sent to CMS, past survey results, and a current tour of the facility. Phase II includes a focused review of concerns identified in Phase I and other tasks that give surveyors information about facility operations. See Figure 14.6 for a listing of these tasks.

    There are seven tasks completed during this survey. Task 1 is completed during Phase I and prior to entering the facility. Tasks 2 through 7 are completed during Phase II and while the surveyors are in the facility.

2. The Traditional Extended Survey is performed after a Traditional Survey when **substandard quality of care** is found in **resident behavior** and facility practices, quality of life, and/or quality of care. Resident behavior means that any resident care by the staff "must be based on a detailed assessment of physical, psychological and behavioral symptoms and underlying causes as well as potential situational or environmental reasons for the behaviors" (CMS, 2013a, p. 15). If the staff cannot explain the rationale for the care, the care

Task 1 – Offsite Survey Preparation

Task 2 – Entrance Conference/Onsite Preparatory Activities

Task 3 – Initial Tour

Task 4 – Resident Sample Selection

Task 5 – Information Gathering

      Sub-Task 5A – General Observations of the Facility

      Sub-Task 5B – Kitchen/Food Service Observation

      Sub-Task 5C – Resident Review

      Sub-Task 5D – Quality of Life Assessment

      Sub-Task 5E – Medication Pass and Pharmacy Services

      Sub-Task 5F – Quality Assessment and Assurance Review

      Sub-Task 5G – Abuse Prohibition Review

Task 6 – Information Analysis for Deficiency Determination

Task 7 – Exit Conference

Figure 14.6   The Seven Traditional Survey Tasks
Source: CMS. (2014a).

may be inappropriate. To be considered substandard quality of care, the scope and severity of the deficiency must be classified as a letter F, H, I, J, K, or L on the Scope and Severity chart. Refer to the Scope and Severity section and Figure 14.9 (CMS, 2014a, p. 88).

3. The Traditional Abbreviated Standard Survey is performed in the following two situations:
   a. Complaint against the facility is investigated. If found valid, facility practices must be corrected.
   b. Change in the organization or management of the facility (e.g., NHA or director of nursing). The survey determines if there is a decline in quality of care due to the change in organization or management (CMS, 2014a, p. 91).

4. The Traditional Partial Extended Survey is performed after a Traditional Abbreviated Standard Survey when substandard quality of care was found in resident behavior and facility practices, quality of life, and/or quality of care (CMS, 2014a, p. 88).

5. The Traditional Post-Survey Revisit (Follow-Up) is performed after the Traditional Survey, Traditional Extended Survey, Traditional Abbreviated Standard Survey, or Traditional Partial Extended Survey(s) to confirm that the facility has corrected deficiencies found in the original survey and that the facility remains in compliance with state and federal regulations (CMS, 2014a, p. 90).

Quality Indicator Survey (QIS) Process

The Traditional Survey was solely used until CMS developed the QIS to improve the consistency, accuracy, effectiveness, and objectivity of the Traditional Survey's results. In 2005, a QIS pilot program was initiated. A national rollout began in 2007, and by December 2011, 26 states had transitioned to this survey process. The most recent state to adopt QIS was South Carolina in 2012. The survey rollout was suspended due to the evaluation results on the benefits of QIS.

Advantages of the QIS survey are more timely and effective feedback, systematic review of requirements and events, and enhanced documentation of the survey through automation. Evaluation results, however, showed no differences in accuracy between the Traditional Survey and QIS. Therefore, no additional states will transition to the QIS process until CMS can improve the QIS process in states where it is currently employed (CMS, 2015b).

There are four surveys used under the QIS model. These surveys gather information and identify nursing, medical, and administrative practices that do not comply with state and federal regulations. The names and purposes of the surveys are as follows:

1. QIS Standard Survey: This survey is completed in two stages. Stage 1 consists of off-site data analysis and data collection at the facility. Surveyors collect data through observations, interviews, and medical record reviews. Stage 2 consists of a systematic investigation that focuses on areas that triggered concerns in Stage 1.

    The QIS Standard Survey consists of nine tasks performed by the surveyors. Task 1 is completed prior to entering the facility. Tasks 2 to 9 are completed in the facility. See Figure 14.7 for activities done in each task and the primary subtasks.

2. QIS Extended Survey: Performed when substandard quality of care is found during the QIS Standard Survey in one or more of the following areas: resident behavior and facility practices, quality of life, and/or quality of care (CMS, 2014a, p. 9).

3. QIS Post-Survey Revisit (Follow-Up): Performed after the QIS standard and/or extended survey to revisit and reevaluate specific care and services cited as not meeting regulatory compliance (CMS, 2014a, p. 10).

4. QIS Complaint Survey Procedures: Performed to investigate any complaints made during the QIS Standard Survey (State Operations Manual, Appendix P—Survey Protocol for Long-Term Care Facilities, 2014, pp. 7–11; CMS, 2014a, p. 11).

Task 1 – Offsite Survey Preparation

Task 2 – Onsite Preparatory Activities and Entrance Conference

Task 3 – Initial Tour

Task 4 – Stage 1 Survey Tasks

      Finalize Sample Selection

      Team Meetings

      Information Gathering

      Admission Sample Review (Medical Record Review)

      Census Sample Review (Includes: Resident Interviews and Observations, Staff Interviews, Medical Record Review and Family Interviews)

Task 5 – Non-Staged Survey Tasks

      Resident Council President/Representative Interview

      Dining Observation

      Kitchen/Food Service Observation

      Infection Control Policies and Practices

      Demand Billing Review

      Abuse Prohibition Review

      Quality Assessment and Assurance Review

Task 6 – Transition From Stage I to Stage II

      Update the Resident Pool

      Review Completion of Stage I

      Review Surveyor-Initiated Residents and/or Care Areas

      Import All Data into the Primary Laptop

      Review the Relevant Findings Report

      Review the QCI Results Report

Task 7 – Stage II Survey Tasks

      Introduction

      Team Meetings

      Stage II Sample Selection (Substituting Residents, Supplementing the Sample)

      Staff Assignments

      Stage II Information Gathering (Stage II Critical Element Pathways, Medication Administration Observation and Unnecessary Drug Review)

      Facility-Level Investigations (Environmental Observation, Resident Funds, Admission, Transfer, and Discharge Review, Sufficient Staff)

Task 8 – Analysis and Decision-Making: Integration of Facility-Level Information and Critical Element Pathways, Analysis of Information Gained, Scope and Severity and Team Decision-Making)

Task 9 – Exit Conference

Figure 14.7   The Nine Quality Indicator Survey Tasks and Main Subtasks

Source: CMS (2014a).

Minimum Data Set (MDS) Survey

The MDS survey was created by CMS in mid-2014 to evaluate the Minimum Data Set Version 3.0 (MDS 3.0) coding practices and their relationship to resident care. Five states have undergone this type of survey; in 2015 CMS plans to expand the use of these surveys nationwide. CMS plans to expand the scope of the survey to include an assessment of reported staffing levels and to verify changes in staffing levels throughout the year. Information obtained from the MDS survey will accomplish more accurate billing practices and help ensure quality of care (CMS, 2014b).

Exit Conference

After the survey is complete, the surveyors hold an **exit conference** to discuss the findings and possible areas of deficient practice. This is a preliminary verbal report given to the NHA and other members of the team. The exit conference, held on the last day of the survey, provides an opportunity for the facility team to discuss the deficiencies with the surveyors and supply additional information that can negate some or all of the findings (CMS, 2014a; State Operations Manual, Appendix P—Survey Protocol for Long-Term Care Facilities, 2014).

Form 2567

The facility receives the statement of **deficiencies** (state and/or federal regulations that were not adequately met by the facility's operations) on a form called Form 2567 within 10 days of the exit conference. Form 2567 contains two sections. The first section lists deficiencies cited by the surveyors as needing correction. Each deficiency is assigned a letter A through L, denoting its scope and severity. Scope and severity are discussed in the next section of this chapter.

The second section of the form is called the Plan of Correction (POC), which reflects

> the facility's plan for corrective action and the anticipated time of correction (an explicit date must be shown). If the action has been completed when the form is returned, the plan should indicate the date completed. The date indicated for completion of the corrective action must be appropriate to the level of the deficiency(ies). (CMS, 1999, p. 2)

The facility must return Form 2567 within 10 calendar days after receipt to the Department of Public Health (Department). The Department or CMS must accept the POC in order for the facility to continue participating in the federal and state certification program. Form 2567 is available on the Nursing Home Compare website (www.medicare.gov/nursinghomecompare; see Figure 14.8) and must also be readily available in the facility.

Scope and Severity

The scope and severity of each deficiency are represented by an assigned letter. The letter can range from A through L. Letter A represents a deficiency with the least severity and scope and letter L the highest. This letter grade is used by CMS to determine the seriousness of the deficiency. See Figure 14.9 (Med-Pass, 2014).

The vertical column on the left of the chart represents the four possible severity levels. The second space from the bottom of this column signifies the lowest severity level and the top space the highest. The spaces at the bottom called Isolated, Pattern, and Widespread designate the scope of the deficiency. An isolated deficiency represents a scope level that impacts one or a very limited number of staff and/or residents or a limited number of locations in the facility. A pattern represents a scope level where staff and/or residents are affected in a limited number of locations. Widespread denotes a scope level that is prevalent throughout the facility and has the potential to affect large numbers of staff and/or residents.

Substandard quality of care is represented in spaces marked by letters F and H to L and gray shaded areas. When a substandard level of care is cited, the facility automatically enters the extended survey.

A **remedy category** is assigned to letters D to L. The remedy category indicates the corrective action required from the facility and can include financial penalties, temporary management as designated by the Department of Health and Human Services, and termination of the CMS reimbursement contract. Letters A to C are not assigned a remedy category because they designate a deficiency that is in substantial compliance with the regulations and is shown on the chart by solid black boxes. The penalty for a letter A is a notice of isolated deficiency and requires a commitment from the facility to correct the deficiency. Letters B and C require a Plan of Correction from the facility to prevent the deficiency from reoccurring. Letters D to L require an action from the facility dictated by the remedy categories. An area with an asterisk denotes that the State or CMS may impose one or more remedy categories along with or instead of termination of the provider agreement when either entity finds that the facility is out of compliance with the requirements of participation (CMS, 2014a; State Operations Manual, Appendix P—Survey Protocol for Long-Term Care Facilities, 2014).

DEPARTMENT OF HEALTH AND HUMAN SERVICES
CENTERS FOR MEDICARE & MEDICAID SERVICES

FORM APPROVED
OMB NO. 0938-0391

STATEMENT OF DEFICIENCIES AND PLAN OF CORRECTION	(X1) PROVIDER/SUPPLIER/CLIA IDENTIFICATION NUMBER:	(X2) MULTIPLE CONSTRUCTION A. BUILDING ______ B. WING ______	(X3) DATE SURVEY COMPLETED
NAME OF FACILITY	STREET ADDRESS, CITY, STATE, ZIP CODE		

(X4) ID PREFIX TAG	SUMMARY STATEMENT OF DEFICIENCIES (EACH DEFICIENCY SHOULD BE PRECEDED BY FULL REGULATORY OR LSC IDENTIFYING INFORMATION)	ID PREFIX TAG	PLAN OF CORRECTION (EACH CORRECTIVE ACTION SHOULD BE CROSS-REFERRED TO THE APPROPRIATE DEFICIENCY)	(X5) COMPLETION DATE

Any deficiency statement ending with an asterisk (*) denotes a deficiency which the institution may be excused from correcting providing it is determined that other safeguards provide sufficient protection to the patients. *(See reverse for further instructions.)* Except for nursing homes, the findings stated above are disclosable 90 days following the date of survey whether or not a plan of correction is provided. For nursing homes, the above findings and plans of correction are disclosable 14 days following the date these documents are made available to the facility. If deficiencies are cited, an approved plan of correction is requisite to continued program participation.

LABORATORY DIRECTOR'S OR PROVIDER/SUPPLIER REPRESENTATIVE'S SIGNATURE	TITLE	(X6) DATE

FORM CMS-2567 (02/99) Previous Versions Obsolete

If continuation sheet Page _____ of _____

Figure 14.8 Form 2567, Statement of Deficiencies and Plan of Correction

	Isolated	Pattern	Widespread
Immediate jeopardy to resident health or safety	J ▨PoC▨ Required: Cat. 3 Optional: Cat. 1 Optional: Cat. 2 ▨	K ▨PoC▨ Required: Cat. 3 Optional: Cat. 1 Optional: Cat. 2 ▨	L ▨PoC▨ Required: Cat. 3 Optional: Cat. 2 Optional: Cat. 1 ▨
Actual harm that is not immediate	G PoC Required* Cat. 2 Optional: Cat. 1	HPoC Required* Cat. 2 Optional: Cat. 1 ▨	I ▨PoC▨ Required* Cat. 2 Optional: Cat. 1 Optional:Temporary Mgmt.
No actual harm with potential for more than minimal harm that is not immediate jeopardy	D PoC Required* Cat. 1 Optional: Cat. 2	E PoC Required* Cat. 1 Optional: Cat. 2	F ▨PoC▨ Required* Cat. 2 Optional: Cat. 1 ▨
No actual harm with potential for minimal harm	A ■No PoC■ No remedies ■ ■Commitment to ■Correct ■ Not on CMS-2567	B ■PoC■ ■ ■ ■ ■	C ■PoC ■ ■ ■
	Isolated	Pattern	Widespread

▨ Substandard quality of care is any deficiency in 42 CFR 483.13, Resident Behavior and Facility Practices, 42 CFR 483.15 Quality of Life, or 42 CFR 483.25, Quality of Care, that constitutes immediate jeopardy to resident health or safety; or a pattern of or widespread actual harm that is not immediate jeopardy; or a widespread potential for more than minimal harm that is not immediate jeopardy, with no actual harm.

■ Substantial compliance

REMEDY CATEGORIES

Category 1 (Cat. 1)	Category 2 (Cat. 2)	Category 3 (Cat. 3)
Directed Plan of Correction State Monitor; and/or Directed In-Service Training	Denial of Payment for New Admissions Denial of Payment for All Individuals imposed by CMS; and/or Civil money penalties: $50 - $3,000/day	Temp. Mgmt. Termination **Optional:** Civil money penalties 3,050-$10,000/day

Figure 14.9   Assessment Factors Used to Determine the Seriousness of Deficiencies Matrix

Informal Dispute Resolution (IDR)

In some cases, the NHA may disagree with a cited deficiency and can choose to file an IDR. "The request must be made within the same 10 calendar day period the facility has for submitting an acceptable plan of correction to the surveying entity." This process is restricted to the current survey and cannot be used for previous survey findings (CMS, 2004a, p. 2).

Summary

This chapter focuses on the nursing and business practices that are necessary to operate a well-managed and high-quality nursing home facility. Specific practices reviewed in this chapter include resident admission and assessment, performance improvement, data management, and survey types and processes.

The text also emphasizes the importance of the NHA as the leader of day-to-day facility operations. In this role, the NHA acts as the key decision maker and communication liaison between residents, staff, families, and state/federal regulatory personnel.

Key Terms

Admission packet: This packet includes information the resident must be given prior to or upon admission, such as the facility house rules.

Advance healthcare directive: A document that expresses the medical wishes of a resident when he can no longer convey them due to a change in medical status.

Clump of eight: A statistically based analysis tool for run charts whereby eight *consecutive* observations in time sequence are either *all* above or *all* below the median, indicative of a process shift.

Common cause variation: The naturally occurring, *predictable* range of a given process's numerical performance due to the presence of already existing process input sources of variation that *randomly* "conspire" to produce any individual numerical result.

Consent to treat: A form that documents that the resident agrees to undergo a medical procedure.

Consistent assignment: When a staff member is assigned to the same resident(s) each shift worked.

Daily NHA rounds: Physical inspections of the facility and discussions with staff and residents regarding operational performance.

Data: A collection of numerical observations generated by a process for which the goal is to draw conclusions to take action.

Deficiencies: State and/or federal regulations that were not adequately met by the facility's operations.

Discharge summary: A document created by a physician or licensed healthcare provider that may accompany a resident upon admission to the facility and gives a summary of the resident's prior medical condition and care.

Do-not-resuscitate form: A form that details the resident's wishes for medical care, such as cardiopulmonary resuscitation (CPR) and ventilator machine use.

Exhaust in-house data: An *initial* strategy for improvement whereby any *already existing* data is used to clarify the situation needing improvement.

Exit conference: Held on the last day of the survey and provides an opportunity for the facility team to discuss the deficiencies found with the surveyors and supply additional information that can negate some or all of their findings.

Facility rules: A list of "behaviors" that all residents should follow to live congenially with others in the facility.

Honoring resident preferences: The process by which staff acts on the resident's preferences.

Human variation: The different perceptions of individuals performing a process that unwittingly add non-numerical variation to any collected data, thereby compromising data quality.

Identifying resident preferences: The process by which residents express their preferences for their daily lifestyle, including waking and sleeping times, meals, and hobbies.

Inclusive decision making: A form of participatory decision making in which no decision is made without staff input.

Managers on duty: The person designated to be in charge in the NHA's absence.

Median: The number at which half the data points fall above the middle point and half below.

Pareto matrix: A diagnostic tool to stratify data into meaningful groups.

Pareto principle: A concept discovered and named in the 1950s by quality expert (the late) Joseph Juran: When looking at an improvement opportunity as a process, he *consistently* noticed that it was only 20% of the process that caused 80% of the problems. His strategy, coined the Pareto principle, is used to isolate a major opportunity within a "vague" situation to focus improvement efforts, making them far more efficient.

Performance improvement: A proactive and continuous study of processes with the intent to prevent or decrease the likelihood of problems by identifying areas of opportunity and testing new approaches to fix underlying causes of persistent/systemic problems.

Plan-Do-Study-Act (PDSA): A process to test an improvement effort.

Preadmission Screening and Resident Review (PASRR): An evaluation tool used in long-term care facilities that aids a person in staying in the least restrictive setting possible while emphasizing resident-centered care.

Process-oriented context: An important framework within which to consider improvement efforts that considers all work as "converting" a series of inputs to create useful outputs.

Quality assurance: A provider program to monitor and study the quality of the services it delivers, and to make recommendations for improvement.

Quality assurance and performance improvement: A combination of quality assurance and performance improvement that is data-driven and proactive in approach and seeks to improve the quality of life, care, and services in nursing homes.

Quality of care: Medical care that maximizes the physical and mental needs of each resident.

Quality of life: The enjoyment and happiness a resident experiences from his life.

Remedy category: Imposed on the facility for cited deficiencies and can vary in corrective action, from in-service training to financial penalties, such as cancellation of the reimbursement contract with CMS.

Resident Assessment Instrument (RAI): A tool used to complete the comprehensive assessment.

Resident behavior: Any resident care by the staff "must be based on a detailed assessment of physical, psychological and behavioral symptoms and underlying causes as well as potential situational or environmental reasons for the behaviors" (CMS, 2013a, p. 15). If the staff cannot explain the rationale for the care, the care may be inappropriate. Examples of behavior causing concern would include "kicking, biting or striking out at others" (CMS, 2014c). The facility has a responsibility to minimize negative behaviors and maximize positive ones such as engaging with other residents or acting as volunteers in the facility.

Resident-centered care: An approach to care that focuses on the resident's preferences and needs. The goal of this type of resident care is to provide a safe and welcoming environment where residents, instead of being told what to do, can freely voice their concerns, make recommendations for improvement, and observe them being put into effect.

Resident-directed move-in: A process in which a resident's preferences are accommodated whenever possible as long as the health and safety of the resident are not at risk.

Resident rights acknowledgment: A form that residents must sign to acknowledge that their individual rights have been explained to them.

Role exit: The process elders may experience when relocating to a long-term care facility and disengaging from social roles and identities that have been central to their lives.

Rounding for relationship: Supervisors build relationships with staff members by being present in their work spaces, asking questions, and following through on requests.

Run chart: A graph in which a process output is plotted in its naturally occurring time order, with the median of the plotted data added as a reference line to determine whether a shift in process performance occurred.

Special cause variation: An outside force acting on a process *in addition to* its normal inputs.

Statistics: A set of numerical techniques designed to analyze data and understand the source(s) of variation for purposes of taking appropriate actions to improve a process.

Stratification: A common cause strategy for improvement by tracing process outputs to a specific source of input (e.g., time of day, day of week, month, doctor doing treatment) to isolate major sources of variation to focus subsequent improvement efforts. This can be done with in-house data or usually be easily designed as a data collection.

Substandard quality of care: Care that does not meet the minimum state and/or federal regulations and cited on the Scope and Severity chart as levels F, H, I, J, K, or L.

Trend: A significant "drift" of seven data points, either upwards or downwards, of process performance.

Variation: Gap between where a process *is* and where it *should be*.

Review Questions

1. Explain four ways the role of the NHA impacts facility operations.
2. Why is a resident-directed move-in important?

3. List three main benefits of QAPI.

4. List three ways data management improves facility operations.

5. Name the reason why a Traditional Extended Survey is performed.

Case Study

Mrs. Moore is a long-time resident of New England. For the past 3 years, she has hiked 1 hour every day. Last year, she fell while hiking and broke her hip. During her hospital stay she developed an infection and was admitted to a skilled nursing facility to resolve the infection prior to going home. The stress from her hip infection combined with living in an unfamiliar place caused Mrs. Moore's underlying cognitive impairment to worsen. Due to her mental and physical status, the family made the decision that she should live permanently in the nursing facility. Mrs. Moore was devastated because she had to leave her home of 45 years. Given her high fall risk and cognitive impairment, the staff felt that Mrs. Moore was unsafe to go outside alone. Being outdoors was an important part of her life, and this restriction negatively impacted her quality of life.

• How may feelings of grief and loss differ for a resident who plans in advance to come to a nursing home facility and one who does not plan such a move, such as Mrs. Moore?

• How would a resident-directed move-in assist Mrs. Moore in her transition into her new living environment?

• Detail the steps required for the development of Mrs. Moore's care plan.

References

Balestracci, D. (2014, April). *How about applying critical thinking to the process of using Rapid Cycle PDSA?* Retrieved from http://archive.aweber.com/davis-newslettr/76Wtr/h/From_Davis_Balestracci_.htm

Balestracci, D. (2015). *Data sanity: A quantum leap to unprecedented results* (2nd ed.). Englewood, CO: Medical Group Management Association.

Berwick, D. (1989). Continuous improvement as an ideal in health care. *New England Journal of Medicine, 320*(1), 56.

Berwick, D. (2002). *Escape fire.* New York, NY: Commonwealth Fund.

Brown, M. G. (1996). *Keeping score: Using the right metrics to drive world-class performance.* New York, NY: Productivity Press.

California Department of Health Care Services. (2015, June). *Pre-admission screening and resident review (PASRR).* Retrieved from http://www.dhcs.ca.gov/services/MH/Pages/PASRR.aspx#PASRRbkgd

Centers for Medicare and Medicaid Services (CMS). (n.d.). *QAPI*. Retrieved from http://www.cms.gov/Medicare/Provider-Enrollment-and-Certification/Survey CertificationGenInfo/Downloads/fiveelementsqapi.pdf

Centers for Medicare and Medicaid Services (CMS). (1999, February). *Statement of deficiencies and plan of correction*. Retrieved from https://www.cms.gov/Medicare/CMS-Forms/CMS-Forms/downloads/cms2567.pdf

Centers for Medicare and Medicaid Services (CMS). (2004, December). *Federal requirements for the informal dispute resolution (IDR) process for nursing homes*. Retrieved from http://www.cms.gov/Medicare/Provider-Enrollment-and-Certification/SurveyCertificationGenInfo/Downloads/SCletter05-10.pdf

Centers for Medicare and Medicaid Services (CMS). (2012, June). *MDS quality measure/indicator report*. Retrieved from http://www.cms.gov/Research-Statistics-Data-and-Systems/Computer-Data-and-Systems/MDSPubQIandRes Rep/qmreport.html

Centers for Medicare and Medicaid Services (CMS). (2013a, May). *CMS's RAI version 3.0 manual*. Chapter 4: Care Area Assessment (CAA) process and care planning. Retrieved from https://nrrs.ne.gov/mds/pdf/11137_MDS_3.0_Chapter_4_V1.10.pdf

Centers for Medicare and Medicaid Services (CMS). (2013b, June). *Rollout of Quality Assurance and Performance Improvement (QAPI) materials for nursing homes*. Retrieved from http://www.cms.gov/Medicare/Provider-Enrollment-and-Certification/SurveyCertificationGenInfo/Downloads/Survey-and-Cert-Letter-13-37.pdf

Centers for Medicare and Medicaid Services (CMS). (2014a). *Medicare state operations manual: Appendix P—Survey protocol for long-term care facilities*. Baltimore, MD: Author.

Centers for Medicare and Medicaid Services (CMS). (2014b, October). Nationwide expansion of minimum data set (MDS) focused survey background. Retrieved from http://www.cms.gov/Medicare/Provider-Enrollment-and-Certification/SurveyCertificationGenInfo/Policy-and-Memos-to-States-and-Regions-Items/Survey-and-Cert-Letter-15-06.html

Centers for Medicare and Medicaid Services (CMS). (2014c). *State operations manual: Appendix PP—Guidance to surveyors for long-term care facilities*. Baltimore, MD: Author.

Centers for Medicare and Medicaid Services (CMS). (2014d, April). *QAPI description and background*. Retrieved from http://www.cms.gov/Medicare/Provider-Enrollment-and-Certification/QAPI/qapidefinition.html

Centers for Medicare and Medicaid Services (CMS). (2015b, May). *Information only: Review and status of Nursing Home Survey—Summary of traditional and Quality Indicator Survey (QIS) findings and issues*. Retrieved from http://www.cms.gov/Medicare/Provider-Enrollment-and-Certification/Survey CertificationGenInfo/Downloads/Survey-and-Cert-Letter-15-40.pdf

Diamond, T. (1992). *Making gray gold: Narratives of nursing home care*. Chicago, IL: University of Chicago Press.

Frampton, S., Gil, H., Guastello, S., Kinsey, J., Boudreau-Scott, D., Lepore, M.,. . . Walden, P. M. (2010). *Long-term care improvement guide*. Derby, CT: Planetree and Picker Institute.

Graneheim, U. H., Johansson, A., & Lindgren, B. M. (2013). Family caregivers' experiences of relinquishing the care of a person with dementia to a nursing home: Insights from a meta-ethnographic study. *Scandinavian Journal of Caring Sciences, 18*(8), 1029–1036.

Juran, J. (2015). *Managerial breakthrough*. New York, NY: McGraw-Hill.

Kinsey, J., & Manning, D. (2015, January). *7 Habits of effective patient centered leaders*. Workshop Session at the West Virginia University Hospital Leadership Development Institute, Morgantown, WV.

Lepore, M., Wild, D., Gil, H., Lattimer, C., Harrison, J., Woddor, N., & Wasson, J. (2013). Two useful tools to improve patient engagement and transition from the hospital. *Journal of Ambulatory Care Management, 36*(4), 338–344.

Med-Pass. (2014). *The facility guide to OBRA regulations, and the long-term care survey process*. Dayton, OH: Author.

National Association of Long-Term Care Administrator Boards. (2003). *NAB study guide: How to prepare for the Nursing Home Administrator's Examination* (5th ed.). Washington, DC: Author.

Saunders, J. C., & Heliker, D. (2008). Lessons learned from 5 women as they transition into assisted living. *Geriatric Nursing, 29*, 369–375.

Silin, P. S. (2009). *Nursing homes and assisted living: The family's guide to making decisions and getting good care* (2nd ed.). Baltimore, MD: Johns Hopkins University Press.

Smith, K., Castle, N., & Hyer, K. (2013). Implementation of quality assurance and performance improvement programs in nursing homes: A brief report. *Journal of the American Medical Director's Association, 14*, 60–61.

Snee, R. (2006). *Process variation: Enemy and opportunity*. Retrieved from http://asq.org/quality-progress/2006/12/statistics-roundtable/process-variation–enemy-and-opportunity.html

Sury, L., Burns, K., & Brodaty, H. (2013). Moving in: Adjustment of people living with dementia going into a nursing home and their families. *International Psychogeriatrics, 25*, 867–876.

TMF Health Quality Institute. (n.d.). *PEPPER Skilled Nursing Facility Program for evaluating payment patterns electronic report* (3rd ed.). Retrieved from http://www.pepperresources.org/Portals/0/Documents/PEPPER/SNF/SNFPEPPERUsersGuide_Edition3.pdf

Acknowledgment

To my dear friend and colleague, Davis Balestracci, for the countless hours you spent teaching me about data and statistics and why it mattered. Your kind mentorship made me a better clinician and I am honored that you consider us colleagues. The data section of this chapter is dedicated to your passion and reflects so much of what you teach in your book *Data Sanity, A Quantum Leap to Unprecedented Results, Second Edition*. (Paige Hector)

CHAPTER 15

FINANCIAL ISSUES AND TOOLS

Robert Miller

Accounting and financial tools and methodologies may not be the most exciting elements in the healthcare profession, but they are critically important. Administrative and clinical professionals and managers need to have a solid working knowledge of these elements to be successful in the current environment. Today healthcare administrators face a variety of challenges that their counterparts of only a few years ago could hardly imagine. In the long-term care arena the growing population seeking these services is straining system capacity, even as payers, notably Medicare and Medicaid, are seeking to restrain the growth in spending for these same services. Understanding and managing the reimbursement process from contracting through billing and finally collections are absolute necessities if a facility is to survive and continue providing services.

This chapter addresses the financial issues and associated tools and methodologies impacting long-term care providers. This includes a description of the various financial instruments, budgets, balances sheets, profit and loss statements used to chart financial performance, and the components of each. We will also examine a number of the key reporting processes used by facilities, and identify the staff members who both produce and utilize these reports in carrying out their management responsibilities. As has been stated elsewhere in this text, health care in the United States today is a big, and growing, business. In order to operate effectively in this arena, knowledge of the critical financial tools used is vital. Understanding how

LEARNING OBJECTIVES

- Identify common financial and management reports and how they are used by healthcare providers.

- Explain staff roles and responsibilities in resident-related payment and reimbursement issues.

- Discuss how the information from these reports can be used by management in the operation of the facility.

- Differentiate between routine revenue and ancillary revenue.

- Explain ways to enhance revenue.

- Discuss the relationship between increased revenue and profit.

- Identify future trends in healthcare financing that may affect costs and reimbursement for long-term care providers.

these business tools are used will enable administrators to maximize reimbursement from government programs, private insurance plans, and other payer sources and better position their organizations for success.

Financial Issues and Financial Tools

This section covers basic financial reports and management tools that healthcare professionals need to understand and utilize in day-to-day operations. Although each facility has its own unique set of issues to address, leadership that demonstrates a comprehensive knowledge of financial reports and tools to answer questions and resolve issues is critical to meet the needs of its residents.

Budgets

Budgets are an important part of the financial health of any healthcare organization. Budgets are an integral part of the planning process that organizations undertake on at least a yearly basis. As a planning tool, the budget can identify both the cost of providing a service and the **revenue** (reimbursement received for services provided) that can be expected to be received for those services. The budget should provide sufficient detail to identify the source of revenue so the administrator can analyze and maximize payer mix. For example, how many Medicare residents versus private pay residents is important to consider because the reimbursement rate differs for both payer sources, which impacts the amount of **gross operating revenue**. Budgets also provide guideposts that identify benchmarks that help the organization stay on track in terms of how much money is being spent and how much money is being generated. This view is important because there must be enough operating revenue to meet current liabilities to keep the organization alive and alert the organization to potential problems by highlighting differences between where the organization planned to be and where it actually is. Budgets are fluid and must flex to circumstances the organization faces. If the organization realizes that a change is necessary, the budget should be adjusted accordingly. If a budget is well thought out and prepared properly, it can help the organization succeed in terms of generating enough revenue to meet its financial obligations.

Budgets should be realistic and achievable. If a budget is not achievable, it has limited or no value. For example, if a budget indicates that revenues for a service should be $1,000 **per unit** (a measure of service, such as an hour of physical therapy or a day in a skilled nursing facility) when the payers that reimburse healthcare providers pay only $100 per unit for that service, the budget is unrealistic and unachievable. If a budget is not realistic regarding current business practices and how the facility operates, it will not be a useful tool for monitoring performance. Similarly, if the budget does not take account of the existing business environment, payers, patient demographics, and so forth, it will be of little value as either a predictive or planning tool.

Budgets should be sufficiently detailed to allow users to assess the difference between the predictive plan and the actual result. Depending on the user, category totals and/or detailed item-by-item analysis may be necessary. An administrator or chief executive officer (CEO) may need to consider only department totals, whereas a department manager will need to analyze each expense and revenue category for his department. Budgets should be reasonably flexible. There will be times when the budget needs to change due to either internal changes—for example, drop in **census**, development of a new program, or service line—or external changes—for example, new facilities coming into the market. If an organization depends on a budget that does not mirror current business practices, then problems can occur. For example, a skilled nursing facility establishes its annual budget based on past years' performance and may assume it will maintain an average daily census of 35 patients. However, 5 months into its fiscal year the hospital system that regularly referred patients to it opens its own SNF and stops referring patients, which causes a drop in anticipated average daily census by six patients. Since the SNF's budget was based on an average daily census that is no longer being met, its revenues will be less, and adjustments to the facility's costs will need to be made. In this example, the most likely source of cost savings would be staffing costs, since these are more closely tied to average daily census than other costs for the facility. If the facility fails to make these adjustments, or does not find another source of revenue to offset the decline in census, it will lose money for the fiscal year, based upon the current budget.

In almost all cases, budgets are developed on a **fiscal year** (FY) basis. The term fiscal year refers to the time period, generally 12 months, that the organization uses for accounting purposes and for preparing financial statements. Traditionally, fiscal years are either from January 1 to December 31 or from July 1 to June 30. The federal government's fiscal year (FFY) runs from October 1 to September 30.

An example of a typical budget for a nursing facility/CCRC is shown in Figure 15.1.

ANYTOWN NURSING and CONTINUING CARE RETIREMENT COMMUNITY BUDGET - FY 2016

REVENUE	Aug-Sep	Oct-Dec	Jan-Mar	Apr-Jun	Total
Total Revenue Bldg A	$ 498,800.00	$ 504,050.00	$ 515,900.00	$ 542,850.00	$ 2,061,600.00
Total Revenue Bldg C	$ 493,900.00	$ 503,650.00	$ 512,100.00	$ 497,134.40	$ 2,006,784.40
Gross Revenue Bldgs. A & C	$ 992,700.00	$ 1,007,700.00	$ 1,028,000.00	$ 1,039,984.40	$ 4,068,384.40
Contract Adjustments	$ (99,270.00)	$ (100,770.00)	$ (102,800.00)	$ (103,998.44)	$ (406,838.44)
NET REVENUE BLDGS A & C	$ 893,430.00	$ 906,930.00	$ 925,200.00	$ 935,985.96	$ 3,661,545.96
Ancillary Services Revenue					
TOTAL ANCILLARY SERVICES REVENUE	$ 30,900.00	$ 34,400.00	$ 33,400.00	$ 31,000.00	$ 129,700.00
TOTAL REVENUE	$ 924,330.00	$ 941,330.00	$ 958,600.00	$ 966,985.96	$ 2,824,260.00
EXPENSES					
Personnel Costs					
Total Salaries & Wages	$ 505,671.00	$ 505,671.00	$ 505,671.00	$ 505,671.00	$ 2,022,684.00
Employee Related Expenses	$ 176,984.85	$ 176,984.85	$ 176,984.85	$ 176,984.85	$ 530,954.55
Total Personnel Costs	$ 682,655.85	$ 682,655.85	$ 682,655.85	$ 682,655.85	$ 2,553,638.55
Professional and Contracted Services					
Total Professional and Contracted Services	$ 37,500.00	$ 37,500.00	$ 37,500.00	$ 37,500.00	$ 112,500.00
Supplies					
Total Supplies Cost	$ 7,140.00	$ 7,140.00	$ 6,705.00	$ 7,140.00	$ 28,125.00
Other Operating Expenses					
Total Other Operating Expenses	$ 175,770.00	$ 175,545.00	$ 175,545.00	$ 175,545.00	$ 702,405.00
TOTAL EXPENSES	$ 903,065.85	$ 902,840.85	$ 902,405.85	$ 902,840.85	$ 3,611,153.40
TOTAL NET REVENUE	$ 21,264.15	$ 38,489.15	$ 56,194.15	$ 64,145.11	$ 115,947.45

Figure 15.1   Budget Example

Budget Development

There are several ways for organizations to develop budgets. The first step is to determine what services are to be provided and how much of the service to provide. Service levels should be matched with reimbursement levels to determine the anticipated service revenue that will be derived. Once this is done, the cost to provide these services is calculated. Calculating costs is generally more difficult than calculating revenue, since organizations must identify both **direct costs** and their **indirect costs**.

Direct costs are those costs directly incurred in providing the desired service—for example, the cost to meet regulatory staffing requirements to provide medical care or the cost of food for patient meals. These costs can be directly tied to providing patient care services, and generally vary with the number of patients being cared for in the facility at any specific time.

At the same time, organizations also have indirect costs, which are incurred by being in business, but which cannot be directly tied to patient care. Examples of indirect costs include utilities, electricity, gas, heating oil, and the costs associated with business and professional liability insurance. In general direct costs can be tied to the provision of care, and increases or decreases occur when the amount of services delivered fluctuates from increases or decreases in census. Indirect costs are fixed at the time of purchase and are not attributed to a patient or a service.

Budgeted costs can also be classified as either fixed or variable. **Fixed costs** do not fluctuate with changes in service levels or the number of patients. Examples of fixed costs include lease or mortgage payments for an organization's buildings or the annual salary of the chief executive officer (this may change if the CEO leaves, but it does not change with the number of patients). As a general rule, fixed costs will remain at their specified level throughout the budget period and do not fluctuate with changes in census. While adjustments to fixed costs may occur, these changes would reflect things such as a renegotiated lease payment or a salary change for a new CEO.

Variable costs include items such as the cost of nurses and aides to care for patients, which we have previously identified as a direct cost. These costs are also variable, since they fluctuate with the number of patients and the number of staff needed to care for them, and thus variable costs will fluctuate with changes in census.

For budget purposes, predicting variable costs is a bigger challenge since these predictions rely on census estimates and assumptions about the costs of providing the expected levels of service. The accuracy and thus the utility of the budget depend to a large extent on the assumptions that are made regarding census levels and the variable costs associated with meeting patient service needs at the assumed levels.

Additive budgeting uses the previous year's budget as the starting point for a new budget. Using this approach enables the organization to begin with assumptions for service levels, number of patients, lengths of stay, or units of rehabilitation. Expenses and revenues are calculated and added into the budget based on the actual (or projected if the fiscal year is not completed) current year budget figures. It is customary to include an inflation factor, a percentage, on the assumption that costs will increase over time. Also, organizations generally include revenue adjustments, on the assumption that they will be able to increase the rates that they charge for their services and the levels of reimbursement that they will be able to negotiate with the payers with whom they are contracted. When including such revenue adjustments, it is important to keep in mind that payers will not want to increase their costs, and thus will seek to limit any increases in reimbursement levels. In fact, as containing healthcare costs becomes increasingly important, insurance plans and government payers can be expected to negotiate for lower rates for providers rather than increases. The pressure to reduce costs will pose additional problems for budget development, since providers may be forced to balance their increased costs for labor and supplies with potentially reduced reimbursement rates.

Zero-based budgeting. While the additive method of budget development is relatively straightforward, it may not afford an organization the chance to examine its basic cost structure. To do this, an alternative budget development method referred to as **zero-based budgeting** is available. This method starts with the assumption that the organization's starting point is the minimum necessary to open the doors. The organization will incur base costs simply by existing, such as a mortgage against its building and utilities needed to allow its physical plant to be utilized. These costs are calculated based upon current levels in the market in which the facility is located, and then the process of adding patients to be cared for, services to be provided, and the amounts of these services begins. This process starts with the costs of providing service for one patient, and is increased from that point. In this process, assumptions are made about the levels of care and ancillary services that will be needed as patient census increases. As patient volume increases and services are added, associated costs and revenues are also added to give stakeholders a preview of the organization's financial viability. By using this approach, the organization can address the questions of need and rationale for costs and services. The zero-based budgeting approach is more detailed and more time-consuming, and therefore not used as frequently as the additive method. For our purposes, it is sufficient to know that both are available.

Whichever budgeting method is used, it is important to evaluate performance to budget on a regular basis. Most commonly, budgets are reviewed on a monthly basis, which includes both expenses and revenues. Performance to the established budget is compared by prior month and prior year as a means of maintaining budgetary discipline. Department managers and senior administration staff participate in these monthly reviews, although department managers are generally required to address only their specific department(s). To effectively evaluate performance, department managers should possess detailed knowledge of their area(s) and be able to recommend changes and corrective actions as needed.

The facility's overall financial performance is the responsibility of the senior management staff, and their understanding of the budget must be broader in scope. Budget performance will also be reviewed on a regular basis with the governing board of the facility. The schedule for this review will be determined by the frequency with which this group meets. These reviews are provided by the facility's administrator or chief executive officer and the chief financial officer, who has responsibility for preparing the monthly financial statements.

Spend-down. Department managers use **spend-down** tools to track how much they have spent for their department as compared to their allowed budgeted amount. This tool starts with the total amount budgeted to be spent in the department during the fiscal year. Expenditures for that department are then recorded and subtracted from the budgeted amount. This procedure allows the manager, at a glance, to see what has been spent in each category and what funds are available in each category for the remainder of the fiscal year.

Capital budget. The **capital budget** is a special tool that identifies "capital" items, items with a cost over a certain threshold, typically ranging from $500 to $1,500, and which have a useful life of more than one year. Capital items include vehicles, hospital beds, electronic medical record systems, construction, and building renovation costs. Depreciation must be considered when an item is a capital expense. Thus, the cost of the item can be amortized (spread) over its useful life. By doing so, the cost of a large capital item, which could cause the organization to show a loss for the fiscal year, is reduced on an annual basis and spread over the useful life of the item, a period of several years. The useful life of an item can be established by asking your organization's accountant or consulting with the Internal Revenue Service. It is important to recognize that the amortized cost of a new building, which may be spread over 15 or 20 years, does not mean that the actual building cost will not be paid upon completion. In these circumstances, the actual cost of a capital item will be paid on delivery or completion, but the budgetary accounting of that expenditure will be spread over a period of years.

Financial statements. **Financial statements** are used to determine and illustrate the financial status of the organization. There are different types of financial statements, so it is important to understand what information is needed before viewing a statement. For example, the **profit and loss (P&L) statement** shows income and expenditures for a certain period of time, with the total expenditures subtracted from the total income to show a positive or negative position for the period in question. Other reports, such as monthly operating reports, detail the financial status, whether it is operating at a profit or a loss, of the operation at a specific point in time (end of the month or year). The **accounts receivable** report, another financial report reviewed on a regular, usually monthly, basis, shows how much money the company is owed for services already provided. The accounts receivable report also includes an "aging" of outstanding accounts, showing how long, in number of days (30, 60, 90, etc.), a particular account has been open. The importance of aging reports will be discussed later in this section.

Profit and loss statements. The profit and loss statement details the revenues and expenses incurred by the company. The revenues minus the expenses is called the **profit**, or, in the case of nonprofit organizations, the **retained earnings**. When an organization reports a profit or positive retained earnings, it simply means that it has taken in more revenue than it has spent to provide its services.

The profit and loss statement is produced on a monthly basis. As the accounting year progresses, the cumulative revenues, expenses, and profit "year to date" are shown, along with results for the immediate past month. At the end of the fiscal or accounting year, the year-end results are shown.

The three components of a P&L statement are revenues, expenses, and profit/loss. In some cases, most often when the organization has contracts that include discounts or, in the case of government programs, when it may bill for services at a higher rate than it will be paid, revenues may be divided into **gross revenues**, or the total amount the organization bills for the services it provides, and **net revenues**, which are funds actually received after **discounts** and **contract adjustments** are made.

Revenues. When a healthcare provider delivers services, it earns money or generates revenue for those services. The provider records a charge (gross revenue) in its accounting books, which records the services it provided. For example, the provider may charge $100 for an hour of physical therapy. However, the amount the provider actually earns (net revenue), the amount the payer will actually pay the provider, may not be $100. In fact, with the exception of a private/cash-paying resident (which is a rare occurrence), payers such as Medicare, Medicaid, and managed care plans pay less than the amount the provider charges. This difference is the result of negotiations (for managed care plans) or simply determinations (government payers). In the current healthcare environment in many areas, where there are a number of providers and facilities competing for patients, payers of all categories (health insurance plans and government agencies) are in a much stronger position than providers. In this circumstance payers can dictate what they will pay for a particular service. An exception to this practice is services not covered by healthcare insurance plans or paid for by government agencies because providers collect what they charge without discounts. In such instances, patients requiring particular uncovered (not paid by insurance plans or government) services have little or no ability to negotiate rates since as individuals they have no bargaining power. The ability of health insurance plans to negotiate favorable rates is solely dependent on their ability to provide a steady flow of patients to providers with whom they are contracted.

This variation in the price of identical services charged to different payers that is seen in health care is very different from the way that goods and services are priced in the "real world." Let's pretend five people walked into Wal-Mart to buy a TV: Ms. Medicare, Mr. Medicaid, Ms. Kaiser, Ms. Blue Cross, and Mr. Cash. All five people pay the same amount for the same TV, the price on the tag. However, if these five "payers" walked into a healthcare provider to buy an hour of physical therapy, they might very well all pay different amounts for the same service, as explained in the following scenario.

For a healthcare provider the amount on the price tag is referred to as the **"usual and customary"** charge and is the amount that Mr. Cash will pay for the service. However, Ms. Medicare may pay only $42.17, Mr. Medicaid may pay only $28.31, Ms. Kaiser may pay only $20, and Ms. Blue Cross may pay only $32 for the hour of physical therapy. The difference between the usual and customary charge and the amount actually collected is called a **contractual allowance** (a discount or amount of money that reduces the original fee to a new amount, which is then collected by the provider). This new amount is below the provider's usual and customary charges and is offered in return for the health insurance plan agreeing to use that provider as a "preferred provider." A **preferred provider** is encouraged by the insurance plan and may be the only provider of some service or services that the insurance plan will use in a particular market or geographic area.

Insurance plans may also require providers to discount their usual and customary charges in order to be included in the plan's network (group) of providers. This benefits the provider because they will have access to a larger patient base. It may seem that contractual allowances are negative because the provider is receiving less net income, but the benefit of a larger patient base and potential need for greater services must be considered as a balancing factor.

As stated earlier, the gross revenue minus the contractual allowance is the amount the provider collects and keeps. This is called the **net income** or the actual amount earned (see Figure 15.2).

The most useful revenue figure on the P&L is the net income because that shows what is actually earned. The P&L statement also offers a useful way to quickly assess the facility's performance to budget, since the net income is one of the key components of the budget. The P&L statement, however, is not a substitute for the budget, since it does not have the detail and specificity in either revenue or expenses that are needed to accurately assess performance and make adjustments when required.

Expenses. Expenses are the amounts the provider spends to purchase items and services in order to operate the facility. For example, food purchased is a product that will be consumed through operations of the facility. In some cases, the expense is not the amount paid and the item may not be used immediately. For example, if a provider buys a piece of equipment, such as a commercial washing machine for $10,000, that washing machine will last a number of years. The provider will record a portion of that $10,000 expense during each accounting period (month or year) over the lifetime of the item purchased to show the cost of using the washing machine during that period. This process is referred to as amortization or depreciation. The expense is called an amortized expense or a depreciation expense. In the latter case, the value of the asset is reduced, depreciated over the useful life of the item. Since the item itself

Revenue:	$25,000.00
Expenses:	20,000.00
Profit:	$ 5,000.00

Figure 15.2   Gross Revenue Calculation

is an asset of the organization, and has a value that can be expressed as a dollar amount, it will be expressed as such when accounting for the assets of the organization.

Profit or Loss

The profit or loss of an organization is the net income minus expenses (see Figure 15.3).

No business, healthcare or other, can survive if a profit cannot be generated. This concept applies to "not-for-profit" organizations because they must also have revenues that exceed expenses, or profit, to stay in business. In not-for-profit organizations the excess of revenues over expenses is referred to as retained earnings. Retained earnings are applied, in some form or another, to further the organization's not-for-profit mission versus for-profit companies, where some of the profit is redistributed to the owners and some of the profit is reinvested back into the organization.

#1 (Showing Profit)

Profit/Loss = Net Income – Expenses

Gross (unadjusted) Income:	$25,000
- Contract Adjustments:	3,000
Net (adjusted) Income:	$22,000
-Expenses:	20,000
Profit:	$2,000

#2 (Showing Loss)

Gross (unadjusted) Income:	$25,000
- Contract Adjustments:	3,000
Net (adjusted) Income:	$22,000
-Expenses:	24,000
Loss:	($2,000)

Figure 15.3   Profit/Loss Calculations

Of course, the need to generate a profit must be balanced against the need to provide quality care. There is a fine line between making a profit in a healthcare organization that allows the organization to survive and carry out its mission and providing quality healthcare services.

Balance sheets. The **balance sheet** is a financial report that tells leadership about the position of the organization at a specific point in time. Unlike the P&L, the balance sheet does not contain information about revenues, expenses, and profit. Rather, the balance sheet has information about the **assets, liabilities**, and **equity** (sometimes called net worth) of an organization.

The assets of a facility are the things of value that a company owns or controls—that is, the asset can be sold, leased, or used in some way in its operations. If a facility owns equipment or a building or has cash in the bank, those things have value and are assets. If a facility has the right to something of value that is not currently in its possession, that item is an asset. For example, if a facility has provided services but has not yet been paid for those services, it has the right to collect the money owed as payment for those services. These monies are called accounts receivable. If a facility has paid a vendor, such as a landlord, a deposit for the right to enter into a building lease, that money is sitting in the landlord's bank account. However, the healthcare provider who paid the deposit still has the right to that money (assuming it lives up to the terms of the lease); therefore, the deposit is considered an asset and part of the accounts receivable. Examples of assets include accounts receivable (money owed to the organization by payers), cash on hand, and the value of land, equipment, and buildings owned by the organization,

Some assets will be **realized**—that is, they will be collected and available for the company to use quickly, like accounts receivable. Some assets may not be available for the company to use for a very long time, such as a lease deposit that will sit in the landlord's bank account until the end of the lease term.

Assets can change in value or have risk associated with them. A change in value would be considered when understanding whether the amount shown for an asset is a historical or original value. Risks would include such things as "**bad debt**," which refers to funds owed to the organization that the organization has determined will not, or cannot, be collected. For example, if a provider bills $1,000 for services rendered and expects to collect that money, it is probably worth $1,000 at the time it was billed. However, if the bill does not get paid and a year has gone by, there is a risk the provider may never get paid and that $1,000 may become an uncollectable account or a "bad debt." While there is no rule that defines bad debt, most organizations will try to collect charges owed to them through their own billing departments or outsourced billing services before paying for an outside collection agency.

Referral of an account to a collection agency, done as early as 90 days outstanding, is the first step to declaring the account a bad debt and writing it off as uncollectable. These collection agencies will attempt to collect the funds owed, charging a percentage of the amount collected for their services. If the collection agency cannot collect the debt after a suitable period of time, 90 to 180 days, the account is declared a bad debt and written off. The write-off will reduce the amount in the organization's accounts receivable category, and may also reduce the tax on earnings liability of a for-profit organization since the amount written off for bad debt may be taken as a tax deduction and thus lower the organization's tax liability. For nonprofit organizations, which do not incur tax liability for accumulating retained earnings, these income tax advantages do not apply.

Liabilities are the opposite of assets. Liabilities are things the facility owes to someone else. If a facility purchased services or supplies but has not yet paid for them, it owes the vendor money. The amounts owed to vendors and suppliers are called **accounts payable**. If a facility borrowed money from a bank or an individual, the facility must repay that loan, which is called **loan payable** or **note payable**. Some liabilities need to be paid quickly, such as the amount owed to the food vendor, while others are paid over a long period of time, perhaps years. Examples of liabilities include accounts payable, short-term and long-term debt, and employee pension expenses.

The equity of a company is the difference between the assets and liabilities. If the value of the assets is higher than the value of the liabilities, the company will have positive equity, sometimes called **net worth**. If the value of the assets is lower than the value of the liabilities, the company will have negative equity.

Cash flow statements. **Cash flow statements** show how much money, typically referred to as **working capital**, an organization has available to pay for personnel or **payroll**, goods and services, and the other costs associated with doing business. This sum of money is, at its most basic, the amount of funds that can be spent at any given time. Although accounts receivable are considered assets, they have not been collected and therefore are not included in the cash flow statement. Cash flow statements provide a means of assessing the organization's immediate ability to fund operations. This statement includes cash or cash equivalents, items that can be converted to cash within 90 days, such as money market funds or securities owned by the organization that do not have restrictions on their sale or liquidation. Cash flow statements are generally divided into three sections:

1. Cash flow from operations

2. Cash flow from investments

3. Cash flow from financing activities (loans)

Financial management. The profit & loss (P&L) statement, balance sheet, and cash flow statement summarize data in a concise and condensed manner. There are a number of detailed reports often referred to as ledgers that contain much greater detail—for example, the general accounts receivable report, which will include summary totals of funds owed to the organization. This report can be divided into ledgers (sub-reports), which may contain information on how much the provider expects to collect on a resident-by-resident basis and how much is owed by each contracted healthcare plan and other payers, such as Medicare. These ledgers, which are aggregated into the accounts receivable report, may have thousands of entries, representing billings to individual residents or to the payers responsible for their costs and charges, which are summarized in the P&L statement and on the balance sheet in only a few lines.

Accounts receivable (A/R). Accounts receivable reports provide details about the amounts owed to the provider. They tell us:

- Which payers currently owe money and the amount that each owes.

- What services the money is related to.

- When each account was billed and how long the amount has been owed.

- The outstanding amounts associated with each resident who has received services.

It is critical for the billing staff and the managers to review the accounts receivable reports on a regular basis, optimally daily, to ensure bills have been submitted in a timely fashion, generally defined as 30 days or less. This should ensure that all charges are accurately billed and that any patient **co-pays** or **share-of-cost** charges are identified and billed to the patient. To ensure that funds that have been billed are actually collected, the billing staff must review all funds received from payers on a daily basis and reconcile these funds to the billed charges. The reconciliation process involves comparing the amount of funds received for each bill to the amount charged on that same bill, making sure that the billed and received amounts agree, and also accounting for any discounts or other adjustments that may have been made to the amount paid. Any discounts or adjustments that have been taken from the billed amount must agree with the amounts allowed for these discounts and/or adjustments in the contract that a payer has with the provider.

As discussed earlier, the longer a bill goes unpaid, the more likely it is that it will never be collected or the amount collected will be less than the billed amount. To help ensure funds owed are collected in a timely manner, it is important to monitor the length of time each bill is outstanding (unpaid). This is done with the **aging report**, which shows how long it has been since a bill was sent to a payer. In health care, the minimum length of time to collect a bill is generally 30 days from the time that a **"clean" claim**, one with no errors, was submitted. In many instances, length of time for payment is set in the contract between the provider and the payer. Contracts may include provisions for discounts if billed charges are paid within a shorter period of time, which will improve the organization's cash flow. Contracts may include penalties in the form of added charges, an interest percentage on the unpaid balance, if the payer fails to send payment within a specified time frame. Both discounts and penalty charges are intended to incentivize payers to pay billed charges in a timely manner, usually defined as 30 days or less from the time that a clean claim is submitted.

Accounts payable. The accounts payable reports show how much the provider owes to the various companies and people from whom it has purchased services and supplies. It details each vendor owed money, what was purchased, and how long the money has been due.

When a provider makes a purchase, the vendor usually expects to be paid within a certain time frame, such as 30 or 60 days (usually spelled out in the contract between the vendor and the provider). If the provider fails to pay in the appropriate time frame, problems may arise, including interest or penalties on the money owed and in some cases the vendor refusing to do business with the provider.

Payroll. Payroll reports show how much the employees have been paid. The detailed payroll ledger combines thousands of individual entries, which reflect the time worked and amounts paid to each employee. This detailed information is summarized as payroll costs, which are included in the profit and loss statement in a few lines.

To provide department managers with the data needed to operate their areas effectively, the payroll reports also include a number of detailed subreports:

- The department each employee works in
- The position title and description for each employee

- The number of hours worked, in a pay period and in the fiscal year-to-date

- The amounts paid and what the employees have been paid for

- Regular time

- Overtime

- Vacation, holiday, or sick time

- Bonuses

- Taxes and employee benefits, such as deductions for health insurance

Salaries, pay to management and department manager-level employees, are based on an annual (yearly) rate, whereas wages are paid to employees on an hourly basis. Related costs, such as payroll taxes and employee benefits, make up a very large percentage of the amount healthcare providers spend to provide services. Therefore, understanding the details associated with payroll is crucial to smooth facility operations.

Management reports. In addition to the basic financial reports described earlier, providers often develop individualized reports that organize data from different sources and help them with specific financial and operational questions. These management reports focus on specific details of the organization's operations and summarize information in concise formats. Doing so presents information that summarizes facility- or department-level performance in a few key data points. Examples include a **dashboard report** that summarizes financial results at a very high level (not much detail). **Key factor reports** summarize **key indicators**, such as **staffing levels (nursing hours worked**) based on the census data (how many residents were served), or other statistical information, such as the number of miles driven per year by the facility's vans when used to transport residents to various functions and appointments.

The data that can be extracted is virtually limitless. The goal with these reports is to aggregate data into formats that can be analyzed efficiently and produce usable information. This process is discussed in greater detail in Chapter 14. Of special note in that discussion is the need to establish appropriate time horizons, collect appropriate data to answer the right questions, and "plot the dots." Of special importance is the necessity of not rushing to interpretations but rather letting the data speak for itself. In this way, you may be able to avoid addressing "issues" that do not need addressing and fixing "problems" that don't need fixing.

Utilization of financial information. Financial information is used in a number of ways to help administrators and department managers monitor and assess performance against the facility's budget. It can also be used to help make decisions on programs to develop, or conversely to eliminate them. The ability to generate accurate and reliable financial information is a prime requirement for the finance department. Without the ability to rely upon the data generated, administrators and managers will be less effective and their decisions may be compromised. In the following section we will discuss how these reports are produced and used to help operate the long-term care facility.

Staff

This section explains how reports are developed and which staff produce them. In some organizations these functions will be performed by staff in the long-term care facility itself, while in larger organizations, with multiple facilities under a common ownership, they will be carried out by personnel working in a central corporate office. In addition, some smaller organizations may choose to outsource these functions or employ contractors who may work on a part-time or as-needed basis. There are many possibilities depending on the particular needs of the facility, so for this section, the focus is on the typical positions and their functions.

The business office. Most long-term care facilities have a finance department, sometimes referred to as the business office, where a variety of staff (who may or may not be accountants) perform the services necessary to keep the facility's finances in order. The typical functions performed in the business office include:

- Processing payroll—the payroll function
- Completion of payments to vendors—the accounts payable function
- Completion of the bills for services rendered—the accounts receivable function

These are very detailed functions where the staff member assigned to a particular functional area must have specialized skills, such as coding for billers, or knowledge of wage and hour regulations for payroll staff. Another example is the accounts payable clerk, who reviews each purchase invoice, assigns it to a specific **cost center**, the term for a budget category that groups expenditures for similar items or uses, schedules it for payment, and writes and sends the check or transmits electronic payments.

The business office staff typically complete the following functions:

- **Resident trust** account maintenance
- **Petty cash** disbursements
- Reception duties

- Administrative assistant duties

- Banking duties, like depositing checks or reconciling bank statements

- Helping department managers access records and details contained in the accounts payable, payroll, and accounts receivable **journals**

Chief financial officer. The finance department (business office) is generally overseen by the facility's chief financial officer (CFO). The CFO, typically a certified public accountant (CPA), has overall responsibility for the finance and accounting functions of the facility. This person is in charge of developing the annual budget, the monthly and annual financial reports, and the various reports submitted to the IRS and corporate licensing agencies. The CFO reports to the administrator or CEO, and also to the **Board of Directors**. Many CFOs actually have dual reporting lines of authority, answering both to the administrator and the Board of Directors. This dual reporting is intended to ensure the independence of the CFO when presenting financial reports to the Board. Establishing a dual reporting authority for the CFO helps to ensure that the Board of Directors receives reports on the organization's financial performance and position that reflect an accurate picture and have not been edited or otherwise manipulated by the CEO or other staff. From a practical standpoint, this often means that the CEO does not have the authority to fire or otherwise discipline the CFO without the concurrence of the Board of Directors. Similarly, the Board will often be responsible for evaluating the performance of the CFO, again to help ensure his independence from outside influence.

Accountants. Accountants, who are also referred to as bookkeepers or clerks, serve vital functions for the facility and ensure all accounting rules, referred to as **Generally Accepted Accounting Principles (GAAP)**, and laws are followed. They might be employed outside the long-term care facility, in a corporate office, or on a contractual basis. A primary task for accountants is to take the data produced by the business office staff and, along with other data, generate profit and loss statements and balance sheets.

There are a number of transactions that require an accountant to take an amount paid to a company and translate it to determine its appropriate classification, such as a capital expenditure or a **recurring expense**. A **journal entry** is created, which includes the account name, the amount owed or spent, and whether it is classified as a **debit (expense)** or **credit (revenue)**. The following is an example of a journal entry.

If the facility buys a piece of equipment for $100,000 and it is expected to have a useful life of 10 years, the facility does not "expense" the cost of the equipment all in 1 year. Rather, the cost of the equipment is **depreciated**, spread out over the life of the equipment (in this example, 10 years). The accountant would set it up so that the $100,000 expenditure is recorded on the balance sheet as an asset and part of it (1/10th) would transfer to the profit and loss statement as **depreciation** (an expense) each year for 10 years. By setting up the expense this way, the organization strives to allocate the initial cost of the equipment over its useful life and match the annual cost of the item against revenue that may be derived from its use.

Accountants also work with statistics, like resident days (census reports) or the number of meals served or even the number of pounds of laundry processed. As these statistics work their way into the reports produced, they are used by the managers for different purposes, such as analyzing efficiency and productivity.

Accountants are also involved in the design and production of management reports, like key factor reports, dashboard reports, spend-down sheets, and other custom reports for managers.

Department managers. Department managers, like the director of nursing or the housekeeping, laundry, or maintenance supervisors, use reports and tools to help manage their departments. They may use the spend-down sheets to determine if their expenses are in line with their budget and examine detailed payroll reports to determine if the amount of labor in these departments is appropriate.

Administrator. The administrator, often called the CEO, has the responsibility of ensuring the facility's overall performance, from the clinical, financial, and regulatory perspectives. This person reports to the Board of Directors and in this capacity needs to see the big picture regarding things like whether the facility made a profit or lost money, or how the facility performed in comparison to the budgets. This person is ultimately responsible for all the operations of the facility, both clinical and administrative, and must be able to answer any question posed. Working closely with staff helps facilitate desired outcomes.

Petty cash. Facilities generally keep a small amount of cash on hand to pay for small items rather than writing a check or using a corporate or personal credit card. Examples of petty cash expenses might be a postage due charge on a package received or to reimburse a staff member for a parking charge he paid when attending an off-site meeting. The petty cash fund is managed by the petty cash custodian, who is often a staff member in the finance department, or a secretary in the corporate office. The amount that a facility maintains in its petty cash fund varies depending on the size of the facility. Amounts generally range from $50.00 to $200.00. The petty cash custodian is responsible for dispersing funds, accounting for those disbursements, and replenishing the fund when it reaches a specified low point.

Revenue Enhancement

The idea of discussing health care as a commodity and determining what the long-term care facility "sells" may seem unusual at first. However, a long-term care facility is a business, and just like any business it has to generate revenue to remain open.

Long-term care facilities typically provide (sell) services that fall into two general categories: (1) routine services and (2) ancillary services. The revenue that is generated from each class of services is usually separated on the financial statements so that administrators and managers can track these revenues to their appropriate categories, the type of service (room and board, physical therapy, etc.), and the payer (Medicare, private insurance, or private pay). Ultimately they will be aggregated into a total revenue figure to measure the facility's total financial performance.

Routine services. Routine services are those services that all residents receive in relatively equal amounts. Another term used for routine services is "room and board" or "room and care." Generally these routine services are sold by the day. In other words, if a resident stays in the facility for one night, he has received one day of room and board. The facility has "sold" one **resident day** or one unit of routine service.

The facility "produces" a unit of routine service for each resident for each night. This unit of service is referred to as a resident day, which is 24 consecutive hours of one resident occupying one bed in the facility. There is an absolute limit to the total units of routine service a facility can produce and sell, which depends on the number of beds that the facility is **licensed** for. If the facility is licensed for 100 beds, it can serve a maximum of 100 residents on any given day. There can be only one resident in a bed at any one time. For 1 year, the facility illustrated in Figure 15.4 can produce and sell a maximum of 36,500 units of routine service (resident days).

Since the facility is limited to a maximum number of resident days (based on the number of licensed beds), how can routine revenue be

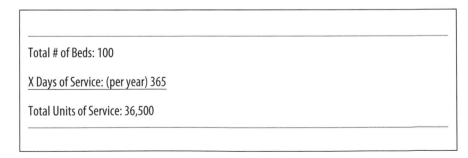

Total # of Beds: 100

X Days of Service: (per year) 365

Total Units of Service: 36,500

Figure 15.4   Maximum Annual Units of Service

enhanced? First, it is important to understand there are different types of routine services based on the acuity (a measure of the degree of severity of the patient's condition) of the patient and the complexity of care needed. Generally, the amount paid for higher-acuity patients requiring more complex routine services will be higher than the amount paid for less complex services. Therefore, if the facility can attract residents with more complex needs, the amount they will be paid will increase.

However, this does not guarantee the profit will increase. If the cost of the more complex services increases (more nursing services), there is likely more staff required to provide the service, which results in higher payroll. Therefore, profit may increase, not change, or potentially go down. It is important for administration to analyze the impact a change in resident complexity or type of services provided will have on both revenue and expenses.

Another consideration is that there is a limit to the number of routine units of service a facility can provide. Some routine services will result in higher payment rates and increased revenues. If the facility provides more units of routine service with the higher payment rates, its routine revenue will go up. However, the facility must analyze the expense side to determine whether there will be a financial benefit from the additional revenue generated.

Ancillary services. **Ancillary services** are those services that are not routinely utilized by, or provided for, all residents. Unlike room and care services, which are provided for all residents and generally come at a set price, ancillary services are provided on an "as needed" basis, most frequently when ordered by a resident's physician. In addition, if residents do receive these services, they are not provided in equal amounts, but only at the levels determined to be appropriate for the resident's condition. Examples of ancillary services include the following:

- Physical therapy
- Occupational therapy
- Speech therapy
- Medical supplies
- Laboratory services
- Radiology services
- Medical equipment

For ancillary services, the process of revenue enhancement is different. Keep in mind that not all residents receive ancillary services and those who do receive these services receive them in differing amounts. However, as with routine services the facility needs to analyze the cost of delivering ancillary services to determine whether they will result in a profit. It is also important to remember that Medicare and other payers will pay only for those ancillary services that are determined to be medically necessary for the patient. Because payment for ancillary services is limited to those that are deemed to be medically necessary, enhancing revenue by increasing the number and/or frequency of these services may be difficult. At the same time increasing the number and frequency of medically necessary and covered (paid for by insurance plans) services may be the best option for enhancing ancillary revenues.

The following examples are provided as a means of illustrating how facilities may try to enhance revenue by increasing or enhancing their ancillary services. For the sake of this discussion we will assume there is a profit margin associated with the delivery of ancillary services.

Level of Services Provided to Residents

The facility can expand ancillary revenue by providing ancillary services to a larger number of residents or by expanding the scope and variety of ancillary services it provides. Examples are provided that illustrate this concept.

Assumptions:

• Currently 10 residents receive ancillary services each day.

• The ancillary service each resident receives is 1 hour of physical therapy (PT).

• The revenue produced for 1 hour of physical therapy is $100.

• The facility admits more residents who need physical therapy.

• The number of residents who receive 1 hour of physical therapy increases to 20 per day.

With these assumptions the financial result shown in Figure 15.5 will occur.

Intensity of Services to the Residents

Another way to increase revenue is to increase the volume of ancillary services already provided. For example, if there are residents currently receiving 1 hour of physical therapy, could they benefit from 2 hours of physical therapy? The resident's physician should routinely assess the optimal level of services provided for the rehabilitation and recovery of the

Currently		
Number of residents receiving physical therapy		10
X <u>Revenue Per Day</u>	<u>$100</u>	
= Total Physical Therapy Revenue per day		$1,000
After Change in Number of PT Units Sold		
Number of residents receiving physical therapy		20
X <u>Revenue Per Day</u>	<u>$100</u>	
= Total Physical Therapy Revenue per day		$2,000
Increase in physical therapy revenue		**$1,000**

Figure 15.5   Physical Therapy Revenue Enhancement Model

resident. This assessment may result in changes in the level of services and intensity of services provided. Continuing the example started earlier.

Assumptions:

- Currently 20 residents receive ancillary services each day.
- The ancillary service each resident is receiving is 1 hour of physical therapy.
- The revenue produced for 1 hour of physical therapy is $100.
- The facility admits residents that need 2 hours of physical therapy each day.

With these assumptions the financial result shown in Figure 15.6 will occur.

A word of caution that bears repeating: Provide only medically necessary services and never consider increasing the volume of services provided simply for the sake of enhancing revenue.

Incentives. Incentive programs are generally reserved for management level employees, and are based upon the facility achieving certain generally budgetary- and performance-related targets. These targets can be either financial in nature, like the facility achieving an established percentage level of profit (or retained earnings) over that projected in the budget, or tied to the facility census, such as maintaining a 100% occupancy rate during the

Currently		
Number of residents receiving one hour of physical therapy	20	
X Revenue Per Day for one hour of PT	$100	
= Total Physical Therapy Revenue per day		$2,000
After Change In Number of PT Units sold		
Number of residents receiving physical therapy		20
X Revenue Per Day for TWO hours of PT		$200
= Total Physical Therapy Revenue per day		$4,000
Increase in physical therapy revenue		**$2,000**

Figure 15.6   Physical Therapy Revenue Enhancement Model 2

fiscal year. Incentive programs can also be used in the short term, such as bonuses for department managers for achieving a zero-deficiency licensure survey. While incentive programs can be a useful means of encouraging high performance, it is important to remember that an incentive that cannot be reached is essentially meaningless.

Future Directions

As with any industry, health care is in the midst of significant changes—in how care is delivered, who delivers it, how it is paid for, and how the various components, facilities, providers, and payers will be organized. In addition, the aging of the baby boomer population, combined with the increased life span seen in many of their parents' generation, is expected to increase the demand for long-term care services in the future. With the average life span in the population increasing, along with the trend to have a more active lifestyle, long-term care facilities will need to change to meet the demands of this emerging population. The impact of these demographic and behavioral shifts on long-term care services and providers, being felt in nations around the world, is discussed in depth in the following chapter. These changes can include integrating long-term care facilities into an expanded continuum of care, including acute care facilities, home health, and home- and community-based services, and even establishing medical home models for an elderly population.

In terms of financial impacts, moving toward a more integrated and holistic model may better position facilities to meet the changing needs of both their current and their future residents, and maintain their financial viability. Some of the changes and potential steps to take to meet these new challenges are addressed ahead.

Level of Care

An emerging trend in long-term care, noted by many administrators, is the increasing acuity of incoming residents requiring higher levels of care once admitted. It is worth noting that individuals entering assisted living facilities are often classed as having a higher acuity on entry than residents who were formerly placed in skilled nursing communities. Likewise, many SNF patients now entering these facilities would have previously been admitted to an acute care or subacute care hospital. This shift in the acuity on admission of the patient population requires administrators to be savvier in the services offered to their residents and in the various reimbursement options available.

Affordable Care Act

The Patient Protection and Affordable Care Act (PPACA), or "Obama-care" as it is sometimes called, is significantly altering the healthcare landscape. The Affordable Care Act addresses Medicare only, and is intended to reduce the rate of growth or "bend the cost curve" in Medicare spending. One component of the PPACA is the provision for the creation of **accountable care organizations (ACOs)** (Centers for Medicare and Medicaid Services, 2015) as one means of achieving cost reductions. ACOs are organizations that combine a wide variety of providers, physicians, hospitals, long-term care facilities, and associated ancillary service providers into integrated networks that assume responsibility for the care of a group of Medicare patients. ACOs are very similar to the HMOs of previous years. ACOs are incentivized to reduce costs by having the opportunity to share in the savings in aggregate costs that they generate for assigned patients.

Impact. The impact of the PPACA on long-term care providers has yet to be determined. Although it was originally intended to include provisions for federally sponsored long-term care insurance, this component was removed before the act's final passage. This was intended to address the increasing cost and utilization of long-term care services. Without these elements, the cost of long-term care is likely to continue to rise (Nawrocki,

2013). It is clear, however, that by encouraging the formation of ACOs, there will be increasing provider consolidation and integration. Also, as the number of Medicare-covered patients assigned to ACOs increases, there will be fewer "unassigned" patients for non-ACO affiliated facilities to serve. The ultimate effect may be to reduce either the number of facilities, which is not likely, given the growth in the number of potential residents with the aging of the baby boomer generation, or the number of facilities that are not part of an ACO. The latter appears to be the more likely scenario.

Strategy. To address the potential impact of the PPACA, facilities will be under increased pressure to affiliate with an ACO. They may also take the approach that increasing their non-Medicare patient/resident population is a strategy to pursue. While Medicare rules limit a facility to participation in only one ACO, these facilities are not limited in the number of non-Medicare, private healthcare insurance contracts and provider organizations they can affiliate with. Increasing their affiliations with these payers, and being willing to discount rates for increased volume, may be winning strategies for some provider facilities.

Summary

Across the healthcare spectrum, there is a growing emphasis on the twin goals of financial performance and the delivery of quality care. While these are not incompatible, the pressure to deliver on each simultaneously means that administrators and managers must be well versed in a variety of financial reporting mechanisms and have a broad knowledge of how their services are paid for. Achieving both of these goals is now the standard that they will be measured against, and that will determine whether their facilities will survive as part of the emerging 21st-century healthcare environment.

To help navigate this changing environment the chapter provides information on how financial data is collected, summarized, and reported. This includes several types of financial statements and various financial reports used by healthcare providers. Some of these reports are very detailed, while others give a broad picture of an organization's financial performance through summarized data. These reports are utilized in a variety of ways by administrators and managers to both assess current facility performance and plan future programs and activities. Along with these financial reports, there is also a discussion of the budgeting process, and different methodologies for developing a facility budget.

The chapter also introduced the various staff members involved in the financial reporting and management of the typical long-term care facility and the activities that these staff members are involved in. Understanding the roles and responsibilities of various staff and departments is vital for effective management and maintaining a facility's financial health and well-being. Finally, there is a discussion of possible methods for enhancing revenues. While these revenue enhancement methods do not guarantee that profit will increase, they do offer insight into some potential strategies that may be pursued. It is important to note that the strategies identified are by no means a complete listing, but are provided as examples that may be utilized. With any such revenue enhancement program it is necessary to be aware of the coverage rules that payers have in place before implementing any revenue enhancement strategy. The impact of aging populations and increased demand for long-term care services is discussed in detail in Chapter 16. The financial strategies discussed in this chapter provide some, but by no means a complete list, of the alternative strategies to address these challenges.

Key Terms

Accountable care organizations (ACOs): ACOs are organizations that combine a wide variety of providers, physicians, hospitals, long-term care facilities, and associated ancillary service providers into integrated networks that assume responsibility for the care of a group of Medicare patients (www.medicare.gov).

Accounts payable: The accounts payable report shows the amounts the organization owes to the various entities from whom it has purchased services and supplies. It details each vendor owed money, what was purchased, and how long the money has been due.

Accounts receivable: Accounts receivable reports provide details about the amounts owed to the organization. They include information on which payers currently owe money and the amount that each owes, the services the money is related to, when each account was billed, and how long each amount has been owed.

Additive budgeting: Additive budgeting is the term used to describe the process of budget development that uses the existing fiscal year budget as the starting point for constructing the budget for the following year. Using the existing budget as a baseline, projections are made that add or subtract percentage amounts to the various budget categories. The assumption is that the existing budget is an accurate starting point for future revenues and expenses.

Aging report: A report that is used to summarize the amount owed to a facility by an individual payer for each patient that it has provided services for. The aging report is measured in days and begins calculating on the day that the organization bills the payer for the services in question. Aging reports are typically calculated in 30 day increments.

Ancillary services: These are services that are not routinely utilized by, or provided for, all residents. These include physical, occupational, and speech therapy services, as well as many others.

Assets: The assets of a facility are the things of value that a company owns or controls—that is, the asset can be sold, leased, or used in some way in its operations. Examples include equipment or buildings that the organization owns or cash in the bank.

Balance sheets: The balance sheet summarizes the organization's financial position at a point in time. It includes all assets, such as cash on hand, accounts receivable (money owed to the organization), and the value of buildings and land. Liabilities are subtracted from assets and include accounts payable (debts the organization must pay), mortgage cost, and bad debt. The balance sheet should show that the sum of all assets and liabilities equals zero.

Board of Directors: A group of individuals having fiduciary responsibility for an organization. The Board of Directors may be paid or unpaid, but in either case they hold ultimate responsibility for the financial health and performance of the organization. The Chief Executive Officer and, often, the Chief Financial Officer, report to, and serve at the pleasure of, the Board of Directors.

Capital budget: The capital budget contains the costs and annual expenditures for those items of equipment, land, and buildings that have a useful life measured in years, or supplies whose cost exceeds a specified threshold. The cost of capital budget items is generally amortized (spread) over several years, thus reducing the impact of these items on the annual budget.

Cash flow statement: Cash flow statements show how much money a company or organization has available to use to pay for personnel, goods and services, and the other costs associated with doing business. It is, at its most basic, the amount of funds on hand at a given time.

Census: The total number of individual patients or residents receiving inpatient services in a healthcare facility in a specified time period.

Typically census is calculated by the day and is referred to as the "average daily census." The census is used as a measure of the facility's activity.

"Clean" claim: A bill for reimbursement for healthcare services provided to a specific patient that is submitted to the payer for that patient and that contains no technical errors that would render the claim unpayable.

Co-pays: The cost required to be paid by a patient by the patient's healthcare plan, or government payer for a specific healthcare service.

Contract adjustments: Any deductions from gross revenue that an organization makes as a result of contract provisions that are included in payer contracts. Adjustments may be the result of the organization making concessions (discounting) or the payer requiring reductions in a provider's rates in order to do business with the payer.

Cost center: A specified department in an organization that incurs specific costs that can be tied directly to the activities of that department.

Credit: An addition to revenue or an amount that the organization is owed for providing goods or services. Credits will be added to other revenue in the net revenue and net worth calculations.

Dashboard report: A financial management report that summarizes financial results at a very high level (not much detail). Dashboard reports may also be used by other departments to provide summary reports of activities and services and monitor performance in various departments.

Debit: A subtraction from revenue or an amount that the organization owes for goods or services. Debits will be subtracted as part of the net revenue and net worth calculations.

Depreciation/Depreciate: The process of subtracting the purchase price of capital acquisitions, land or equipment, over the period of their useful life, measured in years. This process allows the cost of the land or equipment to be accounted for against the revenue that it helps to generate. It does not mean that the full cost is not paid, or incurred if funds are borrowed to make the purchase, upon acquisition of the asset.

Direct costs: Those costs which can be directly tied to the provision of a service or the acquisition of goods and supplies required to provide a service. This can include personnel costs that are directly related to patient care. Direct costs will fluctuate with the number of patients a provider or facility serves and the amount and variety of services that are rendered to those patients.

Discounts: Any adjustments to an organization's rate structure that are provided to payers in return for specified concessions.

Equity: The value of all holdings, including land and equipment and accounts receivable, minus any moneys that are owed to lenders or suppliers. A measure of the actual value of an organization and the amount of cash it could generate if it sold all of its assets.

Financial statements: These statements contain information on the financial performance of the organization. They are produced on a monthly basis and include revenues, expenditures, and comparisons to prior months, the prior year, and the organization's budget. They are the basic tool for financial analysis.

Fiscal year: The fiscal year is an accounting and budgeting period, typically encompassing 12 months and beginning in either January (running through December) or July (running through the following June). Fiscal reporting is used to assess an organization's performance to budget, to projected and expected census.

Fixed costs: Those costs incurred by an organization that do not change with fluctuations in the census or activity levels of the facility. Examples of fixed costs include rent or mortgage payments and amortized costs for capital equipment.

Generally Accepted Accounting Principles (GAAP): The common set of accounting principles, standards, and procedures that companies use to compile their financial statements. GAAP are a combination of authoritative standards (set by policy boards) and the commonly accepted ways of recording and reporting accounting information. GAAP are imposed on companies so that an organization's financial statements are consistent with those produced by other companies and thus can be compared for investment and analysis. GAAP cover such things as revenue recognition, balance sheet item classification, and outstanding share measurements. Companies are expected to follow GAAP rules when reporting their financial data via financial statements.

Gross Operating Revenue: Total funds received from all payer sources for healthcare services provided to patients during a specified period before deducting any discounts or contractual adjustments.

Gross revenue: All funds received by an organization for the provision of services before deducting any discounts or contract adjustments.

Indirect costs: Those costs that are incurred by a facility or organization regardless of the number and/or amount of services that the facility or organization provides. Examples include electricity, rent or mortgage payments, executive salaries, insurance, etc.

Journal: A record, either written or digital, of each and every receipt and expenditure made by an organization. Journals are used as a source for other financial reports.

Journal entry: A recorded entry of a single financial transaction entered into a financial record. Journal entries are used to track expenditures and funds received.

Key factor reports: These reports summarize data that are identified as key indicators of an organization's performance, such as staffing levels (nursing hours worked), average daily census, and per patient, per day revenues.

Key indicators: Performance measures that an organization has determined to be indicative of the organization's ability to deliver its services in an efficient, effective, and profitable manner. Key indicators are used to evaluate and assess performance and to identify areas that need to be addressed for improvement.

Liabilities: Liabilities are the opposite of assets. Liabilities are debts the facility owes to someone else. If a facility purchased services or supplies but has not yet paid for them, it owes the vendor money. These amounts owed to vendors and suppliers are called accounts payable. If a facility borrowed money from a bank or an individual, the facility must repay that loan. This is called a loan payable or note payable.

Licensed: Healthcare facilities are required to be licensed to operate by the various state jurisdictions. Hospitals, skilled nursing facilities, and other providers must be inspected and meet specific criteria in order to be granted a license to operate.

Loan payable (note payable): Funds that an organization owes to creditors for purchases that it has borrowed funds to obtain.

Net income: Net income minus total expenses. This may be a positive or negative number.

Net revenue: All funds received after subtracting all discounts and contracts adjustments. Net revenue minus expenses will give an organization's profit or loss for the particular accounting period.

Net worth: The total of an organization's assets minus its liabilities, the total of all funds it owes to its creditors.

Nursing hours worked: A measure of productivity that includes the sum total of all nursing staff working in a specified time frame, times the number of hours per shift in that time frame. A measure of productivity.

Payroll: The total of all funds due and payable to an organization's employees for work performed during a specified time period.

Per unit: As used in this chapter refers to the revenue received or the cost incurred for providing one unit of a specified healthcare service to a single patient.

Petty cash: A small amount of cash maintained by an organization to pay for incidental expenses under a specified amount. Typically petty cash accounts include no more that $200–500 and are administered by a designated official.

Preferred provider: Refers to a provider or provider organization that has contracted with a health insurance plan or other payer and has been designated by that payer as a provider that its members should use to receive the best rates, or to receive services at a lower rate. Providers who enter such arrangements typically agree to accept reduced reimbursement in exchange for increased access to patients.

Profit: The amount of money that is left to an organization, in a given period of time, after calculating all revenue received from all sources, and deducting all discounts, adjustments, and all costs of providing services. Profit must be a positive number.

Profit and loss (P&L) statements: The profit and loss statement is a financial statement that contains information on revenues and expenses. Revenues minus expenses equal the organization's profit, when revenues exceed expenses, or loss, when expenses exceed revenues. These are one component of the monthly financial statements.

Recurring expense: This refers to expenses that are incurred on a regular, such as a monthly, basis. Recurring expenses can include utility costs, rent or mortgage payments, or payments for outside services to be provided by contractors on a scheduled basis.

Resident day: A measure of performance used to measure activity and associated costs. The resident day equals 24 hours for one resident in a skilled nursing or assisted living facility. Total resident days are calculated by multiplying the total number of residents by the total number of days in the reporting period.

Resident trust: Funds held by a skilled nursing facility in trust for a resident in that facility. Medicare requires that resident trust funds be maintained and that residents have access to their funds. The facility is also responsible for an accurate accounting of the funds received and disbursed on a monthly and annual basis.

Retained earnings: This term is used instead of the term profit when nonprofit organizations refer to the excess of income or revenue over expenses.

Revenue: Moneys received by a provider or provider organization as reimbursement for healthcare services rendered to patients.

Share-of-cost: The term used by Medicare to refer to the beneficiary's required payment for healthcare services provided to the beneficiary. Medicare requires that beneficiaries contribute a certain amount to the cost of the services that they receive.

Spend-down: Spend-down tools track how much how much has been spent in a department. Managers use this to determine whether they are within their operating budget. These tools start with the total amount budgeted to be spent in any department during the fiscal year, and then record each expenditure and subtract it from the total.

Spend-down sheets: A journal or database maintained by the financial office to track the funds remaining when budgeted funds are being expended on a recurring basis (see spend-down).

Staffing levels: The number of staff, of all classes, that are working in a facility or organization in a specified time period. A measure of productivity.

Usual and customary: The reimbursement rate for a service or group of services that a provider will charge to payers before or without discounts or other contract adjustments.

Variable costs: Those costs incurred by an organization that fluctuate with changes in census or activity levels. Examples of variable costs include staffing costs for nurses and aides, food costs, and vehicle gas and maintenance.

Working capital: The term used to identify the funds an organization has available to pay for personnel or payroll, goods and services, and the other costs associated with doing business.

Zero-based budgeting: Zero-based budgeting is a budget development method that starts with the assumption that an organization has a clean slate, and the starting point is the minimum necessary to open the doors. It assumes the organization will incur certain costs simply by existing, which may include a mortgage or loans against its building, and a basic amount of utilities. There will also be certain staff needed to comply with basic regulatory and licensure requirements. These costs are determined, and then the process of adding services and amounts of services begins, including adding associated costs and revenues. This process continues until the organization's expected services and anticipated levels of service are reached.

Review Questions

1. In a P&L statement, net revenue is determined by subtracting _____ from gross revenue.
    a. Liabilities
    b. Equity
    c. Contract adjustments
    d. Variable costs
    e. Capital costs

2. A facility's budget contains the all of the following components except _____.
    a. Accounts receivable
    b. Assets
    c. Personnel costs
    d. Other operating expenses
    e. Employee-related expenses

3. When calculating a healthcare facility's net revenue, the following factors must be included in the calculation: _____
    a. Usual and customary charges
    b. Contractual adjustments
    c. Gross patient service revenue
    d. Liabilities and fund balances
    e. B and C

4. Balance sheets include all of the following except _____.
    a. Equity
    b. Profit margin
    c. Assets

    d. Direct costs

    e. B and D

5. If the value of the assets is higher than the value of the liabilities, the company will have _____ or sometimes called net worth.
   a. Positive cash flow
   b. Positive asset valuation
   c. Positive equity
   d. Positive P/E ratio
   e. Positive earnings position

6. The chief financial officer often has dual reporting lines of authority, to the administrator and the Board of Directors. This dual reporting is intended to ensure that the administrator and the CFO present consistent financial reports to the Board. True or False

7. A facility's indirect costs include all of the following except _____.
   a. Utility costs (gas, electricity, heating oil, etc.)
   b. Professional liability insurance
   c. Patient medications and medical supplies
   d. Professional association fees
   e. Business travel expenses for staff

Case Study

Aurora Skilled Nursing Facility, located in Anytown, has been operating profitably for several years. During that time it has received approximately 35% of its patients from the assisted living center on its campus, while the remaining 65% of its patients are transfers from three local hospitals. Of the hospital referrals, Mercy Hospital sends 20% of the referred patients, Bellevue Hospital sends 25% of the referred patients, and Columbia Hospital sends the remaining 20% of the referred patients. The SNF's revenue per bed/per patient/per day equals $200. In addition, it receives $200 per/patient per/day for ancillary (therapy) services, which are provided for every patient referred from any of the three hospitals. Expenses for the SNF are averaging $188 per bed/per patient/per day for all patients, and $175 per patient/per day for patients receiving ancillary services. For per bed/per day expenses, 35% are considered fixed costs while 65% are considered variable costs. For ancillary services cost, 100% are considered variable costs. Variable costs are directly tied to census.

    Over the past several years, the SNF has consistently maintained an average daily census (ADC) of 96%. Recently Bellevue Hospital announced that it was opening a SNF on its campus as part of its accountable care organization and henceforth would no longer refer patients to Aurora Skilled Nursing Facility. This will have an impact on the Aurora facility.

The Aurora SNF administrator has been asked to prepare an assessment of the impact that the new SNF will have on the facility in terms of census, operating revenues, expenses, and profits. He has also been tasked to develop some alternative strategies to address the expected impacts.

To complete this case study, you will assume the role of the administrator. Please determine the current census, operating revenues and sources, operating expenses, and what the current per month profit is. Then assess the impact of the loss of Bellevue Hospital's referrals on census, revenue, and expenses. Finally, propose two strategies to address the loss of Bellevue Hospital's patients, the cost of each strategy, and the potential impact of each.

References

Centers for Medicare and Medicaid Services. (2015). *Accountable care organizations*. Retrieved from www.medicare.gov

Nawrocki, T. (2013). *How PPACA affects long-term care insurance*. Retrieved from www.lifehealthpro.com/how-ppaca-affects-long-term-care-insurance

Acknowledgment

With gratitude and deep appreciation I wish to acknowledge the assistance, thoughts, and suggestions and necessary criticism provided by Paige Hector, who brought me into this project. This work could not have been completed without her able assistance. To Jim Smith, a colleague, friend and the ablest CFO I have ever worked with, my appreciation for what you taught me. And as ever, I am also, and always grateful to my wife, Dr. Shereen Lerner, for her belief and support.

CHAPTER 16

INTERNATIONAL COMPARISONS AND FUTURE TRENDS IN LONG-TERM CARE

Erlyana Erlyana

As the United Nations (UN) population division reported, population aging is unprecedented, pervasive, and enduring, and has profound implications (United Nations, 2002). The unprecedented changes are happening due to an increase in the proportion of older ages, from 6% of 65+ in 1980 to 15.6% in 2050 and from .9% of 80+ in 1980 to 4.1% in 2050, and declined mortality rates that lead to increased longevity, from 62.4 years in 1980s to 75.9 years in 2040s (United Nations, 2013). In addition, the increased female-labor participation and family structure changes (delayed marriage and lower fertility rates) are also affecting individuals, families, and government in protecting the elders, providing appropriate care, and financing the burden of aging societies. As societies are aging globally, delivering quality long-term care services has to become the priority of any government around the world, particularly in Japan, Germany, Italy, and Republic of South Korea, where the growth of the frailest is the highest and the fastest. This chapter discusses a brief overview of aging trends and long-term care expenditures globally, and reviews long-term care (LTC) financing policies in Japan, Germany, Italy, and Republic of South Korea. In addition, the chapter reviews recent LTC use and future policy direction in the United States. There are some actions that have been implemented, yet much remains to be done.

LEARNING OBJECTIVES
- Describe anticipated growth of long-term care (LTC) needs globally.
- Identify key aging trends and LTC expenditures globally.
- Describe major LTC policies around the world.
- Analyze major differences of several foreign countries' LTC policies.
- Discuss recent trend in the LTC supply and use in the U.S.
- Discuss LTC future policy directions in the U.S.

Growth of Elderly Population

The world population is graying and the need for LTC is expected to increase as people age. In 2050, the global population age 65 and older is projected to triple to reach 1.5 billion, or one in six people. Across Organization for Economic Co-Operation and Development (OECD) countries, the proportion is expected to increase to one in four people (Lafortune & Balestat, 2007). On the other hand, the population of children, 15 years and younger, is expected to increase only by 10%, to reach 2 billion in 2050. As result, in most developed countries, the dependency ratio will continually increase in the next four decades (United Nations, 2013) and people's confidence of living standards in their old age were the lowest in Japan and Italy (Pew Research Center, 2014).

Europe is currently the world's oldest region (Germany and Italy are the countries with the highest median age, on par with Japan). In developing countries or areas Republic of South Korea is one among a few countries that will reach the median age of 50 or higher by 2050. The number of old people is growing very fast globally, however the speed of change in less developed countries was significantly higher than developed countries. The size of the older population in less developed countries was about 100 million in 1950, five times increased to more than 500 million in 2013, and is going to triple to 1.6 billion in 2050 (United Nations, 2013). On the other hand, in developed countries, the size grew from 94 million to 287 million and 417 million respectively (United Nations, 2013).

In Germany, Italy, and Japan, the population that is over 65 makes up more than 20% of their total population, compared with the OECD average of 17.4% (Colombo, Llena-Nozal, Mercier, & Tjadens, 2011), while the Republic of South Korea is one of the fastest aging societies. Its population is aging much faster than other OECD countries. In 2000, South Korean citizens at least 65 years of age made up 7.2% of the population, which grew to 11% in 2010. The proportion is predicted to increase to 37% in 2050 (Kang, Park, & Lee, 2012).

As countries age, the proportion of the oldest old (people aged 85 and over) is increasing as well; the proportion of 80+ is expected to grow from less than 1% in 1980 to more than 4% in 2050 (United Nations, 2013). In Italy, the proportion of people aged 80 and over is projected to be 13.5% of the total population in 2050 (Tediosi & Gabriele, 2010). As the older population is ageing itself, the need of LTC will grow significantly. Across OECD countries, about half of LTC users were aged over 80 years (see Figure 16.1) (Colombo et al., 2011).

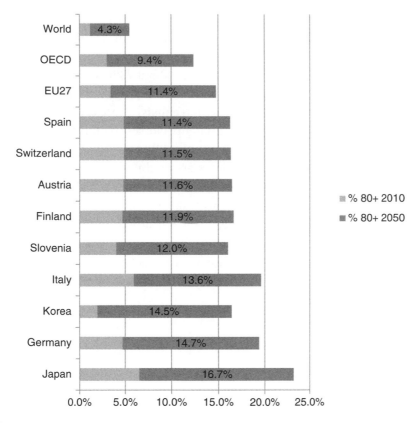

Figure 16.1   Countries with the Highest Share of People Age 80+ by 2050 in Comparison with OECD, EU27, and the World Average
Source: Adapted from OECD (2011).

Increase in Longevity and Disability

In past decades, the world population has gained more than 10 years of life expectancy overall; however, they spend longer years with disabilities caused by injury and illness (Lim et al., 2013). In most parts of the world, the increased longevity was attributable to reduction in infant mortality or maternal mortality death due to improved advanced medicine and public health, living conditions, and levels of education. However, the absence of disability and non-fatal outcomes that improved quality of life should be the ultimate goal. **Healthy life expectancy** (HALE) is a measure of average years of population living in full health with no disability and no non-fatal outcomes. Over the past decades, the rate is also increasing, but it increased more slowly than the increase in life expectancy itself. Over the past two decades, for every 1 year increase in life expectancy, there are only 10 months increased of HALE (Salomon et al., 2013).

According to World Health Survey and Global Burden of Disease report, about 15.6% to 19.4% of world population are living with disability, include both **moderate** and **severe disability** (World Health Organization, 2011). Of those percentages, about 2.2% to 3.8% have severe disabilities, conditions that equivalent to **quadriplegia**, severe depression, blindness, **Down syndrome**, or active **psychosis**. There is no clear conclusive finding on the trend of severe disability globally (Lafortune & Balestat, 2007). A slight declining trend in severe disability was reported in Italy and the U.S., while an increasing trend in severe disability was reported in Japan, Belgium, and Sweden (Damiani et al., 2011; Lafortune & Balestat, 2007). In the Republic of South Korea, although all causes of mortality and severe disability have decreased over time, it was not simply implied that Koreans are healthier (Jang & Kim, 2010). The currently increasing trend of several chronic diseases and aging population were expected to profoundly impact the trends in disability and influence the health care of most countries in the near future.

Increase in Long-Term Care Expenditure

The increasing demand also puts pressure on public budgets throughout the world over the next decades. The LTC expenditure in OECD countries is expected to increase from 6% of GDP in 2006 to 9.5% in 2060 with strong policy actions put in place; without such policies it is projected that the expenditure could reach to 14% of GDP. Major drivers of the increased cost could be divided into demographics, such as age structure and health status, and non-demographic factors, such as income. Rising relative prices, technology progress, and informal long-term care supply also contribute to the increase (OECD, 2013). Given this projection, long-term care spending is more likely to be a major source of concern for most governments. According the 2009–2010 OECD Survey on Long-Term Care Workforce and Financing, of 28 countries that responded to the survey, 85% reported that ensuring financing and fiscal sustainability is the most important policy priority, followed by encouraging home-based arrangement and quality improvement (see Figure 16.2).

There are significant variations in long-term care expenditure per person across countries as well. The spending varies from as little as $42 per person in the Slovak Republic to more than $1,400 per person in the Netherlands (see Figure 16.3).

Ranking	Policy for LTC System
1	Ensuring fiscal and financial sustainability
2	Encouraging home care arrangements
3	Enhancing standards of quality of LTC services
4	Care coordination between health and LTC
5	Providing universal coverage against LTC costs
6	Encouraging informal care
7	Providing coverage to people in need only
8	Sharing financing burden across society or individual responsibility for financing LTC
9	Encouraging formal care capacity and training
10	Immigration for legal foreign born caregivers

Figure 16.2   Top Ten Policy Priorities for LTC Systems in the OECD, 2009–2010
Source: Adapted from OECD (2011).

Country	Per capita Spending (in USD PPPs)
Netherland, Sweden, Norway*	> $1000
Luxemburg, Finland, Denmark*, Belgium*, Iceland*	> $600 but less than $1000
Canada*, France, Japan, Austria*, Germany, United States*	> $400 but less than $600
New Zealand, Australia, Slovenia, Spain, Hungary	> $200 but less than $400
Hungary, Korea	< $200

Note: PPPs stands for purchasing power parities.
* refer to nursing long-term care only.

Figure 16.3   Variation in LTC per capita spending among OECD countries (in USD PPPs)
Source: Adapted from OECD (2011).

International LTC Policies

There are many variations in LTC financing policies across the globe. There are two major categories: public long-term care financing arrangements and private long-term care insurance (Colombo et al., 2011). The public LTC financing arrangements include: universal and comprehensive, mixed system, and means-tested system (Campbell, Ikegami, & Gibson, 2010). Most countries have a higher proportion of publicly financed LTC compared to the United States. Only 4.5% of Americans 65 or older received publicly financed LTC, compared with 10.5% in Germany and 13.5% in Japan. More interestingly, the money was allocated in different ways. In Japan, most of the money was allocated for community services outside the home, in Germany it was allocated for cash allowances, and in the United States it was allocated for nursing home care. Unlike in the United States, Germany and Japan have adopted publicly financed universal long-term care insurance programs. In both countries, everyone contributes (proportionately by income) regardless of the need or availability of family caregiving. They use national standards for eligibility and level of care needed.

Germany

Germany implemented its long-term care national insurance scheme in 1995–1996. The scheme has three fundamental goals: universal protection of the whole population; cost containment; and aging in place embedded in family-oriented support. The universal protection creates national standards for eligibility of support, level of public supports, and type of benefits. All social health insurance beneficiaries are automatically enrolled in the LTC insurance program, and private health insurance beneficiaries are required to purchase LTC insurance. For the eligibility standard, the federal law defines three levels of care dependency based on their functional impairments and required necessary benefits associated with the level of care dependency. In 2002, it added additional benefits for individuals with psychological and cognitive impairments. In 2008, it added levels of support and lowered the threshold of eligibility. The beneficiaries may choose between receiving services or cash benefits or a combination of both cash and in-kind benefits (Da Roit & Le Bihan, 2010).

The German LTC insurance is a social insurance that is financed by contributions and premiums. The contribution is income-dependent and shared equally between employer and employee. After the 2008 Act reform, the contributions are 1.95% of annual income, and 2.2% for childless contributors. The social LTC insurance offers in-kind benefits, including home and institutional care services and cash benefits. Both in-kind and cash benefits have three care levels where the value of the in-kind benefits is about double that of cash benefits. These LTC insurance benefits offer basic care provisions. Recipients are allowed to purchase supplementary private long-term care coverage. In addition to the mandatory contribution, they may need to pay co-payments for formal care that varies across the 16 Lander (states). Social assistance will be available for people with low incomes and special conditions, such as mental illnesses or dementia.

Japan

Japan started formulating its welfare policies for the elderly in the early 1960s. In the beginning the government partially financed nursing home and home care services. The program later was expanded and named "Gold Plan" in 1990. The program was revised again in 1994, and called "New Gold Plan"; in 1997 it became Japan's national long-term care insurance scheme. Implemented in 2000, the scheme requires individuals 40 years or older to pay mandatory monthly premiums. Similar to Germany, Japan has uniformity in eligibility standards and level of needs/benefits across the nation. The LTC services are available for all Japanese citizens aged over 65 years (identified as first category of insured persons) and people under 65 years with age-related illness, such as Parkinson's disease, pre-senile dementia, or stroke (identified as second category insured persons). The insured will receive services based on a long-term care service plan that categorizes five levels of care and the plan will be reviewed regularly. The insurance will reimburse 90% of the costs. The mandatory social insurance in Japan is financed through a mixed source of funding: 45% from taxes, 45% from social contributions (paid by people aged over 40 years), and 10% from cost sharing (Long, 2013; Yong & Saito, 2012).

Despite its success, Japan's LTCI program was threatened by the exponential growth of its cost and declining revenue. The increased costs were most likely caused by longer life expectancy (in 2010, the LE is 79.6 years for men and 86.4 years for women and is projected to increase to 82.4 years for men and 89.1 years for women in 2035), and declining revenues were caused by declining total fertility rate (TFR) (the TFR in Japan is 1.39 in 2011; to have stable population growth the TFR cannot be lower than 2.1). On the supply side, there is a change in family structures resulting in a decline in family caregivers (informal care) that has led to increased need for expensive formal care (Shimizutani, 2014). However, unlike Germany, facing increasing demand and expenditure for LTC, started in 2006, Japan is focusing on implementing a comprehensive community-based integrated care model. It is a community-based system that offers holistic services, such as appropriate living environment and social care in addition to medical services. This model focuses on three main areas: medical care at home, residential facility, and preventative and daily living supports (Tsutsui, 2014). The consumers can select the care services for which they are eligible, and the prices for each service are set by the government. Providers compete by offering convenience and quality services.

Italy

The LTC system in Italy is highly fragmented and with a significant portion funded directly by households. Currently, long-term care health services in Italy are largely regulated at the local level. This regulation also includes the responsibility of helping to fund health services for the disabled and dependent; families help find long-term health services as well if all of the costs are not covered by the government. The public LTC includes three main kinds of formal assistance: community care, residential care, and cash benefits (Tediosi & Gabriele, 2010).

The Italian National Health Service (Servizio Sanitario Nazionale or SSN) manages home health services and other healthcare services provided in residential settings. Health services for the elderly and disabled include outpatient and home services, mental health services, services for patients with addictions, and home visits by health professionals (nurses, physical therapists, specialists, and general practitioners). Personal social services provided at home and social care at residential settings are managed by the local government (municipalities). The cash benefits that can be used to compensate for informal care available for disabled persons are managed by the National Institute of Social Security (INPS). Benefits do not take into account need or age. There is no specific written purpose for these cash benefits. In 2012, the average cash benefit was 492.97 euros a month and in 2010 approximately 10.8% of the disabled used this benefit. The eligibility criteria to receive these cash benefits are determined at the local level (Da Roit & Le Bihan, 2010). Some municipalities also provide cash benefits; therefore, LTC in Italy has a wide variety of levels of supply, funding, and spending.

In Italy, traditional care provided by family members to the elderly has helped keep costs of long-term care funding down for years. The majority of traditional care provided by family members was normally provided by female relatives. The rates of elderly citizens having family to provide at home care has declined with women being more prevalent in the workforce. Seventy-five percent of Italians surveyed felt families were overwhelmed by the burden of having to care for their elderly relative, and 88% of Italians surveyed felt it should be the government's responsibility to care for the elderly. Sixteen percent of households that have a senior citizen provide informal care (out of this 16%, 30% have a disability), which would amount to 4.8 billion euros worth of services. Fourteen percent of households with a senior citizen receive private in-home care (23% of this population have serious limitations). Of all senior citizens, 4.1% require some kind of home health service; however, the need varies greatly by region. Currently 57% of the elderly in long-term care pay their expenses completely out of pocket, 36% pay for a part of their care (47.1% of these patients pay almost half of their expenses out of pocket), and 7% are fully funded by the government (Colombo et al., 2011).

Furthermore, there is a widespread regional difference. In northern Italy, due to high female-labor participation, the public LTC is widely supported. In contrast, LTC in the south is mainly provided by family members with poor public supports. Even though there has been a call for a reform of long-term care since the mid-1990s to strengthen home care, there have not been many significant national changes, only small local changes. The regional priorities and commitments are different and national reform is lacking—the essential level of services is not determined yet.

Italy's ongoing federalist reforms make it difficult to achieve any kind of successful change to its long-term care system since most of it is labeled "in process." Italy does not have a solid foundation upon which to build. Another issue that makes Italian long-term care reform difficult is the vast distribution of wealth. Additionally, long-term care is mainly under local government jurisdiction, so the differences among them make it difficult to have uniform functional policies. Finally, and most critically, Italy's national debt has been a reason national reform of long-term care has been so slow to occur (Gabriele & Tediosi, 2014).

South Korea

Starting in July 2008, the Republic of South Korea implemented national long-term care insurance (LTCI) organized by Ministry of Health and Welfare and administered by the National Health Insurance Corporation (NHIC). The purpose of the LTCI is to reduce the burden of caring for an elderly and/or disabled family member. Eligibility requirements for long-term care insurance are determined by local agents in NHIC according to the assessment sheet that is defined by the LTCI law (Act on Long-Term Care Insurance for the Aged and Enforcement Regulations of Act on Long-Term Care Insurance for the Aged). The program is mainly for people age 65 and older regardless of their income, and it covers both institutionalized and community services in both the public and private sector, depending on the level of need and severity of the patient's conditions. Any prospective beneficiary must be assessed with an interview, which follows a questionnaire as to which of the six categories of need they qualify for (Colombo et al., 2011; Kang et al., 2012). Assistance is given regardless of income and ability to pay (individually or otherwise) (Kang et al., 2012).

The Korean LTC system is financed by contributions of all National Health Insurance participants (covers about 60% to 65% of LTCI spending), subsidies from central government (covers about 20%), and user fees (15% for in-house services and 20% for residential care). For recipients with low income or assets, the user fees are 7.5% for in-house services and 10% for residential care. For welfare recipients, there is no user fee (Colombo et al., 2011). Currently, the program covers about 6% of elders in the population, with 65% of the LTCI beneficiaries receiving home care services and 35% receiving institutional care services. Usage of these services versus long-term care provided by family members was found to be correlated with personal attitudes on this subject (Kim & Choi, 2008). Those who strongly felt that it was their personal responsibility to care for their elderly or disabled family members were less inclined to use any outside services. The majority of Koreans believe that using contracted caretakers is seen as abandonment of family (Kim & Choi, 2008). In addition, South Korea's long-term care insurance has been criticized for focusing on social services and not enough on health services, making it difficult to organize healthcare services to patients in long-term care (Kang et al., 2012).

Future Trends of LTC in the United States

Anticipated Growth of LTC Needs

Accelerated by the aging of the baby boomer generation that started in 2011, the number of elderly Americans (65+) was projected to be 88.5 million (20% of total population) in 2050, up from 13% today. It is more than double its projected elderly population in 2010 (Vincent & Velkoff, 2010). As Americans are living longer, the number of the oldest adults (85+) is projected to be 19 million in 2050, an increase from about 5.8 million in 2010. The total projected dependency ratio increased from 67 in 2010 to 85 in 2050. It means that 100 people in productive age need to give support to 85 people in their nonproductive age (people age 0 to 14 and people aged 65 and over) (Vincent & Velkoff, 2010).

No one wants to use long-term care services, but most people will need them at some point in their lives. As they age, they are likely to experience an increasing number of functional limitations. It was estimated that 7 out of 10 Americans 65+ will need assistance for daily activities for 3 years and 20% will need assistance for an average of 5 years (Kaiser Family Foundation, 2013). In addition, long-term care is not just for older adults. About 43% of community residents who use long-term care service and support were non-elderly (Kaye, Harrington, & LaPlante, 2010).

Trends in Supply and Use

Long-term care can be offered in **institution-based** or at **home-** or **community-based services**.

> As of 2012 in the United States, there were an estimated 4,800 adult day services centers, 12,200 home health agencies, 3,700 hospices, 15,700 nursing homes, and 22,2001 residential care communities. Of these approximately 58,500 regulated, long-term care services providers, about two-thirds provided care in residential settings (26.8% were nursing homes and 37.9% were residential care communities), and about one-third provided care in home- and community-based settings (8.2% were adult day services centers, 20.9% were home health agencies, and 6.3% were hospices)." (Harris-Kojetin, Sengupta, Park-Lee, & Valverde, 2013, p. 9)

Currently, according to the NCHS 2013 Long-Term Care Service Report, the five major types of paid, regulated long-term care services providers served more than 8 million people annually. In 2012, on any given day, there were 273,200 participants enrolled in adult day services centers, 1,383,700 residents in nursing homes, and 713,300 residents living in residential care communities. In 2011, about 4,742,500 patients received services from home health agencies, and 1,244,500 patients received services from hospices (Harris-Kojetin et al., 2013).

Most LTC home- and community-based services are provided by family members. More than two-thirds of Americans believe that they can rely on their family members (Tompson et al., 2013). The family caregivers' roles have been significantly expanded due to the emphasis on home- and community-based long-term care services. However, the supply of family caregivers is shrinking. In 2010 the caregiver support ratio is 7 potential caregivers to 1 high-risk year of 80+. By 2030, the ratio is going to be 4 to 1 and by 2050, the ratio is going to shrink to less than 3 to 1 (Redfoot, Feinberg, & Houser, 2013).

Future Predictions for LTC

Three potential challenges that emerge in the next couple of decades include: (1) the increasing need and declining supply of LTC workers, (2) financial pressure and quality concerns, and (3) widening income and need gaps across population groups (Smith & Feng, 2010). Current efforts are mainly focused on reducing financial pressures, improving quality, and reducing the gaps. The current public and private mix is not sufficient or sustainable to meet the increased demand and to satisfy the level of care needed (Miller, Mor, & Clark, 2010). The gaps also vary across states. Indiana and West Virginia have the worst performance across four dimensions (affordability and access, choice of setting and provider, quality of life and quality of care, and support for family caregivers). Minnesota has the best performance in all four dimensions (Reinhard et al., 2011) (see Figure 16.4).

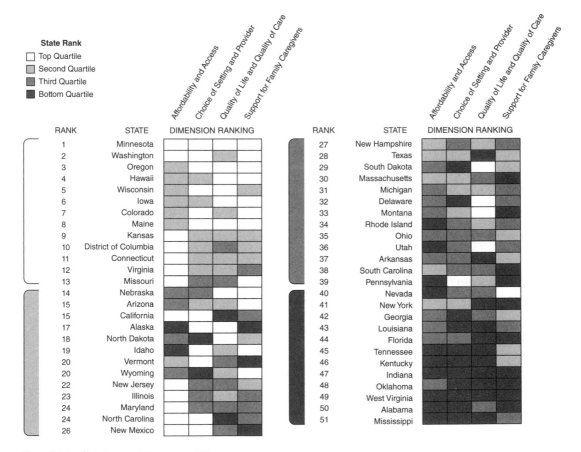

Figure 16.4   State Scorecard Summary on LTC

Source: Adapted from Reinhard et al. (2011).

To anticipate those challenges, there are three main factors that need to be considered. First is the choice of setting. As mentioned before, the focus on de-institutionalized care needs to be continued. Home- and community-based care need to be strengthened and supported. Second is strengthening technology innovation to enable self-care and management. Future efforts need to be focused on sustaining independent living by encouraging healthy and productive aging. Third is creating incentives to facilitate appropriate use across the care continuum, care coordination between medical care and long-term care, and addressing institutional efficiency. Seeking better value for money should be the priority for the future, and stringent regulation enforcement would be needed (Colombo et al., 2011; Mor, Miller, & Clark, 2010).

Summary

As the world population is aging, the need for LTC is increasing dramatically. As the growth of the demand and spending is increasing, there is a need to identify appropriate and timely private and public financing mechanisms to protect our frailest population. A few countries started a mandate for national long-term care insurance, but many other countries adopted only piecemeal regulations on LTC. In the United States, the future trend of LTC is also showing significant increase in demand and spending with no or few public financing mechanisms to support the growth of the needs. There is a long way to go, but there will be a need to start sometime soon in the very near future.

Key Terms

The following terms are important to the chapter. Some of the terms may also be found in other chapters, but may be used in different contexts.

Down syndrome is a genetic condition that alters the course of development. Some common physical characteristics of people with Down syndrome include low muscle tone, small stature, an upward slant to the eyes, and a single deep crease across the center of the palm. See more at http://www.ndss.org/Down-Syndrome/What-Is-Down-Syndrome/#sthash.stbMS4vw.dpuf

Healthy life expectancy (HALE) is a measure of average years of population living with no disability and non-fatal outcomes.

Home- or community-based service refers to services received in the individual's own home or community. It can serve a variety of targeted populations, including people with mental illnesses, intellectual or development disabilities, and/or physical disabilities.

Institution-based service refers to specific benefits authorized in the Social Security Act. It includes hospital services, intermediate care facilities, nursing facility, preadmission screening and resident review, inpatient psychiatric services for individuals under age 21, and services for individuals age 65 or older in an institution for mental diseases.

Moderate disability is defined as one or more IADL limitations. It could be defined as severity Classes III or higher that are the equivalent of having angina, arthritis, low vision, or alcohol dependence.

Psychosis is a symptom such as incoherent speech or disorganized behavior due to hallucinations or delusions.

Quadriplegia is paralysis caused by injury or illness that results in total or partial loss of use of all limbs and arms.

Severe disability is defined as one or more ADL limitations. It could be defined as severity Classes VI and VII that are the equivalent of having blindness, Down syndrome, quadriplegia, severe depression, or active psychosis.

Review Questions

1. What lessons we could learn from LTC policies abroad?

2. Describe future trends in LTC needs in the United States.

3. Describe future trends in spending on LTC in the United States.

4. Discuss potential effective intervention to address the need for LTC in the United States.

Case Study

Other developed countries, such as Japan and Germany, have major reconstructions of their long-term care financing policy. As the United States has started major reform of the country's healthcare system, are we ready to start thinking of ways to restructure our long-term care system and to finance the system? Each major reform requires driving forces and conditions that propel the changes:

1. What are the driving forces and conditions in countries that publicly financed their long-term care system extensively?

2. As for the United States, should we allow opt out of coverage or should we mandate LTC coverage?

3. In addition to strengthening the emphasis on home and community-based care and creating incentives to integrate care across the continuum, is there any other alternative that should be proposed to improve health and quality of life of our elderly population?

References

Campbell, J. C., Ikegami, N., & Gibson, M. J. (2010). Lessons from public long-term care insurance in Germany and Japan. *Health Aff (Millwood)*, *29*(1), 87–95. doi:10.1377/hlthaff.2009.0548

Colombo, F., Llena-Nozal, A., Mercier, J., & Tjadens, F. (2011). *Help wanted? Providing and paying for long term care*. Paris, France: OECD Publishing.

Da Roit, B., & Le Bihan, B. (2010). Similar and yet so different: Cash-for-care in six European countries' long-term care policies. *Milbank Quarterly*, *88*(3), 286–309.

Damiani, G., Farelli, V., Anselmi, A., Sicuro, L., Solipaca, A., Burgio, A., . . . Ricciardi, W. (2011). Patterns of long term care in 29 European countries: Evidence from an exploratory study. *BMC Health Services Research*, *11*(1), 316.

Gabriele, S., & Tediosi, F. (2014). Intergovernmental relations and long term care reforms: Lessons from the Italian case. *Health Policy*, *116*(1), 61–70.

Harris-Kojetin L., Sengupta, M., Park-Lee, E., & Valverde, R. (2013). *Long-term care services in the United States: 2013 overview*. Hyattsville, MD: National Center for Health Statistics.

Jang, S.-N., & Kim, D.-H. (2010). Trends in the health status of older Koreans. *Journal of the American Geriatrics Society*, *58*(3), 592–598. doi:10.1111/j.1532–5415.2010.02744.x

Kaiser Family Foundation. (2013). A short look at long-term care for seniors. *JAMA*, *310*(8), 786–787. doi:10.1001/jama.2013.17676

Kang, I.-O., Park, C. Y., & Lee, Y. (2012). Role of healthcare in Korean long-term care insurance. *Journal of Korean Medical Science*, *27*(Suppl), S41–S46.

Kaye, H. S., Harrington, C., & LaPlante, M. P. (2010). Long-term care: Who gets it, who provides it, who pays, and how much? *Health Affairs*, *29*(1), 11–21.

Kim, H., & Choi, W.-Y. (2008). Willingness to use formal long-term care services by Korean elders and their primary caregivers. *Journal of Aging & Social Policy*, *20*(4), 474–492.

Lafortune, G., & Balestat, G. (2007). *Trends in severe disability among elderly people: Assessing the evidence in 12 OECD countries and the future implications* (OECD Health Working Paper No. 26). Paris, France: OECD Publishing.

Lim, S. S., Vos, T., Flaxman, A. D., Danaei, G., Shibuya, K., Adair-Rohani, H., . . . Andrews, K. G. (2013). A comparative risk assessment of burden of disease and injury attributable to 67 risk factors and risk factor clusters in 21 regions,

1990–2010: a systematic analysis for the Global Burden of Disease Study 2010. *The Lancet, 380*(9859), 2224–2260.

Long, H. (2013). Policy design, basic features and future orientation of the long-term care insurance in Japan. *Economy and Management, 8,* 4.

Miller, E. A., Mor, V., & Clark, M. (2010). Weighing public and private options for reforming long-term care financing: Findings from a national survey of specialists. *Medical Care Research and Review, 67*(4 Suppl), 16S–37S. doi:10.1177/1077558710365886

Mor, V., Miller, E. A., & Clark, M. (2010). The taste for regulation in long-term care. *Medical Care Research and Review, 67*(4 suppl), 38S–64S.

OECD. (2011). *Help wanted? Providing and paying for long-term care.* Retrieved from 10.1787/888932400893

OECD. (2013). *What future for health spending?* Retrieved from http://www.oecd .org/economy/health-spending.pdf

Pew Research Center. (2014). *Attitudes about aging: A global perspective.* Retrieved from http://www.pewglobal.org/2014/01/30/attitudes-about-aging-a-global-perspective/

Redfoot, D., Feinberg, L., & Houser, A. (2013). *The aging of the baby boom and the growing care gap: A look at future declines in the availability of family caregivers.* Washington, DC: AARP Public Policy Institute.

Reinhard, S. C., Kassner, E., Houser, A., Ujvari, K., Mollica, R., & Hendrickson, L. (2011). *Raising expectations: A state scorecard on long-term services and supports for older adults, people with physical disabilities, and family caregivers.* Retrieved from http://assets.aarp.org/rgcenter/ppi/ltc/ltss_scorecard.pdf

Salomon, J. A., Wang, H., Freeman, M. K., Vos, T., Flaxman, A. D., Lopez, A. D., & Murray, C. J. (2013). Healthy life expectancy for 187 countries, 1990–2010: A systematic analysis for the Global Burden Disease Study 2010. *Lancet, 380*(9859), 2144–2162.

Shimizutani, S. (2014). The future of long-term care in Japan. *Asia-Pacific Review, 21*(1), 88–119.

Smith, D. B., & Feng, Z. (2010). The accumulated challenges of long-term care. *Health Affairs, 29*(1), 29–34.

Tediosi, F., & Gabriele, S. (2010). *Long-term care in Italy* (ENEPRI Research Report No. 80). Available at http://www.ancien-longtermcare.eu/sites/default/files/ENEPRI%20_ANCIEN_%20RR%20No%2080%20Italy%20edited%20final.pdf

Tompson, T., Benz, J., Agiesta, J., Junius, D., Nguyen, K., & Lowell, K. (2013). *Long-term care: Perceptions, experiences, and attitudes among Americans 40 or older.* Retrieved from http://www.apnorc.org/PDFs/Long%20Term%20Care/AP_NORC_Long%20Term%20Care%20Perception_FINAL%20REPORT.pdf

Tsutsui, T. (2014). Implementation process and challenges for the community-based integrated care system in Japan. *International Journal of Integrated Care, 14,* e002. Retrieved from http://www.ncbi.nlm.nih.gov/pmc/articles/PMC3905786/

United Nations. (2002). *World population ageing: 1950–2050.* Retrieved from http://www.un.org/esa/population/publications/worldageing19502050/

United Nations. (2013). *World population ageing 2013.* Retrieved from http://www.un.org/en/development/desa/population/publications/pdf/ageing/WorldPopulationAgeing2013.pdf

Vincent, G. K., & Velkoff, V. A. (2010). *The next four decades: The older population in the United States—2010 to 2050.* Retrieved from https://www.census.gov/prod/2010pubs/p25-1138.pdf

World Health Organization. (2011). *World report on disability.* Retrieved from http://www.who.int/disabilities/world_report/2011/en/

Yong, V., & Saito, Y. (2012). National long-term care insurance policy in Japan a decade after implementation: Some lessons for aging countries. *Ageing International, 37*(3), 271–284.

INDEX

Page references followed by *fig* indicate an illustrated figure.

American Diabetes Association, 75
American Geriatrics Society, 350
American Health Care Association, 135
American Indians/Native Alaskans
  Older Americans Act amendment (1973) aging
    services network for, 16–17
  percentage of older adults among, 4
American Legion, 92
American Medical Director's Association, 405
American National Standards Institute (ANSI), 115
American Recovery and Reinvestment Act
  (ARRA), 304
Americans With Disabilities Act Accessibility
  Guidelines (ADAAG), 113
Americans With Disabilities Act (ADA)
  Americans With Disabilities Act Accessibility
    Guidelines (ADAAG) of, 113
  building code requirements of, 112–113, 115
  description of, 22
  federal housing program meeting the standards
    of, 41
  Title I of, 24
  worker accommodations requirements of,
    152–153
  See also Disabilities
Ancillary services
  description and examples of, 489–490
  Medicare Part A, 165
  Medicare Part B, 167–168
  Level of Services Provided to Residents,
    490–492*fig*
  Intensity of Services to the Residents, 490
Anergic cases, 339
Antigens, 338
Anti-Kickback Statute (AKS)
  comparison of the Stark Law and, 252*fig*
  compliance and risk management issues of, 200,
    209, 217–219
  examining the potential violations of, 235
  prohibitions of False Claims Act (FCA) and,
    251–253
Antipsychotics, 376
Anti-supplementation compliance, 220
Anxiety disorders, 347
Approaches or interventions
  care plan goals and, 373–374
  case study on confused resident and, 364
  enhancing feelings of self-worth, independence,
    and choice, 355
  helping with language barriers, 355
  identifying non-drug interventions, 388
  initial orientation/transition to LTC, 353–354

personal possessions and enhancing homelike
  atmosphere, 354
providing regular assessment and care planning
  for, 355–356
staffing levels and consistent care models for,
  354–355
Arab community, 6
Area Agency on Aging (AAA), 46
Area of refuge, 124
Aseptic techniques, 340
Asian community, 6
Asian/Pacific Islander older adult population, 4
Aspiration, 340
Assessment. *See* Nursing home assessment;
  Resident assessment
Assets
  bad debt risk associated with, 480–481
  equity as difference between assets and liabilities
    481
  facility, 480
  Medicaid eligibility and, 169
  realized, 480
Assisted evacuation, 124
Assisted living
  administrators in, 54
  marketing challenges for, 270*t*
Assisted living communities
  care manager evaluation of, 37
  summary of national findings on costs of, 11*t*
Assisted living facilities, description of, 51
Assisted technology programs, 49–50
Association of Households International (AHHI), 87
Asymmetric information issue, 7
At-will employment, 148
Audio impairment, 49
Authorities having jurisdiction (AHJ), 116, 122
Autonomic nervous system, 343–344

B

Baby boomers (1946 to 1964), 33, 137
Bad debt, 480–481
Balance sheets, 480
Balancing Incentive programs, 20
Bargaining unit, 149
Barkan, Debora and Barry, 84
Basic activities of daily living (BADLs), 345, 351
Beatitudes Campus, 92–95
Bed certification, 170–171
Bed hold policy, 434
Bedridden residents, 331–336
Bed side rails, 381

Promotional activities, 291, 292t–293t
Prospective payment system (PPS), 175–176
Prospective payment system (PPS), 171
Prospect registration form, 283
Protected activity, 154
Protected class, 153
Protected health information (PHI)
  admission packet on confidentiality of, 435
  breach of, 248
  Health Insurance Portability and Accountability
    Act (HIPAA) guidelines on, 19, 220–221,
    248–249
  LTC providers and privacy violation of, 230
  staff training on protecting, 144
  See also Medical records; Protected health
    information (PHI); Residents
Provider orders
  description of, 378
  for leave of absence (LOA), 390
  monthly recapitulation (recap) of, 403
  noting the orders, 378
  recapitulation of, 379
  for rehabilitation, 382
  stand-up meeting clinical review of new,
    420e–421e
  verifying the orders, 378
Psychological needs
  anxiety, 347
  depression, 346
  depression and, 346, 347, 370, 373e
  loss and isolation, 345–346
  sleep pattern, 347–348
  specific to older adults, 329
Psychosis, 508
Psychotropic medication
  affect on balance and contributing to falls, 342
  appropriate use of, 213–214
  Centers for Medicare and Medicaid Services
    (CMS)'s national goal of reducing unnecessary
    antipsychotics, 376
  description of, 379
  estimates on older adults taking, 212
  incident report when given without consent,
    379–380
  interdisciplinary approach to, 214
  medical record audit on, 379–382
  Omnibus Budget Reconciliation Act (OBRA)
    limitations on, 348
Public policy
  critiques of, 14–15
  definition of, 7
  impact on long-term care by, 7

rationales and goals for, 7–8
  vulnerabilities of the users of long-term care and
    need for, 8–9
Public policy on LTC milestones
  examples of state-specific laws, 24–25
  federal policies and legislation, 15–19
  important policies affecting LTC professionals
    and paraprofessionals, 22–24
  state and local government policies, 19–22
Public relations
  addressing suspicions and fears, 273
  advertising and promotional activities, 291,
    292t–293t
  case study on marketing and, 298–300
  crisis management, 294–295
  customer service for, 284, 285
  monitoring customer satisfaction, 286
  naming and vocabulary impact on public
    perceptions and, 272t
  preplacement evaluation, 284–285
  resident ambassadors for, 285–286
  social media marketing and, 291, 293–294
  See also Marketing
Public to private gradient, 107

Q

Quality assurance performance improvement
  (QAPI)
  data management necessary to confirm to,
    443–449
  description and official implementation of, 228,
    441
  the five elements of the, 441–442
  policies and procedures (P&P) reviewed in
    conjunction with, 369, 370
  See also Improvement strategies
Quality indicator survey(QIS)process, 456–457
Quadriplegia, 508
Quality assessment and assurance (QAA), 442
Quality assurance (QA)
  description and purpose of, 440–441
  performance improvement (PI), 441
  prior to Omnibus Budget Reconciliation Act
    (OBRA), 441
Quality assurance (QA) studies and audits, 228
quality assessment and assurance (QAA), 442
quality assurance incident reports, 222fig
Quality Measure/Indicator Reports , 442–443
quality of care relationship to, 76–77
See also Performance improvement (PI);
  Surveys